HYPERNUTRITIOUS FOODS

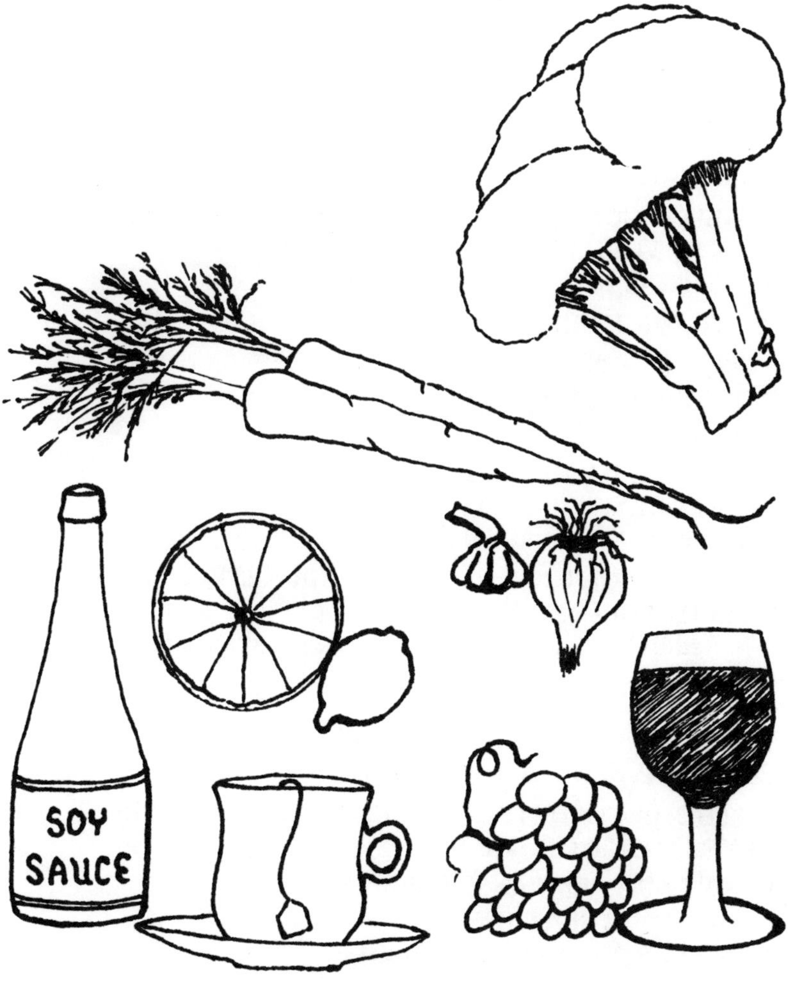

AGRICULTURE AND FOOD SCIENCE
A series of Textbooks, Reference Books and Manuals

---

1. FRUITS OF TROPICAL AND SUBTROPICAL ORIGIN
   Edited by S. Nagy, P. E. Shaw and W. F. Wardowski
2. QUALITY CONTROL MANUAL FOR CITRUS PROCESSING PLANTS: VOLUME II
   J. B. Redd, D. L. Hendrix and C. M. Hendrix, Jr.
3. FRUIT JUICE PROCESSING TECHNOLOGY
   Edited by S. Nagy, C. S. Chen and P. E. Shaw
4. RABBITEYE BLUEBERRIES
   M. E. Austin
5. METHODS TO DETECT ADULTERATION OF FRUIT JUICE BEVERAGES: VOLUME I
   Edited by S. Nagy and R. L. Wade
6. QUALITY CONTROL MANUAL FOR CITRUS PROCESSING PLANTS: VOLUME III
   J. B. Redd, P. E. Shaw, C. M. Hendrix, Jr. and D. L. Hendrix

FORTHCOMING BOOKS

A. TROPICAL AND SUBTROPICAL FRUITS
   Edited by P. E. Shaw, H. Chan and S. Nagy

B. METHODS TO DETECT ADULTERATION OF FRUIT JUICE BEVERAGES: VOLUME II
   Edited by S. Nagy, R. L. Wade and N. Low

C. FOOD ADULTERATION
   Edited by S. Nagy and R. E. Wrolstad

HYPERNUTRITIOUS FOODS

Edited by

JOHN W. FINLEY
Nabisco Foods Group
East Hanover, New Jersey

DAVID J. ARMSTRONG
FDA/NCFST
Summit, Illinois

Steven Nagy

STEVEN NAGY
Florida Department of Citrus
Lake Alfred, Florida

SUSAN F. ROBINSON
American Chemical Society
Washington, D.C.

AGSCIENCE, INC.
103 Arietta Shores Drive
Auburndale, Florida
U.S.A.

AGSCIENCE, INC.
103 Arietta Shores Drive
Auburndale, Florida 33823 U.S.A.
Tel. 941/967-8898, Fax 941/967-1342

Library of Congress Catalog-in-Publication Data
Hypernutritious foods/edited by John W. Finley . . . [et al.].
p. cm.
Includes bibliographical references and index.
ISBN 0-9631397-5-4
1. Nutrition. 2. Diet therapy. 3. Natural foods. I. Finley, John W., 1942 -.
RA784.H97 1996 96-38416
813.2—dc20 CIP

HYPERNUTRITIOUS FOODS/edited by John W. Finley, David J. Armstrong, Steven Nagy and Susan F. Robinson

Current printing (last digit):10987654321
Printed in the United States of America

PREFACE

Health-promoting foods have been labeled with a variety of adjectives, the most common of which are nutraceuticals or functional foods. These foods all generally provide nutrients or other food components thought to enhance health and/or performance of individuals. With all of the descriptors that have been applied to health-promoting foods, the editors have frequently been asked why a new descriptor called "hypernutritious foods"? A good question! Frankly, we felt that a new descriptor was in order that would embrace highly nutritive foods with demonstrated health-promoting attributes, while differentiating itself from dietary supplements and the confusing term, functional food. Dietary supplements can include foods and supplements described as nutraceuticals, medical foods, pharmafoods, designer foods and herbal remedies. It was our feeling that nutraceutical has become a catch-all term that includes a very broad spectrum of foods ranging from foods of demonstrated nutritional enhancement through some foods and ingredients that have not been as carefully scrutinized by the scientific community.

Another frequently used and/or abused term is functional food. We would vehemently argue that all foods are functional in that they provide energy and nutrients essential to body function. Functionality to the food technologist also includes the physical characteristics of an ingredient that result in specific characteristics in a food product. An example is the function of gluten in wheat flour to provide the unique dough characteristics required in bread making. Thus, we would argue that functional foods is not an appropriate term to describe foods that provide nutritional enhancement.

The term "hypernutritious food" is meant to define conventional food with naturally exceptional or enhanced nutritional value. The definition includes foods supplemented with vitamins, minerals, amino acids and other traditional nutrients that are added to enhance the nutritional profile of the food. Hypernutritious foods, in a broader sense, include other food components which have been demonstrated to improve healthy functions of the body, serve to protect against disease or enhance performance of the individual.

Health-promoting substances such as carotenoids can be enhanced through the application of biotechnology. The enhanced products resulting from this technology are excellent examples of food that has been rendered hypernutritious through the enhancement of a specific nutrient. We would also include food enhanced with nutrients to make a processed food nutritionally equivalent to the original raw product. An example of this concept would be a snack food such as an apricot-filled cookie that contains all of the essential nutrients, including vitamin C, that were present in the apricot before processing. In other words this would be a cookie that is equivalent to eating an apricot.

Hypernutritious foods can also be foods that have been altered from the conventional composition to improve their healthfulness. Examples of these foods include low fat comminuted meat products, low fat cookies, low cholesterol eggs and low sodium snacks. In Table 1 examples of hypernutritious foods are listed. From that table it can be seen that a variety of currently available foods fit the hypernutritious food definition, but supplements and foods modified with ingredients of unproved efficacy are excluded from the category.

Adoption of a hypernutritious food category is critical because we believe it may help identify foods where health-related claims can be made. There is growing scientific evidence that many components in foods provide health benefits. Several chapters in this book clearly identify not only the specific components in foods that inhibit cancer but propose mechanisms for the anticancer activity. Eventually food manufacturers will want to communicate the benefits of these components or ingredients to the consumer with health-related claims on labels and in advertising.

In the 1990 NLEA, Congress mandated that the FDA review relationships between certain substances and disease states for

TABLE 1. EXAMPLES OF POTENTIAL HYPERNUTRITIOUS FOODS AND WHY THE FOODS FIT OR DON'T FIT THE CATEGORY

Food	Hypernutritious
Low fat sausage Low fat cookies	Yes, reduced in undesirable fat
Vitamin A & C enriched tomatoes, vitamins through biotechnology	Yes, higher in antioxidants
Low salt cracker or corn chip	Yes, lower in salt or sodium
Tablet containing fish oil	No, dietary supplement
Spread with fish oil	Yes, product enriched with ω-3 fatty acids
Cranberry juice	Yes, reduce risk of bladder infections
Orange juice	Yes, major source of vitamin C; significant source of folic acid
Fiber enriched cereal	Yes, health claim allowed under NLEA
Traditional food with added shark collagen	No, dietary supplement; lacks proof of efficacy
Soy-based dessert	Yes, anti-cancer effect of genestein

the purpose of allowing health claims. Table 2 provides the list mandated by Congress and the claims currently authorized by the FDA after the review process. The FDA has allowed claims for the substances where the preponderance of scientific evidence has supported the specific claim. The other potential claims were not approved pending development of more evidence to establish a relationship between the nutrient and the disease. In addition to the claims for specific food components, the FDA also allows the following health claims for foods rather than specific components:

> Diets low in fat and high in fiber-containing grain products, fruits, and vegetables reduce the risk of cancer.

> Diets low in saturated fat and cholesterol and high in fruits, vegetables and grain products that contain dietary fiber (particularly soluble fiber) reduce the risk of coronary heart disease.

TABLE 2. FOOD SUBSTANCES AND DISEASE RELATIONSHIPS MANDATED FOR FDA REVIEW AND CLAIMS AUTHORIZED BY THE FDA

Substance	Disease	Claim allowed
Calcium	Osteoporosis	Yes
Lipids	Cardiovascular disease	Fat and CHD* Cholesterol and CHD
Lipids	Cancer	Fat and cancer
Sodium	Hypertension	Yes
Folic acid	Neural tube defects	Yes
Dietary fiber	Cancer	
Dietary fiber	Cardiovascular disease	
Zinc	Immune function in elderly	
Antioxidant vitamins	Cancer	
Omega-3 fatty acids	CHD	

*Coronary Heart Diseases

> Diets low in fat and high in fruits and vegetables (foods that are low in fat and may contain dietary fiber, vitamin A, and vitamin C) reduce the risk of cancer.

The health claims allowed under the NLEA are an excellent start, however, many in the food industry feel that we can go much further. The consumer is developing an increased interest in the health consequences of the foods that they consume. As a consequence of this interest, food manufacturers want to communicate the health benefits of current or new products. It is therefore likely that the industry will continue to request additional health claims. In this book the basic technology to support future health claims of foods and ingredients that can improve health are reviewed. We feel that *Hypernutritious Foods* and other books like it will provide a vehicle to communicate the scientific basis for the efficacy and safety of new food ingredients.

John W. Finley
David J. Armstrong
Steven Nagy
Susan F. Robinson

Contributors

ARMSTRONG, DAVID J. FDA/NCFST, Summit, Illinois.
BARNES, STEPHEN. Department of Pharmacology, University of Alabama at Birmingham, Birmingham, Alabama.
BENNINK, MAURICE R. Department of Food Science and Human Nutrition, Michigan State University, East Lansing, Michigan.
BINNIE, WILLIAM H. Department of Biomedical Sciences, Baylor College of Dentistry, Dallas, Texas.
BLOCK, ERIC. Department of Chemistry, State University of New York at Albany, Albany, New York.
BRACKE, MARC E. Department of Radiotherapy, Nuclear Medicine and Experimental Cancerology, University Hospital, Gent, Belgium.
BRUYNEEL, ERIK A. Department of Radiotherapy, Nuclear Medicine and Experimental Cancerology, University Hospital, Gent, Belgium.
CARSON, KAREN. Food and Drug Administration, Washington, D.C.
CERDA, JAMES J. Gastroenterology, Hepatology, and Nutrition, Shands Clinic, University of Florida, Gainesville, Florida.
CHEN, LAISHUN. Laboratory for Cancer Research, Rutgers—The State University, Piscataway, New Jersey.
CHILDS, NANCY M. Department of Food Marketing, Saint Joseph's University, Philadelphia, Pennsylvania.
COWARD, LORI. Department of Biochemistry, University of Alabama at Birmingham, Birmingham, Alabama.
DOUGLASS, JUDITH S. TAS, Inc., Washington, D.C.
FINLEY, JOHN W. Nabisco Foods Group, East Hanover, New Jersey.
FOLTS, JOHN. Department of Medicine, University of Wisconsin, Madison, Wisconsin.
FRANKEL, EDWIN N. Department of Food Science and Technology, University of California, Davis, California.
GERMAN, J. BRUCE. Department of Food Science and Technology, University of California, Davis, California.
GORDON, JOHN. Food and Drug Administration, Washington, D.C.
GUO, INGRID Y. Department of Biomedical Sciences, Baylor College of Dentistry, Dallas Texas.
HASEGAWA, SHIN. Western Regional Research Center, USDA, Albany, California.
HEIMBACH, JAMES T. TAS, Inc., Washington, D.C.
KENNEY, PATRICK M. LKT Laboratories, Inc., St. Paul, Minnesota.

CONTRIBUTORS con't.

KIRK, MARION. Comprehensive Cancer Center Mass Spectroscopy Shared Facility, University of Alabama at Birmingham, Birmingham, Alabama.

LAM, LUKE K. T. LKT Laboratories, Inc., St. Paul, Minnesota.

LEE, MAO-JUNG. Laboratory for Cancer Research, Rutgers—The State University, Piscataway, New Jersey.

MAREEL, MARC M. Department of Radiotherapy, Nuclear Medicine and Experimental Cancerology, University Hospital, Gent, Belgium.

MILLER, EDWARD G. Department of Biomedical Sciences, Baylor College of Dentistry, Dallas, Texas.

MONTANARI, ANTONIO M. Scientific Research Department, Florida Department of Citrus, Lake Alfred, Florida.

NAGY, STEVEN. Scientific Research Department, Florida Department of Citrus, Lake Alfred, Florida.

PETERSEN, BARBARA J. TAS, Inc., Washington, D.C.

PORTER-WRIGHT, JO L. Department of Biomedical Sciences, Baylor College of Dentistry, Dallas, Texas.

ROBINSON, SUSAN F. American Chemical Society, Washington, D.C.

ROUSEFF, RUSSELL L. Citrus Research and Education Center, University of Florida, Lake Alfred, Florida.

SEVER, BROOKE E. TAS, Inc., Washington, D.C.

SHANK, FRED R. Food and Drug Administration, Washington, D.C.

SMITH, ROBERT E. Nabisco, Inc., East Hanover, New Jersey.

TEISSEDRE, PIERRE L. Centre de Formation et de Recherche en Oenologie, Universite de Montpellier, Montpellier, France.

VENNEKENS, KRIST'L. Department of Radiotherapy, Nuclear Medicine and Experimental Cancerology, University Hospital, Gent, Belgium.

VERMEULEN, STEFAN J. Department of Radiotherapy, Nuclear Medicine and Experimental Cancerology, University Hospital, Gent, Belgium.

WALZEM, ROSEMARY L. Department of Molecular Biosciences, University of California, Davis, California.

WANG, ZHI Y. Laboratory for Cancer Research, Rutgers—The State University, Piscataway, New Jersey.

WATERHOUSE, ANDREW L. Department of Viticulture and Enology, University of California, Davis, California.

WAYLETT, DARIN K. TAS, Inc., Washington, D.C.

WEISBERGER, JOHN H. American Health Foundation, Valhalla, New York.

WIDMER, WILBUR W. Scientific Research Department, Florida Department of Citrus, Lake Alfred, Florida.

YANG, CHUNG S. Laboratory for Cancer Research, Rutgers—The State University, Piscataway, New Jersey.

ZHANG, JILUN. LKT Laboratories, Inc., St. Paul, Minnesota.

ZHENG, GUO-QIANG. LKT Laboratories, Inc., St. Paul, Minnesota.

Contents

1

The Processed Food Industries Perspective on Functional or Hypernutritious Foods

Robert E. Smith
John W. Finley

The new world of functional or designer foods could take dietary considerations out of doctors offices and place them on the shelves of supermarkets. Science has extended life, so consumers are more interested in the quality of life; they desire not to just maintain it, but to improve it and they are being bombarded with nutritional information about the health benefits of food components. That presents the food industry with a challenge: How to produce hypernutritious foods in a scientifically justifiable and responsive manner. The responsibilities and potentials for the food industry in the push to provide hypernutritious food products are discussed as well as the responsibilities of regulatory groups, consumer groups, and the scientific community.

Traditionally, foods are thought of as carriers of calories and essential nutrients to support bodily functions. In recent years some foods have been purported to provide therapeutic value or to impart disease resistance. Functional foods is one descriptor that has been applied to such foods. However it could be argued that all foods which supply calories and essential nutrients are functional. Foods with therapeutic or preventative attributes have been described using a number of adjectives some of which are reported in Table 1.1. It would appear from the assigned title that we will be using the descriptor "hypernutritious foods" throughout this book.

From the list it is clear that the demarkation between foods and pharmaceuticals has become extremely blurred. Most of the adjectives in the Table imply a preventative, pharmaceutical benefit or an enhanced performance attribute for the food. In other portions of this book the policy issues, biomedical issues, risk/benefits, label claims and consumer expectations surrounding these types of foods will be discussed. Some of the implications would suggest that everything from known nutrients to "fairy dust" should be included in the food supply. The role of this chapter is to discuss what happens when the scientific and regulatory world of hypernutritious foods meets the everyday world of the food manufacturer and, most importantly, the consumer.

The food industry perspective with respect to hypernutritious foods reminds me a little of a famous study by the London Zoo. In the zoo they used soothing music to enable a lion and a lamb to live together in the same cage. A visitor asked how the experiment was going and the zoo's scientist said, "It's going extremely well, however, just every now and then we have to replace the lamb." This is similar to the market issues surrounding the commercial delivery of functional or hypernutritious foods.

There is little question that in some forms functional foods could play a significant role in the American food supply. However, we would simply be replacing lambs if we confined the issue to the science that creates them and the regulatory issues that would allow their use.

Functional foods must find their way from the shelves into the consumers houses. They must be accepted by the public and consumed with some regularity if they are to have a meaningful impact on the American diet. Two critical market issues must

TABLE 1.1. DESCRIPTORS OF FUNCTIONAL FOODS

medicinal foods	super foods
neutraceuticals	longevity foods
functional foods	pharmaceutical foods
prescriptive foods	pharma foods
neutraceutics	designer foods
nutritional foods	medifoods
fitness foods	foodiceuticals
therapeutic foods	hypernutritious foods

be considered. First, the inevitable questions surrounding the safety of functional foods must be answered to the satisfaction of the regulatory agencies and realistically to consumers and to advocacy groups. Secondly, functional foods must be integrated into the food supply and the overall diets of consumers. Unless we can deal with both issues we will fall far short of the full potential that this emerging science promises.

Our arrival at the door step of the functional food era came in a fairly linear, if uneven series of steps. These steps are outlined in Table 1.2. Nutritional science has long been aware of the link between nutrition and disease. The initial focus and classic evolution of the science of nutrition was focused on nutritional deficiencies and the steps to overcome the deficiencies in the population. For example, in the 18th century it was found that providing an ample supply of citrus fruit warded off scurvy on sailing ships. Once the nature and impact of nutritional deficiency disease were understood, and once the food supply became generally safe and nutritious, medical interest in the health properties of the food supply began to wane. The next major step in the evolution of nutritional science occurred in the 1950s, when science shifted to the isolation of micronutrients in foods. Many of these micronutrients such as selenium were implicated in the prevention of chronic illnesses. The next evolutionary wave took place in the 60's when research focused on gaining insight into the mysteries of cellular metabolism.

In all of these steps there was limited focus or understanding of the interplay between foods, metabolism and health. The results of the research began to bring nutrition-related life threatening situations and nutrition related mortality under control. The next step then as shown in Table 1.2, was an emphasis on the relationship of nutrition to the quality of life. Modern nutrition had succeeded in bringing the bulk of the population to where they *should* be nutritionally. The next step was to accelerate them toward what they *could* be. It was at this point that food manufacturers began to get really interested in the opportunities of selling nutrition as a benefit rather than a necessity. It provided the long sought push to sell foods for what was in them rather than for what they lacked.

From the food industry's point of view **NUTRITION** comes in two very important parts. First is the obvious responsibility of the industry to furnish a wholesome and nutritious food supply. The second is to get the population to use it properly. To accomplish this, a public framework of research, communication, counseling and promotion must be established to encourage the use of diets which not only support good health, but which confront threats of age, environment or chronic illness.

Introducing the concept of hypernutritious foods brings us a big step forward. Now we are introducing foods or ingredients into the diet which can modify the human response to chronic diseases. These foods could take dietary considerations related to chronic disease out of the laboratory and deposit them on the shelves in the supermarket. There is, of course, a very important partner in all of this scientific awareness and progress. It's the good folks in the food industry who put these new and unique foods on the shelves. There has been enormous progress in nutrition science and food processing since Charles Post promised that his new Postum product would build red blood. This business went on from the Postum success to found General

TABLE 1.2. THE EVOLUTION OF FUNCTIONAL FOODS

nutritional deficiencies
nutrients and chronic disease
nutrition and cellular metabolism
nutrition and quality of life

Foods Corporation. A similar story evolved at Kellogg's. With all of the new knowledge that has been developed since that time, foods that offer the potential to improve health, offer even more fascination and potential for marketers and consumers alike.

It is important, however that we present a consistent story to the consumer with what is good and what is not. Frequently claims are made, refuted and then restated. A good example of this shifting consensus surrounded the value of oat bran. With oat bran we stepped forward, stepped back and stepped forward again leaving consumers hopelessly confused. Initial research results on the health benefits of oat bran were exciting and offered great promise. Later results suggested that it was similar to other fiber sources while still providing health benefits. Later it was again shown that oat bran was perhaps better than some other sources of bran. Unfortunately, many times reports of benefits and even claims are reported in popular press before being published in peer reviewed scientific publications. The public has little hope of sorting these out.

For the past 20 years or more, the food industry has been fortifying, supplementing, and removing nutrients at an unprecedented scale. We have altered starches, sweeteners, and fats to produce foods with reduced calories and increased fiber. Don't forget however that we as nutritional scientists can't even agree on how to measure fiber. For example should starch which is poorly digested by human amylases and is fermented by colonic bacteria be considered fiber? What about other sources of soluble fiber which are also fermented? If we as scientists can't agree, how can the consumer be expected to understand the resulting claims and counter claims.

One can speculate that mother nature would be pleased with what is happening to most of her fundamental creations. It is said that if you want to lead, find a parade and get in front of it. The food industry has grabbed the baton on the march toward new health awareness. Nutritional and medical sciences have extended the life span. The delivery of nutritious, wholesome and safe foods to all consumers has been so successful that they are taken for granted. Now, consumers are more interested in foods that will improve their quality of life. They want to run faster, jump higher, think clearer and not only live longer, but live better longer. The expectation is not only to maintain good health, but to improve ones health through self prescribed dietary intervention. This presents the food industry with what business planners like to call, "a non-trivial challenge." Today the food industry and the scientific community are faced with a formidable and often conflicting *to do list*. Our knowledge of the holistic impact of specific nutrients or foods and their impact on health, performance and resistance to chronic disease is limited. As can be seen by other chapters in this book there is a considerable body of encouraging results which offer great promise to the industry and ultimately to the consumer. However, we are also faced with highly confining regulations dealing with products and their advertising. There is no question that we have to produce healthier foods based on sound scientific evidence, define healthier diets, educate the consumer, and serve them up to a more demanding consumer in an industry of eat-or-be-eaten competition. It is also of equal importance that the foods taste good. If they don't taste good the consumer simply will not buy them, at least a second time. All of this attention, the billions being invested in fundamental and applied research and the marketing of the results is already leading to both hope and controversy. The ultimate winner will be the American consumer who will have easy access to a diet that will result in better health.

The knowledge being shared in this book will hopefully lead to more products that apply this knowledge. Improved understanding of the molecular biology of nutrition will allow modification of the food supply in concert with a better definition of health needs. The price of this progress is an initial period of confusion based on legitimate scientific debate and the scientific process to establish a firm understanding and on the basis for modification or supplementation of foods or diets. This is a necessary process of new discovery and advancement of scientific knowledge. We must be cautious however to avoid situations of potential misunderstanding or in worst cases fraud and dangerous practices.

Clearly the majority of the industry and the scientific community have a stellar record for integrity and quality. In addition to the responsibility of the industry, both the FDA and the

FTC monitor activities to assure regulatory compliance. An important step in consumer education is the Nutrition Labeling and Education Act. This act pivots the basis for fair labeling of nutrient content of foods and clear definition of what sort of health or composition claims can be made for a specific product. Enforcement and education are really palliatives; the most serious issue to address is the conflict between the cultures of foods and drugs. Which does what and when? Nowhere is the conflict between food and drugs more apparent than in the area of hypernutrious or functional foods.

At the beginning of this chapter I used the equivocal language of *could* and *might* in describing the potential of hypernutritious foods. As a scientist and a representative of a major food company you might wonder about my personal view of these foods. Am I for them? To which I respond with an unequivocal . . . ***Maybe!***. The answer depends on how the hypernutritious or functional foods are defined and how they are to be sold. There is a large potential for misuse of modern nutritional science, to cash in on this period of uncertainty until the efficacy and safety of components and ingredients are scientifically verified. This is enough of a problem, however, there are also issues of legality and definitions, safety and philosophical conflict and the temptation for marketing abuse. I am not suggesting outright fraud, but we must be concerned about the creative manipulation of scientific fact to gain a market advantage. As we move into the era of designer foods we are confronted with the fundamental question of what is a food and what is a drug.

The Food, Drug and Cosmetic Act defines a drug as the intention for *"use in the diagnosis, cure, mitigation, treatment, or prevention of disease in man or animals and substances other than food that are intended to affect the structure or any function of the body in people or animals"*. The complication is that the new functional or hypernutritious foods will increasingly fall within some of these definitions. This ambiguity will lead to confusion with regard to health claims. The result is a marketing conundrum that says you can do it, but you can't say it. But if you can't say it, who will buy it? And from a marketers standpoint if no one buys it, you might as well forget it. This leaves us in a gray area where caution will win over real communication. Health claims for food, will necessarily be restricted to claims for interactions between diet and disease. This clearly leaves the issue of implied claims as an even larger question mark.

From the industry perspective, at the core of the hypernutritious foods conundrum, is the implication, by definition, that these new foods are better than other foods. They are better even though the other foods may look the same, smell the same and taste the same. The truth of the matter is that **all foods are functional.** Additionally, virtually all the descriptors mentioned in Table 1.1 have the potential for misleading connotations. Thus, we must come up with clear definitions of these foods. The definition must be something that stands apart from the FDA's definitions, but still communicates the real health advantages of the new foods. This clearly is not a trivial task. If we are to claim that a functional or hypernutritious food is better than another food, then the criteria must be defined. Whose criteria do we use? Scientific consensus? That is an extremely difficult goal to achieve, especially when some groups, for their own benefit will remain outside. FDA decree? Public perception? Who knows?

Right now, despite FDA's clear message from Congress, nobody knows and that is going to have to change. Let's put that issue aside for a moment and for further discussion refer to the chapter by Shank et al. in this book. Assuming for a moment that the criteria for claims and the definitions can be agreed upon and we develop a new hypernutritious food which is clearly different from its parent. Does this mean that we have to treat the new product as something new in the food supply? The more successful we are in making distinctions, the more we are going to raise questions. We might develop a new product that is equivalent to walking on water, but we are likely to find advocacy groups waiting on the other side with the torpedoes of opposition turned to full throttle. A classic example is the opposition Monsanto faced with bovine somatotropin. Here milk produced with a naturally occurring, totally safe bovine growth hormone was dumped on the streets of New York. Ben and Jerry assure the world that milk produced from cows receiving BST will not be used in their ice cream. When talking about special interests, I'm reminded of Elbert Hubbards venerable definition of a news editor, as a man "whose business is to separate the wheat from the chaff and to see that the chaff is printed".

To return to our dilemma, on one hand the FDA has said that new functional foods will be treated like any other foods. But on the other hand, they say that the greater the difference in the food, the more concerns could be raised concerning its safety. While this is not illogical, industry must be clever in how it projects its products.

A joint expert committee of the FAO-WHO has proposed that a new food can not be any less safe nor should it be expected to be more safe than its traditional counterpart. This also sounds very reasonable. But, what are the criteria? The only way to know for sure is to do an initial chemical comparison and look for any metabolic information. If any genetic modification is involved in a product to be consumed, the complexity is an order of magnitude greater. There may be a need for extensive animal studies particularly if questions are raised in earlier studies. Finally, if the new food is *very* different from the parent foods, clinical trials would be required. That means that it is time for the FDA to offer "New Food Applications" regulations just as they do "New Drug Applications" permitting human studies. In the arena of safety, it is important to remember that a functional food will almost certainly alter the pattern of nutrients in that food, which is likely to alter our perspective of a balanced diet. Where do functional foods fit in the 90's Food Pyramid? For example, increasing calcium in a wide range of foods could result in hyperalimentation with calcium, upsetting the normal mineral balance. Results demonstrating the advantages of antioxidants are truly exciting. But, how much is too much? Wholesale additions of Vitamin C, beta-carotene, Vitamin E, methionine and other precursors raise the threat of reaching toxic levels in certain individuals.

The point is that the promise of functional or hypernutritious foods is so great, the marketing opportunities so compelling, that the average diet could quickly go into functional food overload. Perhaps that is not a problem, perhaps it is. We simply do not know. One only hopes that we all act as responsibly as we did in the vitamin rush of the 70s, when 100% vitamin supplements were voluntarily restricted to some breakfast cereals.

The final problem we face in functional foods is part philosophical, part promotional and part emotional. By focusing on the curative or preventative powers of selected foods, we reinforce the ill-considered notion of "good foods . . . bad foods". These are always good and these are always bad, ignoring the reality that nutrition is a matter of overall balance rather than a concrete list of do's and don'ts. A market of consumers bent on self-improvement through foods will almost certainly confuse the advantages of products A, B or C with the needs for an overall healthy diet regime.

A real opportunity exists with new hypernutritious foods, but it must be approached with broad vision. Diet can impact health in more ways and to a greater degree than we even know now. But we must be careful not to lose this opportunity by making it a casualty of a war between new foods and old foods, functional and nonfunctional, good and bad. Drawing such arbitrary battle lines will severely impede progress. We need to step toward this new world of opportunity with a sound and consistent approach. That approach is that "food is food". Assurances of human health come not from the individual foods we eat, but the combination of all of the foods in the total diet.

The positioning and presentation of foods in the market must also be done with extreme care. A focus on functional foods, neutraceuticals or hypernutritious foods can send a dangerous message to consumers. We are living in an age when fear of foods is rampant with consumers. They are told they should eat less fat, sodium and less sugar. All foods that are fun are bad. Introducing claims about the advantages of hypernutritious foods or neutraceutricals implies a specific health or medicinal benefit. They imply that the nutrients or foods may be pharmaceuticals, they're not. What they are is a path to a better nutritional balance in our diets.

As implied earlier, I would like to suggest that what we have been calling functional foods, we call "enhanced foods", and be very clear to the public how they have been enhanced. It is not the role of the food industry to convert foods into pharmaceuticals, and I certainly object to the notion of using foods as mere carriers of pharmaceuticals. It is our job to feed this country with safe, wholesome foodstuffs and to encourage the eating of a balanced diet by all individuals. If we are certain that the population is overeating foods which might lead to a nutritionally unbalanced diet, we should consider fortification of those foodstuffs to overcome such the nutritional deficiency. Let me suggest a few examples:

Snack Foods—Why not supplement to improve the total nutritional profile of the product and eliminate the so-called empty calorie issue.

Convenience Foods—Supplement to so-called conventional foods, replace nutrients as fully as possible.

Enhanced Foods—Supplement with nutrients that have proven beneficial health attributes, are safe and do not have a conventional carrier in the food supply.

Fundamentally we should expend research effort and resources to learn how basic foodstuffs can be enhanced in the context of healthier diets, rather than leapfrog into the creation of novel foods as carriers of pharmaceuticals. This appears to be a prudent approach to nutrifying foods so that we can make haste slowly!

Our position is centered on three key points. First, there is strong agreement that foods can be modified or supplemented for any *valid* nutritional or dietary reason. The food industry has been doing this for years. For example fortified flour, removal of trypsin inhibitors, reduced sucrose and calories in many foods, reduced and replaced fat with lower calorie alternatives etc. The technology, the knowledge and the infrastructure are in place to take food improvement to a new paradigm. The second point is a strong disagreement with the common notion "good food . . . bad food". We must continue to consider the whole diet, and support intensive research, particularly in the area of nutritional interactions, the relationship between nutrients and chronic disease, and the optimum supplementation programs for various classes of foods. The third point is the successful employment of modern biology in improving diets. These benefits must be clearly and consistently communicated to our consumers to help them make best use of these advances. The food industry, the pharmaceutical industry, the scientific community, the regulatory agencies, consumer groups all must work together more closely and intensively than in the past. The recent policy concerning the products of biotechnology issued by the FDA is an excellent beginning for this cooperation. Borrowing several pages from the biotechnology saga could help us frame a useful strategy for *nutritionally enhanced foods*.

By developing a consensus on the key points above, we would then be in a position to recommend to the regulatory agencies certain guidelines that would be followed in the labeling and health claims for enhanced foods. Lets consider some examples.

First—Demonstration of safety of the enhancement. This is paramount to any change in a foodstuff.
Second—Any enhancement would require a scientific consensus of the efficacy to support the proposed claim.
Third—Enhancements should be rationally related to the specific foodstuff.
Fourth—Health claims should be in the context of the total diet rather than individual foods.

To reach acceptance of these general guidelines by the food industry, medical practitioners, consumer groups, etc., a mechanism such as the Keystone dialogue could be used. Following such agreement, these guidelines could be offered to the regulatory agencies as a basis for rule making. The challenge, of course, is scientific consensus. It would be our hope that the scientific consensus could be garnered through independent scientific bodies such as the LSRO of FASEB, FEMA or the Food and Nutrition Board.

It is said that we have three basic states of activity in life. To wonder what happened, to watch things happen and to make things happen. I submit that we must make things happen. A new era of enhanced foods cannot be allowed to dawn on us before we're fully awake! We lose one of the most important opportunities in this century for the improvement of diet and health. And, we'll lose it to over-promise, under performance and consumer confusion. We need to get started now, and we need to start working cooperatively to turn the promise of enhanced foods into the reality of improved nutrition and improved quality of life.

2

Hypernutritious Foods: Policy Issues

Fred R. Shank
Karen Carson
John Gordon

In a 1990 address Dr. Samuel Thier observed that the focus of nutrition has evolved from prevention of deficiency diseases in the 1940s toward the prevention or treatment of chronic illness and disability in the 1990s. With this evolution, the line between food and drugs is becoming blurred and the relationships between nutrient and other food components and disease conditions is being touted on the labels of food in the market. Moreover, research is creating ingredients with which to formulate foods with specific health benefits. How should these products be evaluated; what test testing methods? How do we provide for an orderly flow of products with specific health benefits to the market? How best to educate consumers about the diet/disease relationships so they are not misled about the scope of health benefits and to assure that they use products properly? These are only a few issues that must be resolved to realize benefits of applied nutrient/disease research.

Two significant events occurred in 1990 that set the stage for further developments of concepts, not agency policy, on hypernutritious foods. The first was Dr. Samuel Thier's 1990 Keynote address at the Institute of Food Technologists' annual meeting. In that address, Dr. Thier, who was then President, Institute of Medicine, National Academy of Sciences, traced the progression of nutrition science over several centuries. He pointed to the short steps from the concept of nutrition as deficiency, and nutrition as excess, to the evolution of a broader view—the concept of optimum nutrition.

Traditionally, diet is thought of in a biological role, enhancing normal development and aging. Now we have begun to think of it in a health role, first as a preventer of disease or debility, then as a treatment for disease (1).

We are now entering difficult terrain where we begin to see food as drugs and drugs as food. As we begin to develop nutrient substitutes and new food formulations, we must take a critical look at conducting trials of foods as we have trials of drugs. And associated with that, we must worry about whether those kinds of evaluative processes will negatively affect the innovative process. These factors position nutrition in the center of major public policy debates in the areas of health.

The second event of 1990 was the Nutrition Labeling and Education Act (NLEA). These two events have helped form the thoughts on hypernutritious foods expressed in this chapter. In the April 1993 issue of Food Processing, Fran LaBell described what a supermarket might be like in the year 2010. ". . . a shopper at a food and nutrition supermarket stops to check with the store's nutritionist before gathering up his purchases. They include plenty of vegetables seasoned with garlic, high-fiber bread and breakfast muffins, as well as fish oil supplement capsules—all safe and government-approved products. The shopper knows he is increasing the probability that he will not develop the debilitating heart disease that claimed his father, and that he will not have to endure chemotherapy for colon cancer as his mother has. Into his shopping cart are going food products and products made from food components that are designed to keep him healthy" (2).

Is this scenario far-fetched? Look at food labels just 15 years ago and compare them with labels on products in today's stores. Maybe the scenario is not so far-fetched after all. Much has changed in those 15 years. Technological advances in nutrition, genetics, molecular biology, food science, among other scientific disciplines, enable researchers to identify both detrimental and potentially beneficial relationships between nutrients and diseases and between specific food components and disease. Consumers are much more knowledgeable about the composition of the foods they consume and about the relationships between diet and health. Public health officials recognize the need to provide consumers with current, scientifically sound information about the composition of foods and about the health benefits. They are seeking ways to provide that information so consumers can easily understand and use the information in making daily dietary choices.

Still, we are light years away from pushing a basket down an aisle in the 2010 supermarket. At the outset, there must be a fundamental change in how we perceive the role of food and our well-being. Traditionally, we've viewed food as a source of essential nutrients and energy necessary to maintain good health. The supermarket of 2010 described earlier, contains foods that go beyond maintaining good health to preventing or reducing the risk of certain diseases. Beyond this basic sociological change in the role of food, the science base supporting the benefits of specific food components and the development of products must be substantially expanded. Likewise, public education and regulatory programs must be developed that provide the greatest breadth of readily usable information and move safe products into the marketplace rapidly.

This chapter will briefly:

* Review the essential requirements for health claims as the agency has implemented the regulations under the authorities of the Federal Food, Drug, and Cosmetic Act (FD&C Act) and NLEA,

* Take a look at the issue of hypernutritious foods, including what types of products are encompassed by this category of foods and a brief look at how countries other than the U.S. are dealing with these foods,
* Discuss some of the critical issues that *may* be limiting the further development of these foods, and
* Discuss the authors' perceptions of what needs to be done and how we might work together, not only at this conference but in the future to continue to provide for more healthful foods and to foster the future of hypernutritious foods.

With refinement of the science demonstrating diet/health relationships and the resultant development of unique products specifically designed to ameliorate the negative relationships and accent the positive relationships, a series of questions arise. All segments of the food and public health community must consider how to produce, market, educate consumers on the use, and where necessary, regulate this unique category of products if the American public is to reap the benefits.

HEALTH CLAIMS

An initial step in this direction was the development of regulations designed to permit the use of health claims on food labels. FDA began this effort with a proposal on use of health claims in 1987. Congress furthered this effort by including a provision in the NLEA giving FDA the authority to establish regulations permitting health claims for nutrients in conventional foods and in dietary supplements. The following are the seven requirements for a health claim:

1. Significant scientific agreement
2. Totality of publicly available scientific evidence
3. Safe and lawful
4. Claim must be generic
5. Food must be part of total daily diet
6. Food cannot possess any nutrient in an amount that increases risk of disease
7. Claim must be complete, truthful, and not misleading

Significant Scientific Agreement

The requirement for significant scientific agreement among experts qualified by scientific training and experience to evaluate claims characterizing the relationship between nutrients and a disease or health-related condition is a legal requirement of the NLEA (3). Congress intended this standard to be strong and for FDA to have a high level of confidence that a health claim is valid. This does not mean that unanimous agreement is required or that every expert in the field approve or agree with the claim. It does mean that a sound scientific standard must be met. Congress gave FDA responsibility for defining the criteria to meet that standard and these may be found in the regulation on General Requirements for Health Claims (4). While a sound body of scientific evidence establishing the relationship between a substance and a disease or health-related condition is required, there is some flexibility in how that relationship may be demonstrated and the agency has provided some guidance on that (5). For example, no specific set of studies, either type or number, is required, however, various weights are given to various types of studies; clinical, epidemiological, and animal studies. Human data are given the greatest consideration and they must be generalizable to and preferably obtained from the U.S. population. Combinations of studies can compensate for deficiencies in any one type. The overriding principle is demonstration that there are consistent results from different types of well-conducted human studies by different investigators in different populations. In studies conducted using animal models, consistency of results between animal studies and human studies will be considered and interpreted in light of available evidence on the biological mechanism of the substance-disease relationship, evidence of a dose-response relationship, and similarity of the test substance with the nutrient or food component of interest. Judgements on the overall quality of available data will be based on:

* Appropriateness of the study design,
* Consistency across different types of studies and laboratories,

* Conclusions derived from the total body of evidence, and
* The generally recognized scientific procedures and principles that are most appropriate to the issues being considered.

Totality of Publicly Available Scientific Evidence

As a second requirement for a health claim, the claim must be based on the "totality of publicly available scientific evidence" (3). This standard also comes directly from the law—the NLEA. In implementing this standard, FDA adopted criteria that permit the agency to make case-by-case determinations on the scientific validity of a claim, giving greater weight to studies that are more persuasive. The standard for claims on foods is less stringent than the comparable drug requirement for "substantial evidence" that the drug will have the effect it purports to have. The intent of Congress was a more flexible standard. Information that is not publicly available may be submitted in support of a claim, but the agency will make it publicly available when the claim is authorized.

Safe and Lawful

The third requirement—that the substance a claim is made about is "safe and lawful"—comes from the safety provisions of the FD&C Act (6). The NLEA states that a health claim may only be made for a food that does not contain any nutrient in an amount that increases to persons in the general population the risk of a disease or health-related condition that is diet related, taking into account the significance of the food in the total daily diet (7). FDA believes this provision voices Congress' concern that a substance that is subject of health claim be used in a manner that is safe. Since the NLEA did not alter agency responsibility for assuring the safety of foods, it would be inappropriate to authorize a claim for a substance without assurance that it is safe at the levels it may be used and in compliance with the food safety provisions of the Act. "Safe and lawful" can be based on one of the following (8):

1. Demonstration that the substance is generally recognized as safe (GRAS) (9), or
2. Listing of the substance as GRAS, affirmed as GRAS (10) or independent determination of GRAS (11), or
3. Listing of the substance as a food additive regulation (12), or
4. A prior sanction or approval granted by FDA or USDA (13).

If none of these criteria are appropriate, the petitioner for a claim must submit data and information to demonstrate safety.

Claim Must Be Generic

Provisions of NLEA require that health claims enable the public to understand the information in the context of the daily diet (14). FDA has expressed the view that product- or brand-specific claims place the emphasis on that specific product or brand rather than the diet as a whole. Moreover, such specific claims imply that other products containing the same food component may not have the same effect on the disease or health-related conditions, thus misleading consumers" (15). To date, all of the health claims authorized for use have been generic claims. It must be noted that there is no specific requirement in the Act that prohibits authorization of product- or substance-specific claims in cases where all other requirements are met. Therefore, it is not unreasonable to anticipate that, as the body of scientific data about diet/health relationships grows, this "requirement" may very well be eliminated as the larger body of information makes possible more specific claims which may apply to only one product or product formulation.

Food Must Be Part of Total Daily Diet

The fifth requirement for a health claim is that the substance or food that is the subject of the claim must be part of the total daily diet. This requirement also comes directly from NLEA. The concern underlying this requirement is that consumers, in order to understand the importance of diet/health information provided in a claim, must also understand how the substance or food fits into their daily diet and at what point consumption is not expected to provide additional health benefit. For a substance to have significance within the context of the daily diet, it must be a food or a component of food and must retain its food attributes at the consumption levels that are necessary to justify the claim. Food attributes are taste, aroma, nutritive value, or any of a myriad technical effects of food ingredients, such as thickening, antioxidants, emulsifiers, and antimicrobial agents (16).

Food Cannot Possess Any Nutrient In An Amount That Increases Risk of Disease

The sixth requirement is that a food that contains a nutrient in an amount that increases the risk of disease may not bear a health claim. Again, this is a requirement of NLEA. Nutrients categorized as potentially increasing the risk of disease are fat, saturated fat, cholesterol, and sodium and regulations setting disqualifying limits of these nutrients have been established (17). Congress intended that health claims would not merely provide information on particular substance/disease relationships, but that they would help individuals maintain healthy dietary practices. Health claims on foods with disqualifying levels of the above mentioned nutrients make it more difficult for consumers to choose healthy diets, leading to increased risk of diet-related disease. Thus, a food with a high fat content may, in most cases, not bear a health claim for any food component it contains (7).

Claim Must Be Complete, Truthful, and Not Misleading

The final requirement, that a health claim must be "complete, truthful, and not misleading", comes directly from the requirements of the FD&C Act (18), specifically, section 403(a)(1). Labeling may be misleading if it omits significant information needed to properly interpret the claim (19). So, to meet this requirement, it may be necessary that a health claim include information about the influence of other factors, in addition to the affect of the substance the claim is being made about, on the disease- or health-related condition. For example, the affect of gender, race, and age have a bearing on the development of osteoporosis so these factors must be included in the health claim about calcium and osteoporosis. Inclusion of contributing factors in health claims constitutes the "adequate disclosure of significant information" (20) a consumer needs in order to understand the claim and make informed choices. However, inclusion of multiple factors may lead to quite lengthy health claims, such as the claim for folic acid and neural tube defects[1]. It should be noted that this claim is currently being revised, taking into consideration its length.

AUTHORIZED HEALTH CLAIMS

FDA has authorized the use of several health claims on food product labels, four of which are nutrient-specific, and proposed a fifth claim for the relationship between folic acid and neural tube defects. The authorized nutrient/disease claims are for:

* Sodium and hypertension (high blood pressure),
* Calcium and osteoporosis,
* Dietary saturated fat and cholesterol and coronary heart disease, and
* Dietary fat and cancer

In addition, there are several authorized diet/disease or health-related condition claims.

FDA recognizes that the currently approved health claims and the criteria by which the appropriateness of each claim is determined are just the first steps in a process that will evolve over time. It is anticipated that use of the petition process to

---

1.NCFST/IIT Scientific Symposium: HACCP: A Dialogue on Critical Issues. May 8-10, 1995.
Oakbrook, Illinois. "Women who consume adequate amounts of folate daily throughout their childbearing years may reduce their risk of heaving a child with a birth defect of the brain and spinal cord. Such birth defects, while not widespread, are very serious. They can have many causes. Adequate amounts of folate, a B vitamin, can be obtained from diets rich in fruits, dark green leafy vegetables and legumes, enriched grain products, fortified cereals, or a supplement. Women who have had a child with a spinal cord birth defect should consult a physician before becoming pregnant. Folate consumption should be limited to 1,000 μg per day."

establish new health claims will help streamline this process, as well as identify new nutrient or food component/disease relationships based on new scientific developments.

With that groundwork, the universe of "hypernutritious foods" being examined in this book can now be defined. Over the past 10 to 15 years several terms have been used to describe products specially formulated or produced to have particular health benefits.

DEFINITIONS OF TERMS

"Designer foods" may be defined as products tailored to meet specific health needs. Among these might be included the products in which macroingredients, such as fat replacers, are used to reduce the fat content of foods or products in which constituents such as cholesterol are mechanically removed or genetically engineered out of the food.

The term "nutraceutical" was proposed by the Foundation for Innovation in Medicine to encompass any substance considered a food, which provides medical or health benefits, including the prevention and treatment of disease (21). Such products may range from isolated nutrients, dietary supplements, and diets to genetically engineered "designer" foods, herbal products, and processed foods such as cereals, soups, and beverages.

"Phytochemicals" is a term used to describe naturally occurring chemicals in fruits and vegetables that are nutritionally, physiologically, and/or medicinally highly active (22). These substances are thought to reduce the risk of cancer when ingested in proper quantities.

The term "pharmafoods" has been coined to describe any edible product for human consumption, designed, produced, packaged, and sold to consumers, that claims to achieve a well demonstrated health benefit, whether therapeutic, prophylactic, or disease risk reducing (21).

"Foods for Specified Health Use" (Japanese term; formerly known as functional foods) have been described as products with the following characteristics: they are normally consumed in ordinary diets (not as pills or supplements), derived from natural ingredients, should be consumed as part of the daily diet, and have a particular health function (23).

The term "functional foods" is widely used and may be defined as ". . . foods similar in appearance to conventional foods and intended to be consumed as part of a normal diet, but have been modified to subserve physiological roles beyond the provision of simple nutrient requirements" (24).

These products, whatever term is used to describe them, may be produced by the addition of a variety of ingredients. Among these are additives, such as an isolated active ingredient from one food that is concentrated and added to another food; processing aids, such as enzymes produced by biotechnology; or microbiological organisms, such as probiotics (a live microbial food supplement which beneficially affects the host). Or they may be completely novel foods.

The list of terms presented here by no means includes all the names used to categorize the variety of products encompassed by this book. Often the terms are used interchangeably. For the purposes of this discussion, the term "hypernutritious foods" will be used to describe all these products.

DRIVING FORCES

The concept of hypernutritious foods and their place in the diet has been gaining momentum in the last several years. This may be attributed to five interrelated factors that mesh societal trends with scientific advances and industrial growth on a global basis.

First, advances in medical science are resulting in increasing reports of associations between specific food components and specific metabolic responses in individuals. Second, there is a growing affluent sector of the world population that is educated and conscious of the role of diet in promoting good health. Third, advances in food technology are providing the food industry with increasingly sophisticated methods of controlling and manipulating the physical structure and chemical composition of food products. Fourth, there is a growing appreciation for the value-added and market potential of hypernutritious foods. And fifth, growth of the global market. Overall, the trend toward development of hypernutritious foods and inclusion of these foods in healthful daily diets has experienced significant growth in the last few years.

In the past decade, a significant amount of research and product development has occurred to identify specific components of foods that may have health benefits. That knowledge and science has been used in the development of new products which are either modifications of existing foods or completely new foods. New and traditional techniques for producing and manufacturing foods provide routes to development of hypernutritious products.

For example, if an increased intake of a particular phytochemical, such as found in garlic or rosemary, is desired, this can be achieved by a variety of methods. Conventional plant breeding can be used to increase the level of the phytochemical in garlic or rosemary. Biotechnological techniques can be used to introduce that phytochemical into other frequently consumed fruits and vegetables. The phytochemical can be isolated with milling or extraction techniques, or can be chemically synthesized, and added to other processed foods. Some of these techniques require FDA evaluation (e.g., biotechnology, extraction, and chemical synthesis) and others do not (e.g., conventional plant breeding and milling) (25). The variety of potential products that may be manufactured using these or combinations of these and other techniques is infinitesimal.

CLASSES OF HYPERNUTRITIOUS FOODS

In general, however, hypernutritious foods fall into four major categories. First, existing foods which have a health advantage over similar foods. An example of this type of product is high beta-glucan barley or oats which research suggests will lower blood cholesterol more effectively than currently available cultivars (26, 27). A second category, processed foods which have been modified include reduced fat and salt products or fiber-enriched and beta-carotene (antioxidant)-enriched products. Food ingredients specifically designed to be added to foods to replace undesired components or to add desired components constitute the third category of hypernutritious foods. An example of ingredients that might fall into this category are modified starches as replacements for fat or probiotics, such as *Lactobacillus acidophilus*, as an added ingredient in foods. The fourth category of products is novel foods produced by biotechnology to produce high biological functionality, for example, genetic manipulation of a plant to either eliminate a carcinogenic component or increase the level of an anticarcinogenic component.

Many food manufacturers argue that the concept of "hypernutritious foods" should not be limited to specially modified foods or to conventional foods "enriched" with an extrinsic food component identified as having health benefits, but should extend to a variety of conventional foods.

HOW BROAD IS THE UNIVERSE?

Attribution of health benefits to specific foods or nutrients is not new. The following list gives a few examples:

Diet / Health Benefits Continuum

* Calcium builds strong bones
* Cranberry juice and proper urinary tract function
* Prunes and normal bowel function
* Fermented milk drinks and probiotic function
* Vegetables, antioxidants, niacin and lowered lipid levels
* Calcium and osteoporosis
* Folic acid and neural tube defects

"Calcium build strong bones" is a structure/function statement, that is, it conveys information about how calcium intake affects the structure or function of some system in the human body.

Cranberry juice is another example of a food attributed with health benefits. There is some research demonstrating cranberry juice may play a role in maintaining proper functioning of the urinary tract and particularly in reducing the number of infections in susceptible individuals. This effect may be due to the juice increasing the acidity of urine, thus inhibiting microbial growth, although another mechanism may be responsible (28).

A variety of fermented milk products, including yogurt, are claimed to demonstrate a probiotic functional effect by improving the quantity and quality of the microflora in the human intestinal tract. This effect is said to be particularly beneficial after antibiotic therapy which often destroys or alters the normal intestinal microbial environment. In addition, lactase-deficient individuals can benefit from calcium-rich sources of dairy products by consuming fermented dairy products without suffering symptoms of lactose intolerance (29).

Many more products with purported health benefits have been developed in countries outside the U.S., particularly in those countries that have a regulatory mechanism in place to accommodate the research and marketing of these foods.

Japan was at the forefront of the hypernutritious food movement with a 1984 government initiative. In July 1991, regulations were approved for "Foods for Specified Health Use" (FOSHU). The Japanese government is considering requiring sales of FOSHU products only in certified stores staffed by FOSHU nutritionists. No FOSHU products were approved in the first 18 months of the regulations. Table 2.1 lists some examples of FOSHU and the type of label information required (23).

The concept of hypernutritious foods has stimulated interest in other countries and in the international community as well. While Japan is the only country with a regulatory structure for these products, discussion has proceeded to various levels in other countries, as described in Table 2.2 (24). This table illustrates two things: first, the tremendous interest around the world in the development of hypernutritious foods; and second, universal recognition that scientifically supportable health claims, as a means of providing consumers with key health information, are an essential factor in the development of these products.

So, the circle closes back at health claims. The importance of health claims cannot be overemphasized, at this point in the development of hypernutritious foods, as the most important, accessible tool for providing consumers with sound information about the benefits of foods and their relationship to health. However, the underlying science demonstrating the relation-

TABLE 2.1. COMMERCIAL FOSHU PRODUCTS AND HEALTH CLAIMS

Product	Label information
Low Phosphorus Milk (L.P.K.) (Moringa Milk Industries)	A milk powder suitable for nutrition therapy of patients with chronic kidney malfunctions. On market since 1988 and sold to dialysis patients in hospitals and by home delivery routes.
Calcium 160 (Takara Shuzo)	A soft drink containing CCM (calcium citrate malate) *Permitted claim:* Suitable as calcium intake for diets deficient in calcium, the calcium is highly absorbable by man. *Cautions on intake:* 100 ml of this product contains 110 mg of calcium. Adults require calcium in their diet. A daily intake of 600 mg from foods is considered to be a suitable intake.
Goodent Chewing Gum (Lotte)	Contains palatinose and maltitol. *Permitted claim:* Dental caries worry-free gum. *Cautions on intake:* Does not prevent dental caries caused by other foods.
Meilogo granules (Meiji Seika)	A table top sugar consisting of fructo-oligosaccharide *Permitted claim:* Promotes the growth of bifidus bacteria in the gut, keeps your insides in good condition. *Cautions on intake:* Eating excess has an effect on the physical constitution and physical condition, such as a loosening of the bowels.

TABLE 2.2. COMPARISON OF INTERNATIONAL REGULATIONS

Country	Standard for functional foods	Position on health claims
Australia	Under review	Not permitted, to be reviewed as part of the review of the Food Stds. Code
Canada	No regulation	Not permitted
Japan	FOSHU	Permitted only within the FOSHU context
New Zealand	No regulation	Not permitted
Sweden	No regulation	Specific claims permitted
United States	No regulation	As addressed in NLEA
Codex	No regulation	Not permitted
European Community	No regulation	Not permitted

ship and validating the benefit must first exist before the tool can work.

UNAPPROVED CLAIMS

The NLEA directed FDA to consider 10 nutrient/disease relationships. Among the health claims FDA considered for approval, but didn't approve are claims about:

* Antioxidant vitamins and cancer (30)
* Zinc and immune function in the elderly (31)
* Omega-3 fatty acids and coronary heart disease (32)

These claims were not approved because the fundamental scientific evidence to support the claim is not available. Either there is not sufficient data on which to base an evaluation of the food component/health relationship or a well-reasoned claim, as in the case of zinc and immuno-function in the elderly. Or, the limiting factor might be that a direct association between the substance and the disease or health condition cannot be identified with existing scientific data. Examples of the latter are associations between antioxidant vitamins and cancer and between fiber and cancer, although the data do show relationships between consumption of diets high in foods containing these constituents and reduced risk of cancer. The current science cannot clearly differentiate the effect of the nutrient on the health effect from the combined influence of other food constituents in combination with the nutrient on the health effect.

Global interest in hypernutritious foods means global trade in these products. Health drinks developed under the Japanese regulations, known as "smart drinks" and "memory drinks", contain vitamins, oligo-elements, and amino acids and claim to aid memory and intelligence. Some of these products are appearing in the United States and European marketplace under names such as "Rise and Shine", "Memory Fuel", and "Fast Blast" (33). The success of these and other hypernutritious foods is dependent on legislation which facilitates marketing on a global scale. Until this legislation is enacted, mainstream marketing cannot really begin.

CRITICAL ISSUES

As we consider some critical issues related to the requirements for health claims mentioned earlier, it is not the authors' objective to in any way weaken the standard for health claims. The objective is to clarify how the standard is being used and to work within the "spirit" of the standard to develop a better program that accommodates consumer needs as well as those of industry and public health officials. Passage of the NLEA and development of regulations defining the requirements for health claims have crystallized criticism of the U.S. regulatory framework for hypernutritious foods. And that is fair, but it is essential to bear in mind that the legislation was intended to apply to conventional foods, primarily. However, it also provides a framework for future discussions and necessary changes to accommodate the development and marketing of safe, effective products and provide accurate information to consumers.

One other point must be kept in mind in considering the critical issues surrounding health claims. The law within which

FDA functions is grounded in two concepts; one of foods and the other of drugs. Under the present law, if a substance is used for the cure, mitigation, treatment, or prevention of disease, it is considered a drug and is subject to regulation as a drug. Without a doubt, the legal distinction between a food and a drug is far clearer than is the understanding of nutrition science necessary to support a decision one way or the other.

Critical Issue: Significant Scientific Agreement

The requirement for *significant* scientific agreement has triggered considerable criticism. In the words of Mr. Stephen McNamara, Esq., "it appears that the agency is unwilling to authorize claims that talk about preliminary data or anything short of an absolute and unequivocal finding that a particular food bears a favorable relationship with a particular disease" (2). From the perspective of Dr. Stephen DeFelice of the Foundation for Innovation in Medicine, hypernutritious products must be effective, or probably effective, as demonstrated by published clinical trials. Clinical studies must be published in respected clinical journals, but they do not necessarily have to demonstrate definitive clinical activity, such as the effect of vitamin C in patients with scurvy. Strong suggestive data are sufficient as we have seen with a mineral such as magnesium, which inhibits platelet aggregation and reduces insulin resistance in certain diabetics, Dr. DeFelice suggests (34).

Critics ask what "significant" means and question whether it is reasonable to apply the standard evenly across the board. At the time FDA was developing its health claim regulations, a few staff members of the FTC, citing the changing body of research on diet and health and poor understanding of consumers' response to information, considered the type of health benefits and the level of scientific agreement required for a nonmisleading label claim. They concluded that a consensus standard is appropriate in some, but not all, situations. Where the harm to consumers is large and the benefits small if the science proves to be wrong, then a consensus of opinion may be appropriate. Where the harm is small, adherence to a scientific consensus will unnecessarily stem the flow of useful information to consumers. The outcome of this FTC staff paper was the argument that a "standard that requires various levels of substantiation, depending on circumstances surrounding the claim, is likely to better encourage the dissemination of truthful nonmisleading health claims" (35).

Critical Issue: Totality of Publicly Available Information

There are a number of issues embraced in this requirement for a health claim. The first is the totality of scientific evidence. To scientists and public policy officials, the meaning of this requirement is clear and it is doubtful that anyone would take issue with this concept. Simply stated, this means that all of the data must be considered and the weight of the evidence will prevail. It means that one cannot blindly select only that evidence that promotes a particular position.

The requirement that data and information supporting a health claim be publicly available in the scientific literature leaves no leeway for use of proprietary data to support a claim. Thus, development of hypernutritious foods is stifled because innovators are provided with no protections or incentives to expend resources. There are no economic incentives for people to do good basic research. Another problem is that results of any proprietary research submitted in support of a health claim would be made publicly available upon authorization of the claim. Moreover, under current regulations, as soon as FDA authorizes a health claim, the claim is available for all manufacturers to use.

Critical Issue: Safe and Lawful

Safety.—We're seeing an increasing body of research that indicates that nutrient intakes at higher than traditional levels may have health benefits. At increased intake levels, however, questions of safety arise. At the June 1994 NIH Consensus Conference on Calcium and Osteoporosis the impact of calcium intakes higher than RDI levels (i.e., 1,000 mg/day) was considered. Two major conclusions of relevance to this discussion were that: a large percentage of Americans do not consume recommended levels of calcium and calcium intakes up to 2,000 mg/day appear to be safe for most people (36). Some segments of the population, for example, those susceptible to kidney stones, may be adversely affected by elevated calcium intakes. The issue is how to provide the desired amount of calcium without having adverse health consequences.

Legality.—Levels of safe use of a substance, can be established, if necessary, through food additive or GRAS procedures once the data are available to support that process. Once again, the concepts of "food vs. drug" are critical issues impinging on the types of claims that might be made.

Critical Issue: Generic Rather Than Product Specific Claims

The requirement that health claims be generic in nature and not specific to individual products is another source of criticism. Current laws in Japan permit exclusivity in the use of a claim for a specified length of time, by developers of hypernutritious products. The effect is to encourage private sector expenditure of resources and expertise to develop products with specific health benefits and the scientific data to support claims for those products. As the segment of the hypernutritious foods industry focused on development of products specially formulated to deliver specific health benefits grows, it is anticipated that demands for a suitable mechanism facilitating the use of product-specific claims will increase.

Critical Issue: Context of The Daily Diet

The requirement in the law that a health claim must provide information about the substance/disease relationship *within the context of the daily diet* triggers criticism because, at least in some cases, the quantity of information required to accomplish this is so extensive that another, that the claim not be misleading, is exceeded. This may pose a problem down the road when the relationships between specific food components, such as various constituents of garlic, and health are sufficiently elucidated to warrant a health claim. How will consumption of this food component be reasonably evaluated in terms of the daily diet where garlic is usually consumed in only small amounts, if at all. As Mr. Stephen McNamara, Esq. has stated, we can't turn vitamin C into a drug just because someone does some research showing it has disease preventive value (2).

Critical Issue: Disqualifying Nutrient Levels

As mentioned earlier, language in the law provides that a health claim cannot be made on a food that contains "any nutrient in an amount which increases . . . the risk of a disease or a health-related condition". Hence, the calcium/osteoporosis claim may not be made on many cheeses. Although cheese is a rich source of calcium, it also contains significant levels of fat, saturated fat, cholesterol, and sodium. The issue here is how narrowly or broadly the definition of "increasing the risk of a disease or a health-related condition" is to be defined.

In the late 1970s, the agency recognized that substances that are useful in the diet may also have adverse effects when mannitol, a sugar alcohol, was approved as a food additive. The regulation stipulates that the label of a food which may result in the daily ingestion of 20 g of mannitol must bear the statement "Excess consumption may have a laxative effect" to inform consumers of potential adverse affects (37). The issue of disqualifying nutrient levels will, no doubt, be subject to future debate as policies governing hypernutritious foods are further developed.

Critical Issues: Complete, Truthful, and Not Misleading

A look at the model claim for folic acid and neural tube defects rather succinctly sums up this issue (38):

> "Women who consume adequate amounts of folate, a B vitamin, daily throughout their childbearing years may reduce their risk of having a child with a neural tube birth defect. Such birth defects, while not widespread, are very

serious. They can have many causes. Adequate amounts of folate can be obtained from diets rich in fruits, dark green leafy vegetables and legumes, enriched grain products, fortified cereals, or a supplement. Folate consumption should be limited to 1,000 μg per day from all sources."

It is apparent that, in some cases, there may be a level at which the quantity of information required to fully inform consumers must be balanced against whether the sheer length of the message discourages consumer use of the information.

As science advances and relationships between nutrition and diseases are better understood, health claims can be made less cumbersome. As we gain more experience in consumer education and how consumers use label information we will be able to construct more effective messages. But a word of caution. As the messages begin to promise too much and they tend to mislead the consumer, our greatest asset for further development of hypernutritious foods will be lost. That asset is consumer confidence. We must be able to deliver what we promise.

SUMMARY

These criticisms raise issues fundamental to the future development of the hypernutritious foods industry in the U.S. and to conveying relevant information about the health benefits of these foods to consumers. Solutions to these criticisms and situations shaped by the health claim requirements are entertained in Table 2.3. There is currently no mechanism for exclusive health claims based on proprietary research comparable to the provisions in the law for drugs. The NLEA mandates that "publicly available scientific evidence" be used to support health claims for food and the Agency has stated its strong preference for such claims not to be brand specified. Proponents of hypernutritious foods complain that this removes the financial incentive for companies to invest in research and development of products with positive health benefits. How can this be resolved? Perhaps a change in the law will be required or a new law which provides some of the incentives inherent in the Orphan Drug Act.

TABLE 2.3. POSSIBLE SOLUTIONS

Issue	Situation	Solution
Significant scientific agreement	what standard?	Data
Totality of publicly available scientific evidence	Proprietary research	Revised Law
Safe and lawful	Not high quantities that would cause harm; Food, food additive, or GRAS	Data
Claim must be generic	Product specific	Consensus
Food must be part of total daily diet	Food vs. Drug	Consensus
Food cannot possess any nutrient in an amount that increases risk of disease	Negative attribution	Consensus
Claim must be complete, truthful, and not misleading	Cumbersome	Consensus

Continued discussion to attain a satisfactory consensus about scientific substantiation of health claims is needed. Should the "significant scientific agreement" standard be strictly interpreted, as it is now, or is a standard that requires various levels of scientific substantiation, along the lines suggested by the FTC, is more realistic? An integral part of this discussion is how to convey information about the level of scientific substantiation along with the substance/health-condition information in the health claim in a way that consumers may understand and use the information.

When these two issues are resolved in a way that facilitates the development and marketing of hypernutritious foods and provide scientifically sound diet and health information to consumers, the other issues will fall into line. They can be resolved by maintaining dialogue between health professionals, regulators, and industry with the goal of reaching consensus. The Keystone National Policy Dialogue on Food, Nutrition, and Health, currently underway, is just one mechanism to facilitate this communication. FDA has the capability to approve product-specific health claims now, but not the resources this would entail under the current regulatory structure.

The bottom line is science. Today, we do not have the science to support health claims, particularly for unique products, nor do we have the mechanisms for developing that data. Without the essential scientific foundation, the 2010 supermarket, replete with hypernutritious foods is an unlikely reality in the United States. Before that supermarket can be a reality the view of traditional foods must change, scientific advances must occur, regulatory systems must grow and develop, and consumer education systems must grow and develop. Achieving these four requires the concerted, cooperative efforts of scientists, industry, consumers, and public health officials.

BIBLIOGRAPHY

1. THIER, S. O. "The Sciences of Nutrition". *Food Technol.* 1990, *44*(8), 26-34.
2. LABELL, F. "Foods of Tomorrow Part I: Experts ask policy change on health claims". *Food Proc.* 1993, *54*(4), 52-57.
3. DHHS. "Federal Food, Drug, and Cosmetic Act, As Amended". U.S. Government Printing Office: Washington, DC. 1995. Section 403(r)(3)(B)(i).
4. DHHS. "Title 21, Code of Federal Regulations, Parts 100-169". U.S. Government Printing Office; Washington, DC, April 1994. Section 101.14.
5. FDA. "Food Labeling; General Requirements for Health Claims for Food: Final Rule", *Fed. Regist.* January 6, 1993, *58,* 2506.
6. DHHS. "Federal Food, Drug, and Cosmetic Act, As Amended". U.S. Government Printing Office: Washington, DC. Sections 201(s), 402(a)(1) and (a)(2), and 409.
7. DHHS. "Federal Food, Drug, and Cosmetic Act, As Amended". U.S. Government Printing Office: Washington, DC. Section 403(r)(3)(A)(ii).
8. FDA. "Food Labeling; General Requirements for Health Claims for Food: Final Rule", *Fed. Regist.* January 6, 1993, *58,* 2502.
9. DHHS. "Title 21, Code of Federal Regulations, Parts 170-199". U.S. Government Printing Office: Washington, DC. April 1994. Section 170.30.
10. DHHS. "Title 21, Code of Federal Regulations, Parts 170-199". U.S. Government Printing Office, Washington, DC, April 1994. Section 170.35.
11. DHHS. "Federal Food, Drug, and Cosmetic Act, As Amended". U.S. Government Printing Office; Washington, DC. Section 201(s).
12. DHHS. "Title 21, Code of Federal Regulations, Parts 170-199". U.S. Government Printing Office: Washington, DC. April, 1994. Section 172.5.

13. DHHS. "Title 21, Code of Federal Regulations, Parts 170-199". U.S. Government Printing Office: Washington, DC. April, 1994. Section 181.1 and 181.5.
14. DHHS. "Federal Food, Drug, and Cosmetic Act, As Amended". U.S. Government Printing Office: Washington, DC. Section 403(r)(3)(B)(iii).
15. FDA. "Food Labeling; General Requirements for Health Claims for Food: Final Rule", *Fed. Regist.* January 6, 1993, *58,* 2511.
16. FDA. "Food Labeling; General Requirements for Health Claims for Food: Proposed Rule". *Fed. Regist.* November 27, 1991, *56,* 60545.
17. DHHS. "Title 21, Code of Federal Regulations, Parts 100-169". U.S. Government Printing Office: Washington, DC. April 1994. Section 101.14(a)(5).
18. DHHS. "Federal Food, Drug, and Cosmetic Act, As Amended". U.S. Government Printing Office: Washington, DC. Section 403(a)(1).
19. DHHS. "Federal Food, Drug, and Cosmetic Act, As Amended". U.S. Government Printing Office: Washington, DC. Section 201(n).
20. FDA. "Food Labeling; General Requirements for Health Claims for Food: Proposed Rule" *Fed. Regist.* November 27, 1991, *56,* 60552.
21. ANON. "Trendspeak". *The Food Channel.* 1994, *6*(12), 3.
22. LIN, R. I. "Phytochemicals and Antioxidants". *In Functional Foods: Designer Foods, Pharmafoods, Nutraceuticals*; Goldberg, I., Ed.; Chapman & Hall: New York, 1994; Chapter 17.
23. MINISTRY OF HEALTH AND WELFARE (Japan). "List of Foods Approved for Specified Health Use." Office of Health Policy on Newly Developed Foods. 1994.
24. NATIONAL FOOD AUTHORITY. "Functional Foods: Policy Discussion Paper". Canberra, Australia, July, 1994.
25. HATHCOCK, J. N. "Safety and Regulatory Issues for Phytochemical Sources: 'Designer Foods'". *Nutr. Today.* 1993, *28*(6), 23-25.
26. MCINTOSH, G. H.; WHYTE, J.; MCARTHUR, R.; NESTEL, P. J. "Barley and Wheat Foods: Influence on Plasma Cholesterol Concentrations in Hypercholesterolemic Men". *Am. J. Clin. Nutr.* 1991, *53*(5), 1205-1209.
27. RIPSIN, C. M.; KEENAN, J. M.; "The Effects of Dietary Oat Products on Blood Cholesterol". *Trends Food Sci. Techno*l. 1992, *3*(6), 137-141.
28. AVORN, J.; MONANE, M.; GURWILTZ, J. H.; GLYNN, R. J.; CHOODNOVSHIY, I.; LIPSITA, L. A. "Reduction of Bacteriuria and Pyuria after Ingestion of Cranberry Juice". *J. Am. Med. Assoc.* 1994, *271*(10), 751-754.
29. SANDERS, M. E. "Lactic Acid Bacteria as Promoters of Human Health". In *Functional Foods: Designer Foods, Pharmafoods, Nutraceuticals;* Goldberg, I., Ed.; Chapman & Hall: New York, 1994; Chapter 14.
30. FDA. "Food Labeling: Health Claims and Label Statements: Antioxidant Vitamins and Cancer: Final Rule". *Fed. Regist.* January 6, 1993, *58,* 2622.

31. FDA. “Food Labeling: Health Claims and Label Statements: Zinc and Immune Function in the Elderly:Final Rule”. *Fed. Regist.* January 6, 1993, 58, 2661.
32. FDA. “Food Labeling: Health Claims and Label Statements: Omega-3 Fatty Acids and Coronary Heart Disease:Final Rule”. *Fed. Regist.* January 6, 1993, 58, 2682.
33. ANON. “Designing Foods”. *Inform.* 1993, 4(4), 344-352.
34. DEFELICE, S. L. “Nutraceuticals—Opportunities in an Emerging Market”. *Scrip Mag. 1992, Sept.*, 14-15.
35. IPPOLITO, P. M.; MATHIOS, A. D. “The Regulation of Science- Based Claims in Advertising”. *J. Cons. Pol.* 1990, *13,* 413-445.
36. NIH. “NIH Consensus Statement: Optimal Calcium Intake”. 1994, *12*(4).
37. DHHS. “Title 21, Code of Federal Regulations, Part 170-199”. U.S. Government Printing Office: Washington, DC. April 1994. Section 180.25(e).
38. DHHS. “Title 21, Code of Federal Regulations, Parts 100-169”. U.S. Government Printing Office: Washington, DC, April 1994. Section 101.79(d)(1).

3

The Business and Public Policy Issues of Commercializing Nutraceuticals and Hypernutritious Foods

Nancy M. Childs

Government, research and health agencies have recommended eating habits for health promotion and disease prevention. An explosion in technology is allowing scientists to develop "superfoods" with potentially strong preventative or therapeutic properties. This situation generates major market opportunities and policy issues for relevant industries that generate, and government agencies that regulate, these new products. A descriptive business dynamics model is presented for this emerging industry which identifies the macro-drivers that advance the U.S. market for these products. Using this model, this chapter will identify and examine key issues enabling this industry to succeed. Several public policy issues critical to the development of this category are elucidated.

Looking ahead to the twenty-first century for the evolution of hypernutritious foods, four broad trends seem apparent. First, one sees a convergence, a blurring of boundaries, between nutritional, pharmaceutical, and food science. Secondly, a merging of consumer and professionally indicated products seems likely. Consumers are gaining confidence in addressing and resolving issues of health maintenance for themselves. Hypernutritious foods are a consumer driven category. Thirdly, in preparation of these products, there will be a merging of clinical and epidemiological documentation. Familiar food products with new uses based on benefits just recently understood and documented, as may potentially be provided by tea, soy, and other phytochemicals, will demand new combinations and formats of epidemiological and clinical trials and animal study documentation to demonstrate significant scientific agreement. Achieving this agreement may be a process unique for each product in recognition of its particular risk/benefit profile. Lastly, there will be a gradual repositioning of federal agency roles and functions as the FDA continues to expand its role in nutrition and public health education. It will join other agencies in promoting the integration and interdependence of diet and health, foods as medicines.

This chapter will seek to address the key issues accompanying the evolution of this new category of foods for health. A macro-environment and business model will be presented to describe key factors driving the commercialization of this category. Past research issues will be summarized, and the identification of seven business and seven public policy concerns will be presented.

CURRENT FACTORS AND KEY ISSUES FOR HYPERNUTRITIOUS FOODS

Three current factors summarize the present situation for hypernutritious foods. First, there appears to be universal agreement on an academic, regulatory, industry, and consumer level that diet and nutrition are critical control factors in the pursuit of good health. There is an accelerating emphasis on preventive medicine to maintain good health. These two factors are juxtaposed by the FDA's inability to keep up with the technical advances, commercial development, and consumer demand for such products because of the agency's declining resources and expanded responsibilities.

Key issues for discussion accompany the transformation from a simpler separate drug and food paradigm to a new more complex paradigm where hypernutritious foods are developed and marketed for their potential role in health maintenance. Key issues of the past, for the regulatory agency, focused on safety and efficacy. Today, these responsibilities are joined with numerous additional concerns for public health and concerns in the marketplace. These include communication: What can we say? Where can we say it? Economic issues split between the maximization of public health and recognition that product development is pursued in the private sector to obtain a fair return on investment. There are questions regarding product access, both in terms of retail channel and role of physician indication. Major medical and nutrition paradigm shifts are occurring from deficiency to prevention and from therapy to prevention. In recognition of the immense advances in science and growing understanding of the human genome, there is a nutritional paradigm shift expected from addressing population norms to focusing on individual needs.

INTRODUCING A MACRO-ENVIRONMENT MODEL

Seven factors are critical to the momentum driving the successful commercialization of this category. They are shown in Fig. 3.1 and listed below:

* Consumer Trends
* Private and Public Health Agencies
* Health Care Trends
* Food Industry
* Pharmaceutical Industry
* International Factors
* Scientific Discovery

The macro-environment and business model discussed in this chapter assumes continued scientific discovery and documentation in support of hypernutritious foods and does not attempt to summarize these specific discoveries.

CONSUMER TRENDS

Hypernutritious foods are and will remain a consumer driven category. The baby boomer mentality and mortality drive interest in this category. This group is action oriented and comfortable seeking solutions for problems. They generate marketplace response that is then available to the larger population. They are comfortable with self-medication and are responsible for increased interest in natural childbirth, lamaze, homeopathy, mid-wives, and other alternative medicine practices. They are comfortable with self-diagnosis with test-kits and rely on OTC remedies. Their health concerns are underscored by their discovery, once in their forties, that youth is not eternal. Terminal illness of parents, relatives, friends, and cultural icons remind baby boomers of their mortality. The experience of terminal illness in familial circumstances is a double barreled blow of both the specific disease with its genome-based hereditary implications and the cost of the terminal demise, both in quality of life and pocketbook.

Consumers have gained tremendously in their nutrition savviness, learning from government educational campaigns, private sector advertising, and a high level of attention in the media. While their level of nutrition knowledge has improved, it is not optimal. Lastly, consumers are driven to a health maintenance vigilance because they are absorbing significantly more health care cost each year with growing co-payments, deductibles, and premiums.

PRIVATE AND PUBLIC HEALTH AGENCIES

Government nutritional policy recommendations, as promulgated by government public health agencies and government funded institutions, have been accelerating during the past five

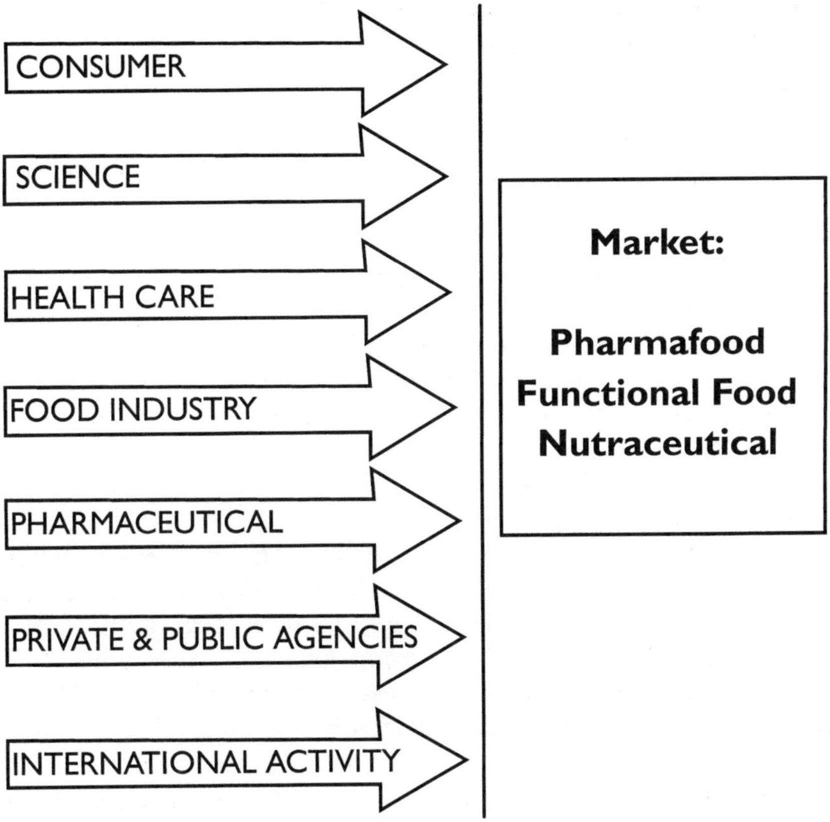

FIG. 3.1. MODEL OF BUSINESS DYNAMICS IMPACTING THE PHARMAFOOD/NUTRACEUTICAL MARKET IN THE UNITED STATES.

years. There is no universal message. While there are numerous proclamations relating diet and health, it is more cacophony than harmony. The trend and the emphasis, if not the specific message, are however reinforcing. Highlights of the past five years include the following:

1988 Surgeon General's Report on Nutrition and Health

1989 Academy of Science Nutrition Guideline

1991 Institute of Medicine Food Guidelines
1991 National Nutritional Monitoring Act

1992 USDA Food Guide Pyramid (DHHS)
1992 NCI 5-A-Day Program

1993 NLEA enacted
1993 FDA Nutritional Content for Restaurants proposed

1994 RDA re-examination proposed
1994 Dietary Supplement legislation passed

Of the many messages, the National Nutritional Monitoring Act is notable because it institutionalizes change in nutrition regulation. The NLEA mandates that the FDA, for the first time, undertake public health education and to approve health claims, thereby, acknowledging that food impacts health. In addition, re-examination of the RDA, which is likely to increase RDA recommendation levels, gives further credence to the role of food in maintaining good health.

It has been twenty-five years since the landmark White House Conference on Nutrition, held in 1969, where nutrition was first formally recognized for its role in obtaining and maintaining good health and not simply avoiding nutritional deficiencies. Another landmark era seems worthy of recognition at this unmarked twenty-fifth anniversary. Such high profile attention, a natural extension of the Clinton emphasis on health care, would catapult the hypernutritious food category to consumer, medical, and media attention.

HEALTH CARE TRENDS

Due to the Clinton health care reform dialog, health care received an exhaustive discussion and review in 1994. Costs are exploding at an alarming rate and demographics of an aging population portend even greater acceleration of health care usage and cost. The managed care (HMO) institution is the increasingly prevalent treatment delivery model which controls cost and optimizes patient care. With the HMO emphasis on preventive medicine and its ability to set treatment protocol for physicians that encompass nutritional and dietary recommendations, such as diet as the primary treatment protocol for cholesterol reduction, HMOs will continue to rely on nutrition as a preventive modality to reduce costs.

FOOD INDUSTRY

Food companies can be characterized as efficient consumer marketers capable of building brands sustained by repeat purchase. They possess immense R&D and packaging capabilities for creating good tasting products. For decades, the food industry has vitamin fortified, polyunsaturated, sugar substituted, artificially flavored, preserved, decaffeinated, calcium added, fat reduced, fiber added, and made other improvements to the American food supply while delivering good taste and value to the consumer. Astute attention to consumer demand is assigned greater importance by the food industry than government nutritional proclamation.

As an industry, characterizations include relatively high cash flow and low R&D expenditure, steady volume with stable margins, and a business sustained by mass markets. They seek value-added opportunities to sell new products to their same customers.

PHARMACEUTICAL INDUSTRY

Formerly, an extremely profitable industry operating within a regulated environment, the pharmaceutical industry today is undergoing immense structural changes that result in major price and margin pressures. Industry consolidation and alliances both drive and result from increased price pressure and competition. The novel molecule as a new drug entity is no longer enough; the new entry must pass a cost effectiveness model and demonstrate improved quality of life for government approval and acceptance in a drug formulary. Generic competition is growing at a rapid rate. Drugs are rapidly diverted to OTC conversion as approval permits. The OTC route was viewed with skepticism a few years ago, but has found enthusiastic endorsement with the discovery that the lower OTC price point is accompanied by phenomenally greater volume generation.

Clearly, full consumer access to a product outperforms the gatekeeper pathway through the physician for the ethical product.

Noteworthy are several major United States pharmaceutical operations, such as Merck and Pfizer, along with European and Japanese enterprises, which have food ingredient divisions that are well positioned to bring core research and clinical testing competencies to the hypernutritious foods category. Their technology and other value-added services complement the food industry needs in product development for this category. They are seeking new market opportunities to leverage existing strengths.

INTERNATIONAL FACTORS

Hypernutritious foods appear to be a global product opportunity and have experienced significant market activity in other markets of the developed world. Notably these include Japan, Europe—particularly Germany, New Zealand and South Africa. Participants in these markets are gaining product experience and collecting market data for possible submission for approval in more rigorous regulatory environments. Certainly, the United States market with its huge size and high expenditure on health products is an enticing opportunity.

International market development has been encouraged by numerous factors including older demographics and national health care programs seeking lower cost and preventive solutions. Asian and European cultures value herbal and natural remedies and accept a food and health relationship. Nutrition is a part of the medical curriculum and health claims for food products may be more specifically permitted. In some countries reimbursement, to varying degrees, is permitted for such products and provides added incentive to develop and market hypernutritious and nutraceutical products.

PROPOSED BUSINESS MODEL

A business model capturing the key driver of each of these sectors is displayed in Table 3.1. The model indicates strong

TABLE 3.1. BUSINESS MODEL OF KEY FACTORS IN THE HYPERNUTRITIOUS FOOD MARKET

Component	Driver
Consumer	Quality of Life Cost Savings
Private & Public Agencies	Improve Public Health Deliver Nutrition Education
FDA	Safety, Efficacy, Trust Outdated Structure, New Mandates, Multiple Priorities
Health Care Industry	Cost Containment
Food Industry	Value-added opportunities
Pharmaceutical Industry	New Markets
International Activity	Leverage International Experience to US Market
Nutrition Science	Public Research—Generic, Private Research—ROI Concern

motivation and momentum among the many participants to participate in the hypernutritious and nutraceutical category. On the macro level described by the model, there appear to be strong trends and motivations for the category to evolve, from the consumer level through to the government policy agenda. The model also identifies some areas of potential policy disagreement.

Research Findings

Earlier research by the author, while investigating food and pharmaceutical industry activity in the category, documented several findings. Primary concern for both industries focused on vocabulary confusion for the category. A small proclivity for the terms "medical foods" and "nutraceuticals" was reported among the pharmaceutical firms, whereas preference for "functional foods" and "nutritional foods" was found among the food industry. Importantly, both industries showed high interest in the category, but were intending to stay in their familiar territory in their method of addressing and developing the category. This suggests a rigidity that invites opportunities for other players.

Their concerns focused on regulations and the expense of clinical trials. Additionally, all acknowledged that the media has become the prime communication channel to the consumer for science and products.

Business Issues

The successful commercialization of hypernutritious foods, within the macro-environment described, raises several business issues on the micro, or market, level.

Brand Development.—The importance of brand development and marketing activity will be proportional to the degree the product can make a proprietary, differentiated claim. A generic claim does not guarantee exclusivity in the market place and permit a competitive advantage like a patent or proprietary claim. If a proprietary claim, or patent-like exclusivity, is not provided then brand development becomes essential for success. The product will differentiate itself on marketing and promotion points of difference, such as packaging, price, product form and flavor, positioning, point of sale, spokesperson, and media weight. These are not product or science based points of difference. Like a Gatorade product, brand mystique will be built relying on the physical prowess of a spokesperson such as Michael Jordon, and not documented science. Under this scenario money is diverted to marketing campaigns at the expense of research.

Clinical Trials Format.—The clinical trial format is important for two reasons: first is the cost and time factor, and second is the resultant generic or proprietary claim and its implication for a sustainable competitive advantage. At present NLEA health claims are ***generic*** and pertinent to a category of foods, such as vegetables, that meet prescribed criteria. The NCI designer foods research is also category based. Product or molecule specific trials resulting in proprietary claims are limited to the FDA approval process for drugs only and not to foods or health claims for foods.

The issue of generic or proprietary claims and product or category trials determines, ultimately, if the category will be characterized by price competition or product competition. Without protected differentiation, the category will see price competition emerge as there is little sustainable competitive advantage. What does emerge will be the marketplace power of the enormous consumer goods companies who have the ability to leverage immense marketing know-how, distribution strength, and retailer relationships to assure their product is available to the consumer. This scenario projects the consumer advantages of price competition and increased awareness of the product's benefit resulting from a heavy marketing campaign. While proprietary products produce less direct competition, and hence less price competition, the proprietary incentive with higher investment return promises more product research and development. It also attracts more entrepreneurs to the market.

Pricing and Market Size.—Fundamentally, pricing expectations will vary by industry. The pharmaceutical industry with its higher internal rate of return hurdles will demand higher price points. Physician-indicated products can solicit higher price points from the consumer. Market size is deceptive. While there are mass market needs, there will be niche market solutions. These health-specific categories will require careful target marketing and target product development.

HMO and Managed Care Environment.—The managed health care environment brings an element of access and control through the endorsement of hypernutritious foods and nutraceuticals. The documented success of these products in prolonging good health and preventing disease will justify their inclusion in a preventive care regime. Their purpose will be to achieve cost containment for the HMO, the corporate client, and the individual. Utilization of these products could result in reduced insurance premiums and lower deductibles. Enforcement issues are addressed through partial reimbursement, HMO tracked coupon usage, and HMO private label products.

Role of Other Players.—The food ingredient suppliers, biotech ventures, international participants, herbal manufacturers, and nutritional supplement manufacturers are potential participants in the category, either directly or indirectly through alliances and partnerships. They may assume significant roles by providing technical support, product competition, market experience, and market data.

Retail Channel Choices.—As research has shown, channel preferences vary by industry. The existing herbal and health food channel is large but fragmented and ignored by the major players examining this market. Channel choices will vary by price points and degree of consumer interest in the category as a mass market or a niche specialty.

Private Label Opportunities.—Private label opportunities will abound, in different formats for different reasons, depending on whether the market evolves on price or product differentiation, and whether the consumer seeks specialized or mass products such as vitamins.

Public Policy Concerns

The business issues discussed above will operate on a micro or market level while many of these same issues impact on the macro level as public policy concerns. The major drivers in the public policy arena appear to be the consumer's growing attention to diet, nutrition and health, the government's expanding commitment to nutrition education, the FDA regulatory structure restricting marketing and health claims, and the FDA's legal separation of food and drug. Seven public policy concerns are presented below:

Investment Dollars Pursuing Marketing Tactics at the Expense of Research Investment.—As discussed above under the business implications of brand development, this concern has many facets. A lack of R&D investment brings fewer product advances. A higher level of marketing activity increases the likelihood of more indirect public health nutrition education through product advertisement. Price competition is to the consumer's short term advantage with a longer term repercussion of fewer product choices.

"Uncontrolled Media" Becomes Marketer.—As briefly mentioned in the section on Research Findings, the media has become the primary communication channel to the consumer for science and product information. As regulations circumscribe the direct discussion of a product's health impact on the label and in marketing promotions or advertising, the information is directed to the consumer through the media. This format allows misinformation and incomplete information to reach the consumer in an indiscriminate way accompanying the legitimate findings. This format permits marketplace bonanzas and disasters outside the marketer's control. It also results in jaded and confused consumers who loose trust in the category's product benefits.

Current NLEA Format.—The new NLEA legislation, as interpreted through regulation, continues the heritage of safety and efficacy. For foods qualifying for NLEA health claim approval, the standard is rigorous and set. At present there is not a flexible or sliding scale of risk and benefit evaluation that encourages products with low risk profiles to market in a more timely, less rigorous and expensive manner. New products, without years or centuries of use in the diet, or without usage experience at megadose levels, engender higher risk levels and therefore a more exhaustive review.

Current NLEA format:

BENEFIT		COST
Extreme Assurance for Safety		Suppressed Nutrition Information
+	vs.	+
Extreme Assurance of Product Efficacy		Media-hyped Misinformation

Formally blocking products, and product information, from market through the regulated channels of label, labeling and advertising forces information to reach the consumer through the unregulated channels of media. Nutrition and product information through this channel is often incomplete or erroneous. Less information, and less complete information, reaches the consumer under this format.

New Clinical Trial Protocol.—A possible response to a cost—benefit approach to product approval is the endorsement of new clinical trial formats and evaluation modes of epidemiologic data and animal studies. The preventive mode requires separate evaluation formats than the treatment mode.

Foreign Competitors Gaining Market Experience.—As foreign competitors gain market experience and data outside the U.S., they are gaining a competitive advantage for entering the U.S. marketplace.

Government Agencies are not Coordinated.—The nutrition public health message promoted by numerous government and government supported private agencies is not identical. In addition to it differing by degree, the message is promoting dietary goals while the FDA regulates the product label of individual foods.

Changing Nutritional Paradigm.—Scientific advances permit an understanding of the human genome on the individual level. The impact of hypernutritious foods and nutraceuticals on individual health states and health proclivities, based on their genome, will become a reality. The nutritional paradigm will change from population norms to individual needs, and this distinction will necessitate a new framework of public health education.

SUMMARY

In conclusion, a macro-environment model suggests numerous factors contributing to the commercialization of a hypernutritious food and nutraceuticals category. The emergence of this category is dependent on the resolution of several business issues involving branding, clinical trial formats, pricing, channels and competitors. The ability to capture competitive advantage is key. The commercialized category operates in an arena of public policy issues regarding the investment outcome dependent on the regulatory framework for labeling, advertising and testing these products. While many issues are catalogued and discussed in this chapter their resolution is dependent on regulatory structure and interpretation. Looking further ahead, as stated in the beginning, the twenty-first century portends the merging of nutritional, pharmaceutical and food science, and products.

BIBLIOGRAPHY

1. *A Comparison of the U.S., European & Japanese Nutraceutical Health and Medical Claim Rules.* New York City: The Foundation for the Innovation in Medicine conference, Jan. 1993.
2. "Amino Acids and Other Dietary Supplements Should be Regulated by FDA." *The Pink Sheet.* 53.6 F-D-C Accession Number 15530224 (11 Feb. 1991).
3. "Are There Pharmafoods in Pharmacy's Future?" *Health Ind. Monitor.* SRI International, third quarter 1988, 1+.
4. "BioTechnica, Inc. in Joint Venture With RJR Nabisco, Inc. to Develop Improved Food Products Through Biotechnology." *Appl. Genet. News* 1987, 8.3, 9.
5. CALFEE, J. E. "FDA Underestimates Food Shoppers." *The Wall Street Journal* 1990, A.
6. "Can an Apple a Day Really Keep the Doctor Away?" *Prepared Foods,* Jan. 1991.
7. CHILDS, N. Ed. Pharmafoods: Is the U.S. Ready? Philadelphia: St. Joseph's Univ., 1992.
8. COLE, M. "When Food Meets Medicine." *Food Manufacture* (UK) 1991, 66(1), 26-28.
9. *Consumer Attitudes Toward Supermarket Pharmacies,* Washington DC: Food Marketing Institute, 1991.
10. "Crossroads '91 Foods of the 90's." *Food Technol.* N. Z. 1991, 26(6), 9.
11. DEFELICE, S. L. "Feeding the Nutraceutical Revolution." *Pharma. Exec.* 1991, 11, 78.
12. *Develop and Market Nutrient Fortified Foods.* Orlando: Institute for International Research, Dec. 1991.
13. EISENBERG, D. M., et. al. "Unconventional Medicine in the United States: Prevalence, Costs and Patterns of Use." *N. Engl. J. Med.* 1993, 328, 246-252.
14. ERICKSON, J. L.; DOGNOLI, J. "Healthy Food Pace Quickens: Leaving Regulatory Forces Behind." *Advert. Age.* 1989, 60(4), 3.
15. "Feasts From the East." *Food FIPP* (UK) 1990, 12(5), 37.
16. "Foods That Bring Better Health." *Futurist* 1991, 25(5), 52.
17. FOX, H. "Functional Foods Are On Their Way." *Food Ind. S. Africa* (UK) 1990, 43(7), 55.
18. *Functional Foods—A new Global Added Value Market?* London: PA Consulting Group, 1990.
19. *Future Issues in the Pharmaceutical Industry,* Philadelphia: St. Joseph's Univ., 1993.
20. "Futures: The Self-Medication Market of the Nineties." OTC Market Report Update USA. Oct. 1992.
21. GANNON, K. "Can Foods Cure Disease? Consumers Want to Know." *Drug Topics* 1991, 135, 32.

22. GARRITY, M. F. "Coming to Grips With the Rx-to-OTC Switch." *Drug Topics* 1989, 58-65.
23. Healthy Wealthy & Wiser: New Products for New Markets. Scottsdale AZ: *Delta Food Group*, Oct. 1992.
24. "Homeopathy—A New Direction." *OTC News and Market Report* (UK) 1992, 52, 403-410.
25. JOHNSON, M. "Firms Test Medical Food." *Marketing* (U.K.) 1990, Apr. 5, 1.
26. LEVINE, B. S., et. al. "A National Survey of Attitudes and Practices of Primary-Care Physicians Relating to Nutrition: Strategies for Enhancing the Use of Clinical Nutrition in Medical Practice." *Am. J. Clin. Nutr.* 1993, 7, 115-119.
27. MCNAMARA, S. H. "FDA's Rules on Health Claims for Foods— Including the New 1993 Regulations, Issued Under the Nutrition Labeling and Education Act (NLEA)." Washington DC: Hyman, Phelps & McNamara, Jan. 1993.
28. MCNUTT, K. "Pharmafoods and Magazines: Education by Default?" *Pharma. Technol.* 1991, 15(8), 57-58.
29. MCNUTT, K. "2013AD: Start Watching Now." *Eng. Foods* 1988, May, 62-63.
30. *Nutraceuticals and Pharmafoods—The Food and Drug Interface.* New Orleans: International Business Communications, Jan. 1991.
31. SENAUER, B.; ELAINE A.; KINSEY, *J. Food Trends and the Changing Consumer,* Eagan Press: St.Paul, MN, 1991.
32. SHEEHY, R. "Taking On U.S. Drug Giants." *Washington Bus. J.* 1986, Nov. 10, 7.
33. *Shopping For Health, A Report on Food and Nutrition.* Washington DC: Food Marketing Institute, 1992.
34. *The Nutraceutical Initiative: A Proposal for Economic and Regulatory Reform.* New York: The Foundation for Innovation in Medicine, Dec. 1991.
35. *The Surgeon General's Report on Nutrition and Health,* Washington DC: U.S. Department of Health and Human Services, 1988.
36. WAGNER, J. "NutraCeuticals—Foods on the Verge of Being Drugs." *Food Eng.* 1990, Mar., 9.
37. WOLF, C. "Functional Foods From Japan." *Food Channel.*
38. WOLF, C. "Pharmafoodicals on the Horizon." *Food Channel* 1991, Dec. 16, 6.
39. YANKELOVICH; SKELLY; WHITE. "Public Attitudes Toward the Use and Regulation of Vitamins, Minerals and Herbs." *Presentation to National Health Alliance,* Sept. 18, 1992.
40. ZEIGLER, R. "Vegetables, Fruits and Carotenoids and the Risk of Cancer." *Am. J. Clin. Nutr.* 1991, 53, 251 S+.

4

Vitamins and Disease Prevention: Update on Optimal Intakes

John H. Weisburger

Vitamins are essential micronutrients available in diverse foods. Committees of the National Academy of Sciences have devised values for the Recommended Daily Allowances (RDA) of each vitamin. The original aim of setting such values was to provide an adequate intake of each micronutrient to avoid deficiency diseases. In most of the developed world, this has been successful since the target diseases are quite rare. Research on etiological and protective factors associated with a number of chronic diseases now shows that a re-examination of the RDA concept is needed to lower the risk of major chronic diseases. This chapter deals with a new definition of the RDA for each essential micronutrient to accomplish this goal.

Anywhere in the world, people are afflicted with a number of chronic diseases including coronary heart disease, hypertension and stroke, adult on-set diabetes, many types of cancer and of growing importance, AIDS. Extensive research on the etiology of each type of disease has indicated that most cases stem from the locally prevailing and personal lifestyle (1-8). It has been shown that tobacco use, especially smoking of cigarettes or chewing of tobacco products in some parts of the world, account for about 35% of chronic diseases, including coronary heart disease, and cancer in the respiratory tract, pancreas, kidney, urinary bladder and cervix. Nutritional traditions involving salted and pickled foods are associated with a high risk of hypertension and stroke and cancer of the esophagus and stomach. Eating habits involving high fat diets are accompanied by a risk for heart disease and cancer of the colon, pancreas, breast, prostate, ovary and endometrium. Such diets also potentiate the effect of smoking on the lung. Importantly, it was discovered that populations who by tradition also consume regularly vegetables and fruits have a lower risk, everything else being equal (12-21). For example, the Mediterranean countries display a lower incidence of heart disease and many types of cancer, as is also true in the Southern part of the United States. In Southern areas of China and Japan, there are fewer cases of stroke and gastric cancer.

Vegetables and fruits contain a variety of micronutrients that may play a role in the protection against chronic diseases. They contain fibers, particularly soluble fibers, that together with insoluble fibers as found in bran cereals, increase intestinal health and lower the risk of heart disease and breast cancer by limiting the enterohepatic circulation of cholesterol, bile acids, and hormones (22-23). In addition, vegetables, fruits, and also tea, include powerful antioxidants, with a polyphenol structure accounting for their beneficial effect. They induce also phase I and phase II enzymes with detoxifying potential for endogenous and xenobiotic substrates (24).

Vegetables and fruits also contain essential micronutrients as vitamins (25-28). Vitamins are defined as being complex organic substances found in many foods that are essential in small amounts for the normal function of the body. Individuals or populations who have a low intake of vitamins may suffer from deficiency diseases. For example, a deficiency of vitamin A affects the function of the eye, leading to blindness, a low intake of vitamin C is a cause of scurvy, vitamin B_1 in low levels is a cause of beriberi, and a low intake of niacin relates to the occurrence of pellagra. Vitamin D is an essential component in calcium availability and metabolism, and a low intake may lead to rickets. With the development, beginning in 1940, of the concept of Recommended Daily Allowances, RDA, by experts in nutrition under the auspices of the Food and Nutrition Board of the US National Academy of Sciences, recommendations were made on specific amounts of each vitamin that would minimize the risk of these deficiency diseases (29). In each case, the amount selected was higher than the minimum, to provide some buffer against inadequate intake under specific conditions. These concepts were implemented not only by improving the nutritional status of individuals through personal action but also through the fortification of widely used foods with specific vitamins. For example, milk contains additional vitamin A and D, and certain breakfast cereals in the United States are fortified with varied vitamins. In the last 50 years, implementation of the RDA concept has been most successful. Deficiency diseases have disappeared, even in the lower socio-economic groups that previously had most of the cases.

Research in the last 35 years has suggested that deficiency diseases were not the only concern where vitamin supplementation might benefit the public. One pioneering study in Norway showed that smokers often had appreciably lower values of plasma vitamin A than non-smokers (30). Part of the explanation is that individuals who smoke frequently have poor nutritional habits. In addition, however, it was found that individuals who smoke display a different biochemical pattern to metabolize chemicals. Cigarette smoke induces metabolic enzymes such as those of the cytochrome P450 system, and the phase II conjugating enzymes, such as glucuronyl transferase. Thus, vitamin A undergoes metabolism to products that no longer serve the vitamin A function. This is true for many other of the fat-soluble micronutrients, including vitamin E and vitamin D. In smokers, such metabolic reactions occur at a higher rate, and hence, account for higher vitamin requirements (31-35). The Recommended Daily Allowance for vitamin E is quite low, 10 IU per day, simply because this excellent antioxidant is found in diverse foods (29). Thus, classical nutritionists comment that deficiencies of vitamin E are nonexistent. In recent years, however, research has shown that vitamin E has a number of extraordinarily beneficial effects as a specific antioxidant, acting together with vitamin C and ß-carotene, in improving antioxidant defenses in the body (36-46).

A number of lifestyle-associated adverse effects stem from cell-mediated oxidative systems. For example, LDL-cholesterol is one of the circulating lipoproteins that act as carriers for cholesterol. It has been found that the specific mechanism underlying its adverse effect is oxidation (46-50). The oxidized LDL-cholesterol damages the vascular system. Active oxygen compounds are also generated through normal physiological reactions that can modify the genetic apparatus of the cell and lead to modified DNA, visualized as the 8-hydroxydeoxyguanylic acid (8-OHdG) component in DNA (51). It is thought that a number of carcinogenic events relate to the production of 8-OHdG in DNA. All of these reactions are lowered by antioxidants, including the antioxidant vitamins individually, or especially when acting in concert. Studies in humans and in animal models have shown that supplementation with vitamin E decreases the risk of atherosclerosis and coronary heart disease (52-56). Vitamin E and vitamin C act individually or together as efficient traps for nitrite in foods, or nitrite formed by the bacterial flora in the oral cavity and in the stomach from environmental nitrate. Current concepts indicate that nitrite may be associated with risk for gastric cancer, as well as cancer of the esophagus in the Far East. Populations on an adequate intake, either through an adequate intake of vegetables, fruits and tea, rich in nitrite-traps and antioxidants, or with supplements of vitamin C or E, have a lower risk of these types of cancer (57-61).

A number of vitamins are essential cofactors on specific enzyme systems (Table 4.1). Thus, it is important for optimal functioning of these varied enzymes that sufficient amounts of these vitamins are available. A number of these vitamins act

TABLE 4.1. FUNCTIONS OF VITAMINS

Water-soluble Vitamins					
Vitamin	Active form	Functions	Enzyme cofactor	Deficiency indicator	Deficiency disease
Thiamine Vitamin B_1	Thiamine pyrophosphate	Decarboxylation α-ketoacids, carbohydrate metabolism	Transketolase	Increased pyrut is blood, Erthrocyte transketolase	Beri-beri, Neuritis cardiovascular, Alcoholic polyneuropathy
Riboflavin Vitamin B_2	Flavin mononucleotide, Flavin adenine dinucleotide, generated with ATP	Respiratory enzymes flavoprotein catalytic systems	Xanthine oxidase dehydrogenases, oxidases, reductases	Reduced erythrocyte GSH reductase, dermatitis, anemia, neuropathy	Non-specific syndromes (See indicators)
Pyridoxine Vitamin B_6	Pyridoxal phosphate, Pyridoxamine phosphate	Amino acid metabolism, decarboxylation, transamination, racemization	Transaminases, decarboxylases	Abnormal tryptophan metabolism, neuritis, seborrheitis, glossitis, stomatitis, blood homocysteine	Non-specific syndromes (See indicators)
Cyanocobalamin Vitamin B_{12}	Methylcobalamin 5-Deoxyadenylcobalamin hydroxycobalamin Bound to intrinsic factor, a glycoprotein	Cell growth, duplication; methionine purine, pyrimidine RNA, DNA biosynthesis (with folate) hematological and nervous systems	Enzymes for 1-carbon and sulphydryl metabolism, in coordination with folate	Deficiency in folate metabolism, methionine biosynthesis; malabsorption syndrome; homocysteine accumulation, abnormal DNA replication	Megaloblastic erthropoiesis, or anemia, pancytopenia, neurologic syndromes, including irreversible neural damage
Folic acid pteroly-glutamic acid	Tetrahydrofolates	Homocysteine to cysteine, serine to glycine, formate and histidine; organization and differentiation	Enzymes for 1-carbon and sulphydryl, purine synthesis metabolism, in concert with vitamin	Alcoholism lowers avail- abnormal hematopoietic system	Megaloblastic erythropoiesis, or anemia; abnormal fetal development; neural tube (cf. vitamin B_{12})

TABLE 4.1. (CONTINUED) FUNCTIONS OF VITAMINS

Water-soluble Vitamins					
Vitamin	Active form	Functions	Enzyme cofactor	Deficiency indicator	Deficiency disease
Pantothenic acid	Coenzyme A	2-carbon metabolism, acetyltransfer; metabolism of carbohydrates, fatty acids, biosynthesis of sterols, porphyrins	Acyltransferases	Adrenocortical deficiencies, neuromuscular degeneration (rare to find deficiencies)	Rarely observed
Nicotinic acid or amide, niacin (biosynthesis from tryptophan)	Nicotinamide adenine dinucleotide (NAD), nicotinamide adenine dinucleotide phosphate (NADP)	Coenzymes for oxidation-reduction enzymes, microsomal, mitochondrial enzymes, dehydrogenases, coordinated with flavoproteins	Oxido-reductases	Dermatitis, diarrhea, dementia (chronic alcoholism)	pellagra
Biotin	Complex with lysine	Carboxylation of acetyl-coenzyme A, carbohydrate/fat metabolism CO_2 fixation oxidative enzyme reactions nitrite trap	Carboxylases acetyl-transfer	Exfoliative dermetitis alopeaa, (patients with malabsorption)	Rare
Vitamin C	Facilitates iron absorption	Several oxidation-reduction enzymes, provides terminal reductive element to other antioxidants such as ß-carotene, vitamin E, sulfhydryl and GSH transferases	Provides coordinated reductive potential to oxidation-reduction enzymes and their associated cofactors	Low plasma vitamin C; perifollicular hyperkeratosis; hemorrhages hematomas, alcohol cigarette use, oral contraceptives, infectious diseases, surgical stress increase requirements, nitrite-related methemoglobinemia	Scurvy

TABLE 4.1. (CONTINUED) FUNCTIONS OF VITAMINS

		Fat-Soluble Vitamins			
Vitamin	Active form	Functions	Enzyme cofactor	Deficiency indicator	Deficiency disease
ß-carotene	ß-carotene and vitamin A, carotenoids	Antioxidant, biosynthesis progesterone, trapsoxiradicals and peroxides	See Vitamin A	See Vitamin A	See Vitamin A
Vitamin A	Retinol, Retinal	Antioxidant, growth and differentiation, eye, bone, reproduction, embryonic development, intercellular communication, gene expression	Rhodopsin biosynthesis, epithelial differentiation, retinol binding protein	Visual defects, night blindness, skin lesions, keratomalacia, deficient pulmonary mucus, fetal resorption, teratogenesis	Fetal or infant deaths owing to incomplete function of epithelial tissues
Vitamin D	Cholecalciferol, calciferol	Regulation of calcium and phosphate metabolism through calcifediol and calcitriol bone synthesis, degradation, magnesium energy cycle, cell duplication, blood pressure regulation	—	Intestinal metaplasia (Diarrhea), increased cancer risk, malabsorption of calcium, magnesium; demineralization	Rickets, Tetany
Vitamin E	α-tocopherol	Antioxidant, stabilizes ubiquinone, acts in concert with carotene, vitamin A, vitamin C, selenium prevents peroxidation, and free radicals, nitrite trap of LDL-cholesterol, fats, DNA, antagonizes metal-catalyzed oxidations	—	Neurological syndromes, reproductive defects; peroxidation, myopathy, cardiac disorders, erythrocyte, instability, vascular reperfusion injury	Rare, except in fetus, newborn

TABLE 4.1. (CONTINUED) FUNCTIONS OF VITAMINS

Fat-Soluble Vitamins					
Vitamin	Active form	Functions	Enzyme cofactor	Deficiency indicator	Deficiency disease
Vitamin K	K_1: 2-methyl-3-phytyl-1,4-naphthoquinone, phylloquinone; K_2: Series of menoquinones; synthetic 2-methyl-1,4-naphthoquinone	Synthesis of blood clotting factors, prothrombins	Microsomal decarboxylase, epoxide reductase	Increased bleeding, gastro-intestinal bleeding, hematuria, congulation defects	Rare, except in newborn

not only as co-factors for enzymes but also can assist in the chemical detoxification of potentially harmful metabolites. For example, it has been shown that moderate to high intake of alcoholic beverages depletes a number of enzymes, particularly the water-soluble vitamins, such as vitamin B_6 and folate (63). One element in the loss of vitamin B_6 could be the reaction of acetaldehyde, a key metabolite of alcohol, with pyridoxamine, forming an inactive Schiff-base (64).

The antioxidant ß-carotene, a pro-vitamin A, has not been part of the recognized list of essential micronutrients. Yet, numerous studies document that carotene and vitamin A can function as effective inhibitors in neoplasia and other chronic diseases (65-83). It has been established, however, that β-carotene is converted metabolically to vitamin A. It is an excellent precursor, because β-carotene has not displayed any indication of chronic toxicity, in part because the modest intestinal absorption of carotene limits the amount of circulating carotene. On the other hand, chronic use of high levels of vitamin A has lead to adverse effects, with emphasis on liver damage. For this reason, there is a recommendation to hold the intake of vitamin A to 10,000 units per day (84-86). In addition, β-carotene has antioxidant functions beyond its action as a source of vitamin A. Carotene can act as a trap for radical reactions. Such oxidative reactions lead to the introduction in carotene of an unbalanced electron structure, and for that reason, it is best to consider the use of carotene together with vitamin E and vitamin C to terminate the effect of reactive radicals through a chain reaction, eventuating in the oxidation of vitamin C.

Based on these and related considerations, outside of the main thrust of this article, it would seem important to revise the recommended daily allowances by new proposals providing amounts of essential micronutrients, with the ultimate aim being the avoidance of chronic diseases (Table 4.2). In many instances, the desirable amounts of vitamins involve higher daily intakes than the conventional RDA. If populations could be convinced to change their lifestyle and consume on a daily regular basis the desirable 5 to 9 fruits and vegetables per day with emphasis on the higher amount, the preventive needs

TABLE 4.2. OPTIMAL INTAKE OF VITAMINS FOR CHRONIC DISEASE PREVENTION

			Fat-Soluble Vitamins					Water-Soluble Vitamins								
Category	Age (years) or Condition	Protein (g)	ß-carotene mg[a]	Vitamin A (µg TE)[a]	Vitamin D (µg)[b]	Vitamin E (mg α-TE)[c]	Vitamin K (ug)	Vitamin C (mg)	Thiamin (mg)	Riboflavin (mg)	Niacin (mg NE)[d]	D-Pantothenate (mg)	Vitamin B_6 (mg)	Folate (mg)	Biotin (mg)	Vitamin B_{12} (µg)
Infants	0.0-0.5	13	3	200	7.5	10-12	5	30	0.3	0.4	5	5	0.3	0.25	0.1	0.3
Children	4-6	24	5	400-600	8-10	30-40	20	60-100	0.9	1.1	12	10	1.5	0.75	0.2	2.0-3.0
Males	11-14	42-50	8	1500	10-12	80-120	45	300-400	2.0-3.0	2.0-3.0	40	20	4.0	0.4-0.5	0.5	10
	25-50	42-50	8	1500	10-12	80-120	80	400	2.0-3.0	2.0-3.0	40	20	4.0	0.4-0.5	0.5	10
	51+	40	8	1500	10-12	80-120	65	400	2.0-3.0	2.0-3.0	40	20	4.0	0.4-0.5	0.5	10
Females	11-14	40-45	8	1500	10-12	80-120	45	300-400	2.0-3.0	2.0-3.0	40	20	4.0	0.4-0.5	0.5	10
	25-50	40-45	8	1500	10-12	80-120	80	400	2.0-3.0	2.0-3.0	40	20	4.0	0.4-0.5	0.5	10
	51+	40	8	1500	10-12	80-120	65	400	2.0-3.0	2.0-3.0	40	20	4.0	0.4-0.5	0.5	10
Pregnant		55-65	10	1200	10-12	100-150	65	500	3.0	3.0	50	30	4.0	0.4-0.5	0.7	12
Lactating	1st 6 months	60-65	10	1500	15	100-150	65	500	3.0	3.0	50	30	4.0	0.5	0.7	12
	2nd 6 months	60-70	10	2000	15	100-150	65	500	3.0	3.0	50	30	4.0	0.5	0.7	12

This table is modified from the Monograph Recommended Daily Allowances, 10th ed. Food and Nutrition Board, National Academy of Sciences, Washington, DC.
[a]Retinol equivalents. 1 retinol equivalent = 1 µg retinol or 6 µg ß-carotene, or 3.3 i.u. vitamin A activity.
[b]As cholecalciferol. 10 µg cholecalciferol = 400 iu of vitamin D.
[c]α-Tocopherol equivalents. 1 mg d-α tocopherol = 1 α-TE.
[d]1 NE (niacin equivalent) is equal to 1 mg of niacin or 60 mg of dietary tryptophan.

could be met through fruits and vegetables. In fact, in the history of mankind, anthropology shows that humans were gatherers of fruits and vegetables for their daily nutritional needs. This tradition has changed with the development of the agricultural industries and especially the relocation of people from rural areas to cities where the gathering of fruits and vegetables was not possible. Also, in the last century, industrialization led to increasing intakes of fatty foods, meats and refined foods in which essential micronutrients were present in reduced amounts. Also, segments of populations acquired singular nutritional habits, such as a diet almost exclusively derived from corn, and associated products. Such manner of imbalanced eating was a cause of deficiency diseases. In addition, consumption of even 9 fruits and vegetables per day fails to meet the recommended, optimal intake of vitamin E by adults of 80-120 units per day. Thus, supplementation of vitamin E, an inexpensive product, is indicated.

Is general supplementation with vitamins necessary? Probably not, if individuals had a lifestyle providing for an adequate consumption of fruits and vegetables (see note on supplementary vitamin E, above). In most instances, however, this goal is not achieved for a number of reasons, including time for preparing meals, as well as the cost of these desirable foods. Thus, moderate supplementation, as suggested in Table 4.2, may be in order. It is important to realize that the fat-soluble vitamins require a certain amount of food, particularly some fatty foods, to ensure their complete absorption. Thus, people that use vitamin supplements should take them after their main meal, essentially fortifying the foods eaten present in the stomach, and increasing their availability to tissues and cells.

In the United States, about one third of men and women are regular users of vitamin supplements. There is less information about other countries, but it seems that the Americans stand out. Within this country, there may be a socioeconomic gradient, and the lower groups seem to be less likely users. Actually, that fairly sizeable part of the population might be better off with supplement use, since their nutritional habits often are poor in vegetable and fruit intake. In fact, there might be merit in public policies providing appropriate multi-vitamins, including adequate amounts of vitamin E, to these groups of people, perhaps as part of the supply of food stamps. This situation also applies to institutional food supplies, such as in hospitals, schools, armed services, and in general, in broad public nutrition programs. Legislation passed by 103rd Congress in 1994, the Dietary Supplement Act, recognizes these micronutrients as part of the dietary supply, and provides for their continuing availability on the open market.

In the sale of drugs and pharmaceuticals, the areas of primary concern are safety and effectiveness. Vitamin supplements are not drugs but are part of an informed nutritional intake. Except for infrequent reports on toxicity with excessive use of vitamins A, D and B_6, there have been few safety problems reported in vitamin users. The late Professor Pauling is said to have consumed 10 grams of vitamin C per day without any obvious adverse effects; he succumbed recently to prostate cancer at the age of 93. The question of effectiveness is important. A number of field studies have shown that short-term vitamin supplementation does not seem to lower the development of cancer of the lung or cancer of the esophagus. These trials were designed more to develop information on the possible therapeutic effect of vitamins. It would seem that vitamin use should be part of a healthy lifestyle with life-long proper dietary habits, exercise and vitamin use, and emphasis on prevention. There are relatively few studies in which vitamin supplementation has been, thus, explored. As noted, populations, who as a rule have nutritional traditions involving regular intake of fruits, vegetables and tea display fewer of the main chronic diseases, including heart disease and cancer. Vitamin C and E act as inhibitors of nitrosation and through this mechanism should decrease the risk of gastric cancer. Yet, it is known that the intake of salted pickled foods or living in area with high geochemical nitrate for the first 20 years of life determines the eventual occurrence of gastric cancer. Hence, it seems likely that any relatively short trial with these two vitamins would fail to display evidence of lower risk. On the other hand, carotene and vitamin A, that may operate through enhancing differentiation and decreasing cell duplication could eventually yield evidence that regular adequate intake would lower the development of clinical cancer (87-89). Experiments in animal models have also indicated that vitamin A may decrease the development of breast cancer. Vitamin D plays an essential role in the proper metabolism of calcium and thus, maintaining bone structure (91-95). Vitamin D analogs begin to be introduced that have shown effectiveness in certain types of cancer. Vitamin B_6 has been found useful in cases of poisoning with certain hydrazines, including the drug isoniazid. Research in my laboratory deals with exploration of the relevant mechanisms.

CONCLUDING COMMENTS

Vitamins are essential micronutrients that were discovered in the first half of this century, because their low intake led to specific deficiency diseases. Introduction of the concept of the Recommended Daily Allowances and ensuring adequate intake of such micronutrients through foods or supplements has been effective in its designed goal to eliminate deficiency diseases.

The current problem is to assess the role of specific vitamins and of mixtures of the essential micronutrients in multivitamin pills in order to lower the risk of the current burden of chronic diseases with such a high cost to individuals and to society. It is clear that vitamins, as used, are safe. About one third of the American people regularly take vitamin supplements, and cases of adverse effects are extremely rare. People consuming the recommended 5-9 servings of vegetables and fruits per day are likely to have an adequate, indeed optimal, intake of vitamins and minerals and other desirable micronutrients, to prevent the major chronic diseases due to lifestyle or environmental factors. The exception would be vitamin E where some moderate supplementation of the order of 80 to 120 IU per day may be desirable. Much has been learned about the role of each vitamin or sets of vitamins in terms of mechanisms of beneficial effects. Thus, there is an underlying body of evidence that adequate intake of vitamins and minerals is part of a healthy lifestyle, designed to lower the risk of major diseases.

ACKNOWLEDGEMENTS

Research in my laboratory is supported by a grant from the Tea Trade Health Research Association, a contract NO1-CN35569 from the National Cancer Institute, and a gift from Texaco, Inc. Ms. Beth-Alayne McKinney assisted effectively in the development of this chapter.

BIBLIOGRAPHY

1. MCGINNIS, J. M.; FOEGE, W. H. "Actual Causes of Death in the United States". *J. Am. Med. Assn.*, 1993, 270, 2207-2212.
2. WHO Study Group, Technical Report Series 797, *Diet, Nutrition, and the Prevention of Chronic Diseases*; World Health Organization, Geneva, 1990, 1-203.
3. Surgeon General's Report, *Nutrition and Health*, Washington, DC, Public Health Service DHHS (PHS) Publication No. 88-50210, 1988.
4. LEVI, F.; LUCCHINI, F.; LA VECCHIA, C. "Worldwide Patterns of Cancer Mortality, 1985-89". *Europ. J Cancer Prev.*, 1994, 109-143.
5. HILL, M. J.; GIACOSA, A.; CAYGILL, C. P. J., Eds. *Epidemiology of Diet and Cancer*, Ellis Horwood:Chichester, Sussex, UK, 1994, pp. 1-411.
6. HOFFMANN, D.; RIVENSON, A.; CHUNG, F-L.; WYNDER, E. L. "Potential Inhibitors of Tobacco Carcinogenesis". *Ann. N.Y. Acad. Sci.* 1993, 686, 140-160.
7. WEISBURGER, J. H.; HORN, C. L.; WYNDER, E. L. "Mechanisms of Nutritional Elements in Prevention of Cancer and Other Chronic Diseases". In *Recent Advances in Clinical Nutrition: 3. Proceedings of the Fourth International Symposium on Clinical Nutrition*, Schlierf, G., Ed.; Smith-Gordon:London, 1991, pp. 83-96.
8. WILLIAMS, C. L.; BOLLELLA, M.; WYNDER, E. "Prevention Cardiology in Primary Care". *Atherosclerosis* 1994, 108, S117-S126.
9. TEMPLE, N. J.; BURKITT, D. P. Eds. *Western Diseases: Their Dietary Prevention and Reversibility*, Humana Press Inc.:Totowa, NJ, 1994, pp. 1-453.
10. WATTENBERG, L. W. *"Inhibition of Carcinogenesis by Minor Dietary Prevention and Reversibility". Cancer Res.* 1992, 52, 2085-2091.
11. DWYER, J. T. "Health Aspects of Vegetarian Diets". *Am. J. Clin. Nutr.*, 1988, 712-738.
12. SHIBATA, A.; PAGANINI-HILL, A.; ROSS, R. K.; HENDERSON, B. E. "Intake of Vegetables, Fruits, Beta-carotene, Vitamin C and Vitamin Supplements and Cancer Incidence Among the Elderly: A Prospective Study". *Brit. J. Cancer* 1992, 66, 673-679.
13. GAO, C-M.; TAJIMA, K.; KUROISHI, T.; HIROSE, K.; INOUE, M. "Protective Effects of Raw Vegetables and Fruit Against Lung Cancer

Among Smokers and Ex-smokers: A Case-control Study in the Tokai Area of Japan". *Jpn. J. Cancer Res.* 1993, 84, 594-600.

14. STEINMETZ, K. A.; POTTER, J. D.; FOLSOM, A. R. "Vegetables, Fruit and Lung Cancer in the Iowa Women's Health Study". *Cancer Res.* 1993, 53, 536-543.
15. STEINMETZ, K. A.; KUSHI, L. H.; BOSTICK, R. M.; FOLSOM, A. R.; POTTER, J. D. "Vegetables, Fruit and Colon Cancer in the Iowa Women's Health Study". *Am. J. Epidem.* 1994, 139, 1-15.
16. BLOCK, G.; PATTERSON, B.; SUBAR, A. "Fruit, Vegetables, and Cancer Prevention: A Review of the Epidemiological Evidence". *Nutr. Cancer* 1992, 18, 1-29.
17. TROCK, B.; LANZA, E.; GREENWALD, P. "Dietary Fiber, Vegetables, and Colon Cancer: Critical Review and Meta-analyses of the Epidemiologic Evidence". *J. Natl. Cancer Inst.* 1990, 82, 650-661.
18. WYNDER, E. L. "Cancer Prevention: Optimizing Life-styles with Special Reference to Nutritional Carcinogenesis". *J. Natl. Cancer Inst.* 1992, 12, 87-91.
19. BAL, D. G.; FOERSTER, S. B. "Dietary Strategies for Cancer Prevention". *Cancer* 1993, 72, 1005-1110.
20. GILLMAN, M. W.; CUPPLES, L. A.; GAGNON, D.; POSNER, B. M.; ELLISON, R. C.; CASTELLI, W. P.; WOLF, P. A. "Protective Effect of Fruits and Vegetables on Development of Stroke in Men". *J. Am. Med. Assoc.* 1995, 273, 1113-1117.
21. VERLANGIERI, A. J.; KAPEGHIAN, J. C.; EL-DEAN, S.; BUSH, M. "Fruit and Vegetable Consumption and Cardiovascular Mortality". *Med. Hypotheses* 1985, 16, 7-15.
22. MICOZZI, M. S.; MOON, T. E. Eds.; *Macronutrients: Investigating their Role in Cancer*, Marcel Dekker:New York, 1992, 477 pp.
23. PARKE, D. V.; IOANNIDES, C.; WALKER, R., Eds. *Food, Nutrition and Chemical Toxicity*, Smith -Gordon:Nishimura, 1993, pp. 1-451.
24. SOHN, O. S.; SURACE, A.; FIALA, E. S.; RICHIE, J.; COLOSIMO, S.; ZANG, E.; WEISBURGER, J. H. "Effects of Green Tea and Black Tea Drinking on Hepatic Xenobiotic Metabolizing Systems in Male F344 Rats". *Xenobiotica* 1994, 24, 119-127.
25. MOON, T. E.; MICOZZI, M. S., Eds. *Nutrition and Cancer Prevention*, Marcel Dekker:New York, 1989, 588 pp.
26. SAUBERLICH, H. E.; MACHLIN, L. J., Eds. *Beyond Deficiency, New Views on the Function and Health Effects of Vitamins*, Ann. N.Y. Acad. Sci., 1992, 669, 1-404.
27. GABY, S. K.; BENDICH, A.; SINGH, V. N.; MACHLIN L. J., Eds. *Vitamin Intake and Health*, Marcel Dekker:New York, 1991, pp. 1-217.
28. BLOCK, G. "Micronutrients and Cancer: Time for action?". *J Natl. Cancer Inst.* 1993, 85, 846-848.
29. National Research Council, *Recommended Dietary Allowances*, National Academy Press:Washington, DC, 10th Ed., 1989.

30. BJELKE, E. "Dietary Vitamin A and Human Lung Cancer". *Int. J. Cancer* 1975, 15, 561-565.
31. EDES, T. E.; KWAN S. M.; BUCKLEY, C. S.; THORNTON, W. H. "Tissue Vitamin A Repletion is Impaired by Exposure to Carcinogen". *Int. J. Cancer* 1992, 50, 99-102.
32. PAMUK E. R.; BYERS, T.; COATES, R. J.; VANN, J. W.; SOWELL, A. L.; GUNTER, E. W.; GLASS, D. "Effect of Smoking on Serum Nutrient Concentrations in African-American Women". *Am. J. Clin. Nutr.* 1994, 59, 891-895.
33. SCHECTMAN, G. "Estimating Ascorbic Acid Requirements for Cigarette Smokers". *Ann. N.Y. Acad. Sci.* 1993, 686, 335-345.
34. TRIBBLE, D. L.; GIULIANO, L. J.; FORTMANN, S. P. "Reduced Plasma Ascorbic Acid Concentrations in Nonsmokers Regularly Exposed to Environmental Tobacco Smoke". *Am. J. Clin. Nutr.* 1993, 58, 886-890.
35. VAN POPPEL, G.; VERHAGEN, H.; VAN'T VEER, P.; VAN BLADEREN, P. J. "Markers for Cytogenetic Damage in Smokers: Associations with Plasma Antioxidants and Glutathione S-transferase mu". *Cancer Epid., Biomark. Prev.* 1993, 2, 441-447.
36. LUBIN, B.; MACHLIN, L. J., Eds. *Vitamin E: Biochemical, Hematological, and Clinical Aspects*; Eds.; Ann. N.Y. Acad. Sci., 1982, 393, 1-506.
37. KNEKT, P. "Vitamin E and Smoking and the Risk of Lung Cancer". *Ann. N.Y. Acad. Sci.* 1993, 686, 280-287.
38. COMPORTI, M.; MAELLARO, E.; DELBELLO, B.; CASINI, A. F. "Glutathione Depletion: Its Effects on Other Antioxidant Systems and Hepatocellular Damage". *Xenobiotica* 1991, 21, 1067-1076.
39. PAOLISSO, G.; DI MARO, G.; GALZERANO, D.; CACCIAPUOTI, F.; VARRICCHIO, G.; VARRICCHIO, M.; D'ONOFRIO, F. "Pharmacological Doses of Vitamin E and Insulin". *Am. J. Clin. Nutr.* 1994, 59, 1291-1296.
40. YANO, T.; OBATA, Y.; YANO, Y.; OTANI, S.; ICHIKAWA, T. "Vitamin E Acts as a Useful Chemopreventive Agent to Reduce Spontaneous Lung Tumorigenesis in Mice". *Cancer Lett.* 1994, 87, 205-210.
41. LONGNECKER, M. P., MARTIN-MORENO, J-M.; KNEKT, P.; NOMURA, A. M. Y.; SCHOBER, S. E.; STÄHELIN, H. B.; WALD, N. J.; GEY, K. F.; WILLETT, W. C. "Serum a-Tocopherol Concentration in Relation to Subsequent Colorectal Cancer: Pooled Data From Five Cohorts". *J. Natl. Cancer Inst.* 1992, 84, 430-435.
42. GAREWAL, H. "Chemoprevention of Oral Cancer: Beta-carotene and Vitamin E in Leukoplakia". *Europ. J. Cancer Prev.* 1994, 3, 101-107.
43. SINHA, R.; PATTERSON, B. H.; MANGELS, A. R.; LEVANDER, O. A.; GIBSON, T.; TAYLOR, P. R.; BLOCK G. "Determinants of Plasma Vitamin E in Health Males". *Cancer Epid. Biomark. Prevent.* 1993, 2, 473-479.
44. VERLANGIERI, A. J.; BUSH, M. J. "Effects of d-a-Tocopherol Supplementation on Experimentally Induced Primate Atherosclerosis". *J. Am. College Nutr.* 1992, 2, 131-138.

45. BOSTICK, R. M.; POTTER, J. D.; MCKENZIE, D. R.; SELLERS, T. A.; KUSHI, L. H.; STEINMETZ, K. A.; FOLSOM, A. R. "Reduced Risk of Colon Cancer with High Intake of Vitamin E: The Iowa Women's Health Study". *Cancer Res.* 1993, 53, 4230-4237.
46. WITZTUM, J. L.; STEINBERG, D. "Role of Oxidized Low Density Lipoprotein in Atherosclerosis". *J. Clin. Invest.* 1991, 88, 1785-1792.
47. ESTERBAUER, H.; DIEBER-ROTHENEDER, M.; STRIEGL, G.; WAEG, G. "Role of Vitamin E in Preventing the Oxidation of Low-density Lipoprotein". *Am. J. Clin. Nutr.* 1991, 53, 314-321.
48. JIALAL, I.; GUNDY, S. M. "Effect of Combined Supplementation with a-Tocopherol, Ascorbate, and Beta Carotene on Low-density Lipoprotein Oxidation". *Circulation* 1991, 88, 2780-2786.
49. PACKER, L., Ed. *Methods in Enzymology: Oxygen Radicals in Biological Systems, Part C & D, Vol. 233 & 234*, Academic Press:San Diego, CA, 1994, 711 pp & 704 pp.
50. EICHHOLZER, M.; STÄHELIN, H. B.; GEY, K. F. "Inverse Correlation Between Essential Antioxidants in Plasma and Subsequent Risk to Develop Cancer, Ischemic Heart Disease and Stroke Respectively: 12-year Follow-up of the Prospective Basel Study". *EXS* 1992, 62, 398-410.
51. KENSLER, T. W.; SIMIC M. G.; TRUSH, M. A. "4th International Conference on Anticarcinogenesis & Radiation Protection". *Cancer Res.* 1994, 54, 1872-2051.
52. JACQUES, P. F.; SULSKY, S. I.; PERRONE, G. A.; SCHAEFER, E. J. "Ascorbic Acid and Plasma Lipids". *Epidemiology* 1994, 5, 19-26.
53. HERBERT, J. R.; HURLEY, T. G.; HSIEH, J.; ROGERS, E.; STODDARD, A. M.; SORENSEN, G.; NICOLOSI, R. J. "Determinants of Plasma Vitamins and Lipids: The Working Well Study". *Am. J. Epidemiol.* 1994, 140, 132-147.
54. DEMAIO, S. J.; KING, S. B.; LEMBO, N. J.; ROUBIN, G. S.; HEARN, J. A.; BHAGAVAN, H. N.; SGOUTAS, D. S. "Vitamin E Supplementation, Plasma Lipids and Incidence of Restenosis After Precutaneous Transluminal Coronary Angioplasty (PTCA)". *J. Am. College Nutr.* 1992, 11, 68-73.
55. FERRARI, R.; CECONI, C.; CURELLO, S.; CARGNONI, A.; ALFIERI, O.; PARDINI, A.; MARZOLLO, P.; VISIOLI, O. "Oxygen Free Radicals and Myocardial Damage: Protective Role of Thiol-Containing Agents". *Am. J. Med.* 1991, 91, 95-105.
56. STALENHOEF, A. F. H. "Clinical Implications of Increased Low-Density Lipoprotein Oxidation in Patients with Hypercholesterolemia". *Nutrition* 1994, 10, 564-566.
57. SLATER, T. F.; BLOCK, G., Eds. "Antioxidant Vitamins and b-carotene in Disease Prevention". *Am. J. Clin. Nutr.* 1991, 53, 189-396.
58. BARONE, J.; TAIOLI, E.; HERBERT, J. R.; WYNDER, E. L. "Vitamin Supplement Use and Risk for Oral and Esophageal Cancer". *Nutr. Cancer* 1992, 18, 31-41.

59. LA VECCHIA, C.; FERRARONI, M.; D'AVANZO, B.; DECARLI, A.; FRANCESCHI, S. "Selected Micronutrient Intake and the Risk of Gastric Cancer". *Cancer Epid. Biomark. Prev.* 1994, 3, 393-398.
60. XU, G. P.; SONG, P. J.; REED, P. I. "Effects of Fruit Juices, Processed Vegetable Juice, Orange Peel and Green Tea on Endogenous Formation of N-nitrosoproline in Subjects from a High-risk Area for Gastric Cancer in Moping County, China". *Europ. J. Cancer Prevent.* 1993, 2, 327-335.
61. DYKE, G. W.; CRAVEN, J. L.; HALL, R.; GARNER, R. C. "Effect of Vitamin C Supplementation on Gastric Mucosal DNA Damage". *Carcinogenesis* 1994, 15, 291-295.
62. WANG, G-Q.; DAWSEY, S. M.; LI, J-Y.; TAYLOR, P. R.; LI, B.; BLOT, W. J.; WEINSTEIN, W. M.; LIU, F-S.; LEWIN, K. J.; WANG, H.; WIGGETT, S.; GAIL, M. H.; YANG, C. S. "Effects of Vitamin/Mineral Supplementation on the Prevalence of Histological Dysplasia and Early Cancer of the Esophagus and Stomach: Results From the General Population Trial in Linxian, China". *Cancer Epid. Biomark. Prev.* 1994, 3, 161-166.
63. LIEBER, C. S. "Biochemical Factors in Alcoholic Liver Disease". *Seminars Liver Diseases* 1993, 13, 136-153.
64. DAKSHINAUMURTI, K., Ed. *Vitamin B_6*, Ann. N.Y. Acad. Sci. 1990, 585, 1-570.
65. BYERS, T.; PERRY, G. "Dietary Carotenes, Vitamin C, and Vitamin E as Protective Antioxidants in Human Cancers". *Ann. Rev. Nutr.* 1992, 12, 139-159.
66. MACHLIN, L. J. "New Views on the Function and Health Effects of Vitamins". *Nutrition* 1994, 10, 507-513.
67. ZIEGLER, R. G.; SUBAR, A. F.; CRAFT, N. E.; URSIN, G.; PATTERSON, B. H.; GRAUBARD, B. I. "Does ß-carotene Explain Why Reduced Cancer Risk is Associated with Vegetable and Fruit Intake". *Cancer Res.* 1992, 52, 2060-2066.
68. LE MARCHAND, L.; HANKIN, J. H.; KOLONEL, L. N.; BEECHER, G. R.; WILKENS, L. R.; ZHAO, L. P. "Intake of Specific Carotenoids and Lung Cancer Risk". *Cancer Epid., Biomark. Prev.* 1993, 2, 183-187.
69. CANFIELD, L. M., KRINSKY, N. I.; OLSON, J. A. Eds. *Carotenoids in Human Health*; Ann. N.Y. Acad. Sci. 1993, 691, 1-300.
70. GAREWAL, H.; MEYSKENS, F.; FRIEDMAN, S.; ALBERTS, D.; RAMSEY, L. "Oral Cancer Prevention: The Case for Carotenoids and Antioxidant Nutrients". *Prev. Med.* 1993, 22, 701-711.
71. TOMINAGA, K.; SAITO, Y.; MORI, K.; MIYAZAWA, N.; YOKOI, K.; KOYAMA, Y.; SHIMAMURA, K.; IMURA, J.; NAGAI, M. "An Evaluation of Serum Microelement Concentrations in Lung Cancer and Matched Non-cancer Patients to Determine the Risk of Developing Lung Cancer". *Jap. J. Clin. Oncol.* 1992, 96-101.
72. SHEKELLE, R. B.; TANGNEY, C. C.; ROSSOF, A. H.; STAMLER, J. "Serum Cholesterol, Beta-carotene, and Risk of Lung Cancer". *Epidemiology* 1992, 3, 282-287, 1992.

73. BOS, R. P.; VAN POPPEL, G.; THEUWS, J. L.; KOK, F. J. "Decreased Excretion of Thioethers in Urine of Smokers After the Use of Beta-carotene". *Int. Arch. Occupat. Environ. Health.* 1992, 64, 189-193.
74. EDES, T. E.; GYSBERS, D. S. "Carcinogen-induced Tissue Vitamin A Depletion. Potential Protective Advantages of Beta-carotene". *Ann. N.Y. Acad. Sci.* 1993, 686, 203-212.
75. HOFFMANN, D.; RIVENSON, A.; CHUNG, F. L.; WYNDER, E. L. "Potential Inhibitors of Tobacco Carcinogenesis". *Ann. N.Y. Acad. Sci.* 1993, 686, 140-160.
76. GOODMAN, G. E.; OMENN, G. S.; THORNQUIST, M. D.; LUND, B.; METCH, B.; GYLYS-COLWELL, I. "The Carotene and Retinol Efficacy Trial (CARET) to Prevent Lung Cancer in High-risk Populations: Pilot Study With Cigarette Smokers". *Cancer Epid. Biomark. Prev.* 1993, 2, 389-396.
77. KARDINAAL, A. F.; VAN'T VEER, P.; KOKI, F. J.; KOHLMEIER, L.; MARTIN-MORENO, J. M.; HUTTUNEN, J. K.; HALLEN, M.; ARO, A.; DELGADO-RODRIGUEZ, M.; GOMEZ-ARACENA, J. "EURAMIC Coordinating Centre. TNO Toxicology and Nutrition Institute, Zeist, The Netherlands". *Europ. J. Clin. Nutr.* 1993, 2, 64-72.
78. GREENBERG, E. R. "Retinoids or Carotenoids: Is There Another Choice?". *Prev. Med.* 1993, 22, 723-727.
79. HARRIS, R. W.; KEY T. J.; SILCOCKS, P. B.; BULL, D.; WALD, N. J. "A Case-control Study of Dietary Carotene in Men with Lung Cancer and in Men With Other Epithelial Cancers". *Nutr. Cancer* 1991, 15, 63-68.
80. STÄHELIN, H. B.; GEY, K. F.; EICHHOLZER, M. "Beta-carotene and Cancer Prevention: The Basel Study". *Am J. Clin. Nutr.* 1991, 53, 265-269.
81. MAYNE, S. T.; JANERICH, D. T.; GREENWALD, P.; CHOROST, S.; TUCCI, C.; ZAMAN, M. B.; MELAMED, M. R.; KIELY, M.; MCKNEALLY, M. F. "Dietary Beta-carotene and Lung Cancer Risk in U.S. Nonsmokers". *J. Natl. Cancer Inst.* 1994, 86, 33-38.
82. MOGREN, H. "Opening Remarks". *Nutr. Rev.* 1994, 52, 1-93.
83. SHIBATA, A.; PAGANINI-HILL, A.; ROSS, R. K.; YU, M. C.; HENDERSON, B. E. "Dietary ß-carotene, Cigarette Smoking, and Lung Cancer in Men". *Cancer Causes Control* 1992, 3, 207-214.
84. HATHCOCK, J. N.; HATTAN, D. G.; JENKINS, M. Y.; MCDONALD, J. T.; SUNDARESAN, P. R.; WILKENING, V. L. "Evaluation of Vitamin A Toxicity". *Am. J. Clin. Nutr.* 1990, 52, 183-202.
85. FALLON, M. B.; BOYER, J. L. "Hepatic Toxicity of Vitamin A and Synthetic Retinoids". *J Gastroenterol. Hepatol.* 1990, 5, 334-342.
86. VAN DAM, M. A. "The Recognition and Treatment of Hypervitaminosis A". *Nurse Practitioner* 1989, 28, 30-31.
87. ZHANG, L-X.; ACEVEDO P.; GUO, H.; BERTRAM, J. S. "Upregulation of Gap Junctional Communication and Connexin43 Gene Expression by Carotenoids in Human Dermal Fibroblasts But Not in Human Keratinocytes". *Mol. Carcinogenesis* 1995, 12, 50-58.

88. SCITA, G.; WOLF. G. “Retinoic Acid and Beta-carotene Inhibit Fibronectin Synthesis and Release by Fibroblasts: Antagonism to Phorbol Ester”. *Carcinogenesis* 1994, 1043-1048.
89. MERCIER, T.; HONIKMAN-LEBAN, E.; CHAUMONTET, C.; MARTEL, P.; SHAHIN, M. M. “Studies on the Modulating Effects of Retinoic Acid and Retinol Acetate Using Dye Transfer and Metabolic Cooperation Assays”. *Fundam. Appl. Toxicol.* 1993, 21, 270-276.
90. FRASER, D. R. “Vitamin D”. *Lancet* 1995, 345, 104-107.
91. MACHLIN, L. J.; SAUBERLICH, H. E. “New Views on the Function and Health Effects of Vitamins”. *Nutrition Today* 1994, 25-29.
92. KELLOFF, G. J.; BOONE, C. W.; CROWELL, J. A.; STEELE, V. E.; LUBET, R.; SIGMAN C. C. “Chemopreventive Drug Development: Perspectives and Progress”. *Cancer Epidemiol. Biomark. Prev.* 1994, 3, 85-98.
93. BENDICH, A.; BUTTERWORTH, C. E., Eds. *Micronutrients in Health and in Disease Prevention*, Marcel Dekker:New York, 1991, pp. 1-504.
94. DICKINSON, V. A.; BLOCK, G.; RUSSEK-COHEN, E. “Supplement Use, Other Dietary and Demographic Variables, and Serum Vitamin C in NHANES II”. *J. Am.Coll. Nutr.* 1994, 13, 22-32.
95. HELZLSOUER, K. J.; BLOCK, G.; BLUMBERG, J.; DIPLOCK, A. T.; LEVINE, M.; MARNETT, L. J.; SCHUEPLEIN, R. J.; SPENCE, J. T.; SIMIC, M. G. “Summary of the Round Table Discussion on Strategies for Cancer Prevention: Diet, Food, Additives, Supplements, and Drugs”. *Cancer Res.* 1994, 2044-2051.
96. Public Health Service, *Healthy People 2000: National Health Promotion and Disease Prevention Objectives*, US Dept. Health Human Services:Washington, DC, 1991.

5

The Potential for Citrus Phytochemicals in Hypernutritious Foods

Wilbur W. Widmer
Antonio M. Montanari

Citrus fruit contain a complex of chemicals with potential health benefits besides ascorbic acid. These include flavonoids, limonoids, coumarins, carotenoids, monoterpenes, organic acids, and pectin. With few exceptions, amounts of these components in commercial juices are minimal due to processing practices or their insolubility in juice. Processing practices set minimum levels because of an impact on flavor, texture or appearance. As a result, the bulk of these components with potential health benefits are processed into cattle feed for sale at 5-10% above the cost of processing. Recovery methods of these beneficial chemicals are being investigated and using recent advances in processing technology, we are looking at ways to enhance the hypernutritious value of commercial and fortified citrus products without adversely affecting quality.

Citrus fruit have traditionally been associated with vitamin C content. Citrus can also be a significant source of folic acid and thiamine (1, 2). Some varieties of tangerine and red grapefruit also contain substantial amounts of pro-vitamin A (1). However, the health benefits derived from the consumption of fruits and vegetables are gradually becoming accepted to go beyond vitamin content and one needs to consider all the components in a food or juice matrix. Besides the above mentioned vitamins, citrus contain one of the largest and most diverse number of phytochemicals of any food. Some of these phytochemicals are now gaining recognition as having important beneficial health effects and are excellent candidates for use in the fortification and creation of hypernutritious foods.

Other constituents beneficial in maintaining health that are present in citrus fruit and processed products include: carotenoids, flavonoids, limonoids, terpenes, phenolic acids, and pectin. Many of these also occur in low value by-products from the citrus processing operation or are concentrated in waste streams. In fact, processing parameters are adjusted to regulate the amounts of these components in processed products to optimize product quality. High levels of limonene or peel oil lend a harsh flavor and a terpeny aftertaste in juice. Limonoid glucosides have little impact on flavor or appearance. The limonoid aglycone limonin, however, is a very bitter compound and will contribute to bitterness in both orange and grapefruit (3). Naringin, a flavanone glycoside, is also a bitter compound found in grapefruit. Excessive naringin levels are also responsible for bitterness in grapefruit products (4). Hesperidin, the predominate flavanone glycoside in orange has no flavor impact. However, it is extremely insoluble in aqueous solutions and precipitation of white hesperidin crystals in juice is a visual defect (4). Pectin is a thickening agent. Excess pectin in juice products can have a detrimental effect on mouthfeel and appearance (5). The methoxyflavones are also bitter components, but they are present in juice at well below their taste threshold (6). Ferulic acid, the major hydroxycinnamic acid present, fortunately occurs largely in the form of glycosides (7). Free ferulic acid will quickly degrade to p-vinyl guiacol when citrus juices are not properly stored (8). P-vinyl guiacol can be detected as a rotten off-flavor when present in the low part per billion level.

As mentioned previously, processing parameters are adjusted to regulate amounts of these components to optimize product quality. While carotenoids and hydroxycinammic acids are important constituents of citrus products, functioning as natural antioxidants (9), better sources for commercial utilization occur and they will not be considered for recovery. The potential exists, however, for recovery of these other valuable phytochemicals to be formulated into hypernutritious foods.

PEEL OILS

Citrus oils have already been approved for food use. They are used as flavoring additives to beverages including orange and grapefruit juices, foods, baked goods, candy, and confections. In a separate chapter of this book, Dr. Lam discusses the cancer chemopreventative action of components found in plant essential oils, one of them being limonene. Limonene has been reported to be an effective cancer preventative agent against the carcinogens nitrosodiethylamine, nitrosoamine urea, tobacco nitrosoamines, and dimethylbenzylanthracene.

Orange and grapefruit essential oils contain 90-95% d-limonene (10). Cold pressed orange and tangerine peel oils analyzed by the authors were also found to contain 0.2-0.3% and 0.5-0.8% total methoxyflavones, respectively. The methoxylated flavones will be discussed later. The Florida Department of Agriculture and Consumer Services (11) reported utilization of oranges, grapefruit, and tangerines for processing in Florida during the 1990-91 season were 6.75, 1.12, 0.17 million tons, respectively. Based on oil content, extraction efficiency, and crop percentages utilized for oil recovery (10), approximately 4,600 tons of orange oil, 880 tons of grapefruit oil, and 100 tons of tangerine oil were produced in this season.

LIMONENE

Another citrus byproduct currently produced during the processing of citrus which could be utilized for incorporation into a hypernutritious food is d-limonene. The citrus industry in Florida produces such a large crop, processors often have more peel than is possible to process. Therefore, peel oil recovery is optimized to produce the maximum amount of oil possible per hour. Approximately 40% of the total oil contained in the peel is recovered. By limiting oil recovery, a citrus oil of higher quality is also obtained over extraction of the maximum amount of possible from a given amount of peel (12). The remaining peel oil is recovered as the byproduct d-limonene during production of cattlefeed from the waste citrus peel. Including peel waste that is not utilized in oil recovery, an estimated 20,000 of tons of limonene were produced by the Florida Citrus industry during the 1990-91 season.

PECTIN

Dr. Cerda (chapter 10) has demonstrated in many research studies the beneficial role of pectin in the diet. Grapefruit pectin can significantly lower blood serum cholesterol and incidence of atherosclorosis. The effectiveness of citrus pectin in lowering blood serum cholesterol and prevention of hardening of the arteries are discussed in detail by Dr. Cerda in chapter 10. The activity of citrus pectin has only been demonstrated for grapefruit pectin at this time. Although pectin was commercially produced from grapefruit peel in Florida up until several years ago, pectin from grapefruit or any other citrus variety is no longer processed anywhere in the United States. With more stringent regulations for disposal of waste water streams, it is no longer cost effective to recover pectin for the traditional use as a food thickening agent. The opportunity exists for utilization of Florida grapefruit pectin in hypernutritious foods, approximately one half of the fruit is waste peel and processed into cattlefeed. Approximately 25 million 85 pound boxes of grapefruit are processed annually (11), producing approximately 300,000 tons of waste peel. Sinclair (13) reported grapefruit peel contains about 3.5% pectin on a wet weight basis. There is a potential annual yield of 10,000 tons grapefruit pectin from waste peel. Should it turn out that orange pectin is active, approximately 60,000 tons of pectin could be recovered from orange peel waste. As the health benefits of pectin become better known, it may again become economically attractive to recover pectin in Florida from citrus peel.

FLAVANONES

The flavonoids are another important class of compounds that are found in many foods. They are some of the most common antioxidants present in fruits and vegetables. Human consumption is estimated to be approximately 1 gram of flavonoids per day (14). The flavanone glycosides naringin and narirutin are the most abundant flavonoids found in grapefruit while hesperidin is the predominant flavanone in orange and tangerine. In lemon and lime, eriocitrin and hesperidin predominate. The structures of these components are shown in Fig. 5.1.

The health attributes associated with flavanones have been somewhat controversial. While it has been recognized for some time that citrus flavanones are not essential vitamins, they are recognized as having therapeutic effects (15). They were first reported to decrease capillary fragility and improve blood flow (16). Further research failed to substantiate that abnormal capillary permeability was due to a deficiency in bioflavonoids. After review, the Federation of American Societies for Experimental Biology concluded that increased capillary permeability was not the cause, but occurred as a result of a disease. In 1950 it was recommended the term "Vitamin P" be discontinued (17).

One problem with research on bioflavonoids is that they are crude mixtures and may be obtained from varieties of lemon, orange, mandarin, or grapefruit. This causes a variation in the composition of bioflavonoid extracts, especially when the composition of minor components is considered. Recent research has been conducted on individual citrus flavonoids purified from the crude extracts. Vlietinck (18) did not find hesperidin or naringin to have any antiviral activity against herpes simplex or polio myelitis type viruses. However, intact flavanone glycosides are not absorbed by humans or other mammals. Intestinal flora in the gut cleave off the disaccharides of hesperidin and naringin.

Citrus Flavanones

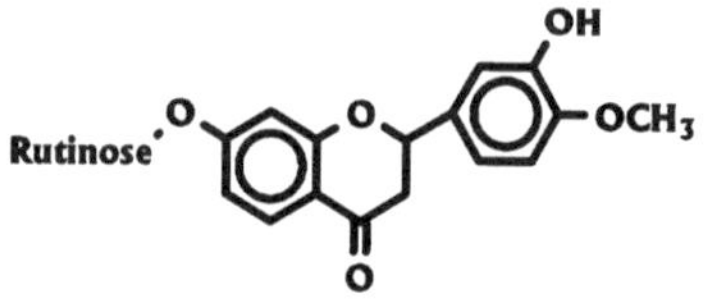

Hesperidin
(Hesperitin-7-rutinoside)

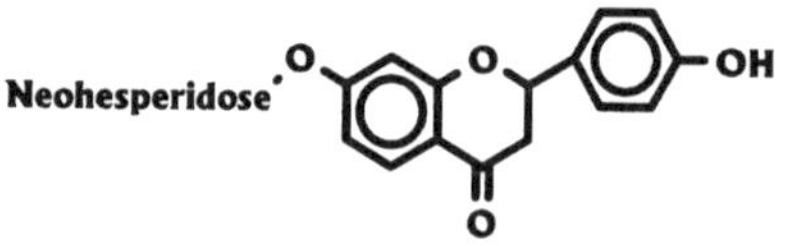

Naringin
(Naringenin-7-neohesperidoside)

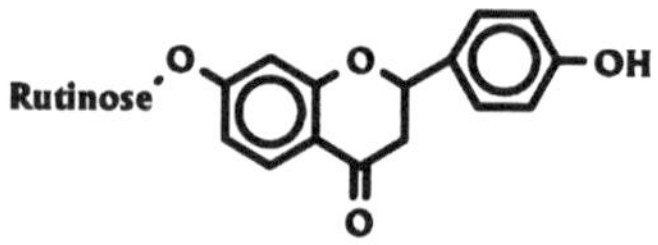

Narirutin
(Naringenin-7-rutinoside)

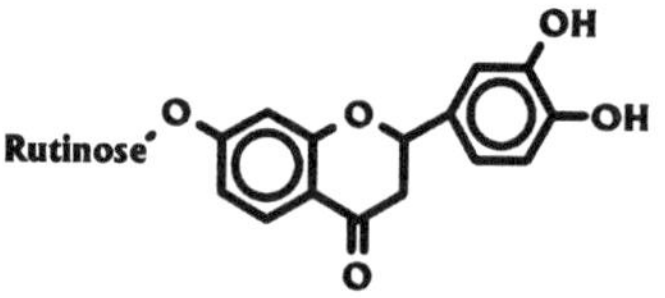

Eriocitrin
(Eriodictyol-7-rutinoside)

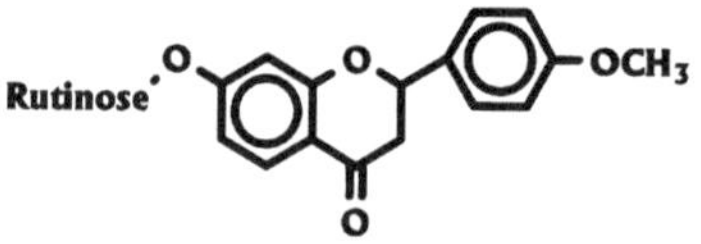

Didymin
(Isosakuranetin-7-rutinoside)

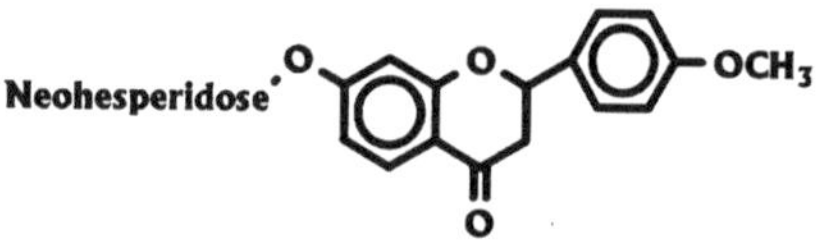

Poncirin
(Isosakuranetin-7-neohesperidoside)

FIG. 5.1. STRUCTURES OF THE COMMON FLAVANONE GLYCOSIDES FOUND IN CITRUS.

The released aglycones hesperitin and naringinin are the flavonoids absorbed (19, 20, 21). The efficiency of absorption of these aglycones, however, is yet to be determined. Hesperitin (aglycone of hesperidin) was shown by Kaul, Middleton, and Ogra (22) to actively inhibit the replication but not the infectivity of herpes simplex, polio and parainfluenza type viruses. Naringinin has recently been found by Carroll of the University of Western Ontario (23) to be more effective than genistein, an isoflavone in soybeans, in inhibition of MDA-MB-435 human breast cell cancer proliferation in vitro. They are currently testing the anticancer effects of naringinin and naringin in vivo in rats.

Naringin has been used as an additive in foods, beverages, and candy as a bittering agent. Hesperidin was briefly used to retard off-flavor formation in some milk products. One or both components are present in a health bioflavonoid complex. Commercial extraction of citrus flavanone glycosides from citrus peel is done with calcium hydroxide. Present at levels of up to 0.4% of the total fresh fruit weight, Florida could potentially produce 300 tons of hesperidin and 50 tons of naringin annually. Currently however, flavanones are only produced on a very limited basis in California by Nutrilite Products Inc. There is an ample supply of these bioflavonoids readily available should market demand become favorable for enrichment in a hypernutritious food.

METHOXYLATED FLAVONES

The citrus fully-methoxylated flavones are an interesting group of bioactive compounds (Fig. 5.2). They are present as minor components in crude extracts of citrus bioflavonoids. Robbins (24) found the isolated methoxylated flavones were much more active than flavanone glycosides in their antiadhesive effects on red blood cells and platelets. They have also been shown by Middleton and coworkers to have anti-inflammatory properties and inhibit histamine release to reduce allergic reactions (25, 26). Bracke discusses the effectiveness of tangeretin in invasive inhibition of human breast carcinoma cells elsewhere in this book (see Chapter 13). Nobiletin and tangeretin were also found by Bracke (27) to have the most potent anti-invasive action of all flavonoids tested on mouse MO4 tumor cells against invasion in normal tissue. Kandaswami and coworkers (28) found nobiletin and tangeretin inhibited human squamous cell carcinoma at all concentrations tested.

Methoxylated flavones are unique to citrus and are present as minor components in the peel oil glands. They are most abundant in tangerines comprising 0.5 to 1% of the peel oil with tangeretin and nobiletin being most prevalent. Smaller amounts of sinensetin, heptamethoxyflavone, tetramethyl scutellarein, and hexamethyl gossypetin are also present.

Citrus Methoxyflavones

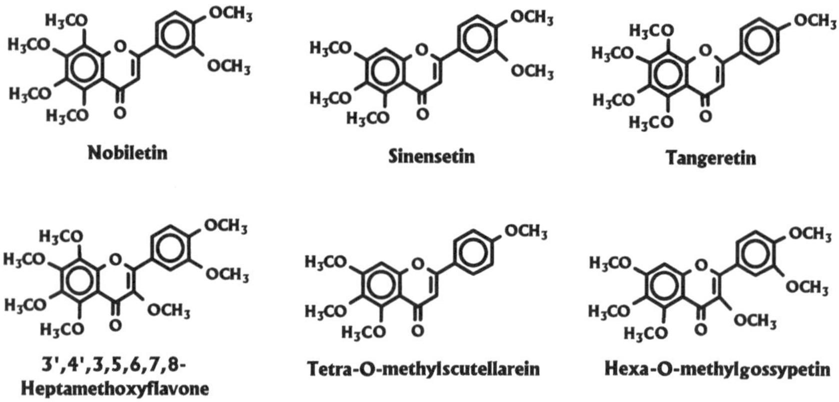

FIG. 5.2. STRUCTURES OF THE COMMON METHOXYLATED FLAVONES FOUND IN CITRUS.

Structures with substitution patterns are shown in Fig. 5.2. In orange oil nobiletin is the major methoxylated flavone with the total flavone content in orange oil being 0.2 to 0.4%.

The methoxylated flavones in the peel flavedo are extracted along with waxes during production of cold-pressed peel oil. Before citrus peel oils are used, they are cooled to precipitate excess surface waxes and methoxylated flavones in a process called winterization. Peel oil is decanted off and the precipitate waste stream containing wax and methoxylated flavones is added to peel waste for processing into cattle feed. An estimated 4,600 tons of orange oil and 100 tons of tangerine oil are produced annually. From the amount of winterization solids estimated to be produced annually in Florida, there are from 0.5 to 5 tons of methoxylated flavones, mostly nobiletin, discarded in waste streams for incorporation into cattle feed. This represents the material which can be easily recovered. Since the methoxylated flavones are associated exclusively with the oil glands in the flavedo, one can further estimate there are at least another 10 tons of methoxyflavones that were never removed from the peel during the oil extraction process. Therefore, a considerable amount of these phytochemicals are available for recovery depending on the demand. At the Florida Department of Citrus, we are continuing to isolate the major and minor methoxylated flavones from citrus so they can be further tested for biological activity.

LIMONOIDS

The limonoids isolated from citrus products have also been found to possess strong anticancer activity. In a separate chapter (Chapter 12), Dr. Miller discusses the cancer chemopreventive activity of the citrus limonoids in relation to structure. The anticarcinogenic activity associated with limonoids has also been well summarized elsewhere by Lam et al. (29). Limonin and nomilin, the two major citrus limonoid aglycones along with several other minor limonoids, are potent inhibitors of forestomach and lung tumor formation induced by benzopyran in mice. They are also effective inhibitors of skin cancer induced by dimethylbenzylanthracene. The preventative action was shown to be associated with induction of the glutathione s-transferase detoxification enzyme system. Limonin and nomilin bound as glucosides have also been found to be potent inhibitors of cancer (30).

Limonoids are abundant in citrus fruit. The highest concentrations occur in the seed with limonin, nomilin and nomilin-17-β-d-glucoside predominating (Fig. 5.3). In the peel, membranes, and juice, limonin and nomilin are the predominate limonoids bound as glucosides. Limonin and nomilin are present as aglycones in citrus juices in low amounts, but are abundant in the seeds (3). Unfortunately citrus seeds are no longer collected during processing as they once were for extraction of citrus seed oil. Citrus limonoids are not produced commercially, and have never been considered commercially valuable. In fact, because of the extremely bitter nature of the limonoid aglycones, a considerable amount of research has been conducted to find ways to reduce their occurrence in Navel orange.

Limonin and nomilin are concentrated within the debittering resin during debittering of grapefruit juice, orange juice, pulp

Citrus Limonoids

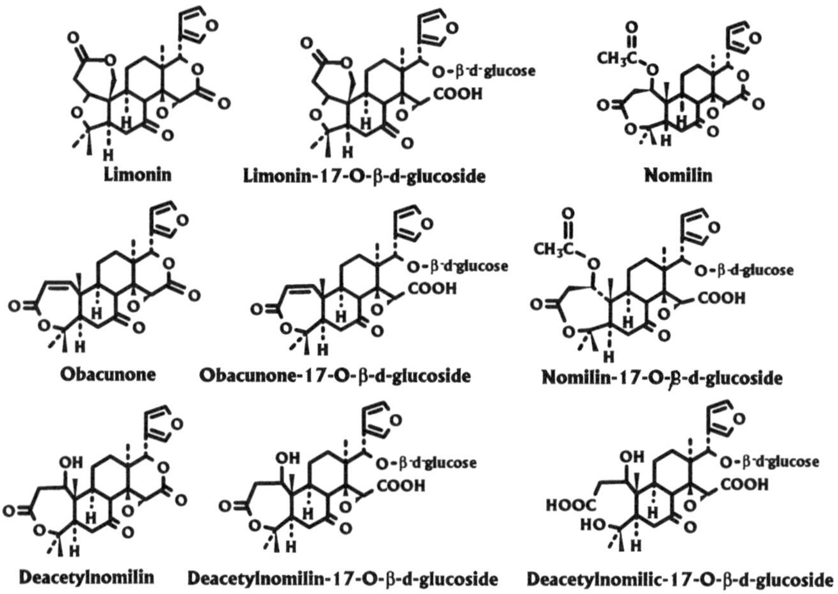

FIG. 5.3 STRUCTURES OF THE COMMON LIMONOIDS FOUND IN CITRUS.

wash and peel wash. These limonoids can be recovered by extraction along with flavanone glycosides. These limonoids, available from the peel and debittering waste streams, could be recovered and utilized for use in hypernutritious foods. However, due to their insolubility in aqueous solutions and extreme bitter nature, the limonoid aglycones probably have little value as a hypernutritious food additive.

CITRUS JUICES

One should also consider the citrus juices with their complex matrix of phytochemicals for incorporation in a base for hypernutrititious foods. Citrus juices are already perceived as a healthy beverage and good source for ascorbic acid, folic acid,

TABLE 5.1 AMOUNTS OF BIOACTIVE COMPONENTS IN AN 8 OZ. OF ORANGE AND GRAPEFRUIT JUICE

	Amount	
Component	Orange juice 8 oz.	Grapefruit juice 8 oz.
Total flavanone glycosides	70 - 190	70 - 190
Hesperitin	20 - 70	12 - 25
Naringinin	2 - 6	28 - 80
Limonene[1]	35 - 110	35 - 110
Limonoid glucosides[2]	59 - 102	33 - 54
Limonin glucoside[2]	38 - 54	22 - 38
Limonin[2]	0.2 - 1	0.7 - 3.5
Methoxylated flavones	0.7 - 2	<1
Pectin[3]	95 - 190	95 - 190
Total Carotenoids[4]	2 - 6	0 - 26
Hydroxycinnamic acids[5]	15 - 20	15 - 24

[1]Data from USDA (33, 34); [2]Data from Fong et al. (31); [3]Data from Baker (5); [4]Data from Stewart (35) for orange and Rouseff et al. (36) for grapefruit; [5] Data from Peleg et al. (7)

thiamine, and potassium (1, 2). The range of other beneficial components present in an 8-ounce glass of orange and grapefruit juices are listed in Table 5.1.

While the amounts of limonoid aglycones are very low in citrus juices, it has been recently discovered that limonoid glucosides are abundant in orange juices at the 200 to 300 ppm level, making orange juice a good source of active limonoids after all (31, 32). The anticarcinogenic activity of the limonoid glucosides is discussed by Dr. Miller in chapter 12 of this book. The most abundant glucosides in orange and grapefruit juice are those bound to limonin and nomilin with smaller amounts of the glucosides of obacunone, deacetylnomilin, and deacetylnomilinic acid (3). An 8 ounce glass of orange juice contains 60 to 103 mg total limonoids and approximately one half this amount in a serving of grapefruit juice (31).

Total flavanone glycoside levels in orange and grapefruit juices range from 70 to 190mg. Approximately 65 to 70 percent of this total in orange juice is hesperidin with smaller amounts of narirutin and didymin. The major flavanone glycoside in grapefruit juice is naringin followed by narirutin, poncirin and didymin. The aglycone of hesperidin is hesperitin, the form that is absorbed by the body. It is present at 20 to 70 mg in an 8 ounce serving of orange juice. Naringinin is the aglycone of naringin and narirutin, it is present in orange and grapefruit juice at 2-6 mg and 28 to 80 mg respectively. The value of 35 to 100 mg d-limonene represents the amount of oil allowed in a grade A juice by the United States Department of Agriculture Standards of Identity for orange (33) and grapefruit juice (34). The most abundant methoxyflavone found in orange varieties is nobiletin with lesser amounts of heptamethoxyflavone, sinensetin and tangeretin. Grapefruit juice contains a very small amount of tangeretin. Although orange juice contains very little pro-vitamin A, the total carotenoid content is 2 to 6 mg (35). In grapefruit juice some of the red varieties can contain up to 26 mg of carotenoids (36). While not all carotenoids have pro-vitamin A activity, they can function as antioxidants (37). Hydroxycinnamic acids can also function as antioxidants (9). While the individual amounts of some of these compounds are below the amount necessary for activity, synergistic effects between components most likely contribute to the total benefit derived from the consumption of citrus fruit and their products.

SUMMARY

Citrus juices, already perceived as a healthy beverage, would make an excellent drink base for addition of bioactive components to make a hypernutritious drink. The commercial production of limonene and citrus oils is already practiced by industry and readily available for use as a supplement in hypernutritious foods. Commercial extraction procedures already exist for pectin and flavanone recovery although they are not currently being utilized. These phytochemicals are currently incorporated into cattlefeed along with the peel waste. Commercial recovery of methoxyflavones is achievable as they are already concentrated in peel oil processing waste streams and could be recovered with a little effort. The limonoid aglycones and glucosides are present in seeds, peel and debittering waste where they could also be recovered and utilized should a demand be created. The size to the Florida Citrus Processing Industry which currently utilizes over 8 million tons of citrus fruit annually allows the opportunity to isolate these valuable phytochemicals in bulk quantities for utilization in citrus products and other hypernutritious foods.

BIBLIOGRAPHY

1. TING, S. V. "Nutrients and Nutrition of Citrus Fruits". In *Citrus Nutrition and Quality*; Nagy, S.; Attaway, J. A. Eds.; ACS Symposium Series No. 143; American Chemical Society: Washington, DC, 1980; Chapter 1.
2. FELLERS, P. J.; NIKDEL, S.; LEE, H. S. "Nutrient Content and Nutrition Labeling of Several Processed Florida Citrus Juice Products". *J. Am. Diet. Assoc.* 1990 90, 1079-84.
3. HASEGAWA, S.; MIYAKE, M.; OZAKI, Y. "Biochemistry of Citrus Limonoids and Their Anticarcinogenic Activity". In *Food Phytochemicals for Cancer Prevention I: Fruits & Vegetables;* Haung, M. T.; Osawa, O., Ho, C. T.; Rosen, R., Eds.; ACS Symposium Series No. 546; American Chemical Society: Washington, DC, 1993; Chapter 15.
4. ROUSEFF, R. L. "Flavonoids and Citrus Quality". In *Citrus Nutrition and Quality;* Nagy, S.; Attaway, J. A., Eds.; ACS Symposium Series No. 143; American Chemical Society: Washington, DC, 1980; Chapter 5.
5. BAKER, R. A. "The Role of Pectin in Citrus Quality and Nutrition". In *Citrus Nutrition and Quality*; Nagy, S.; Attaway, J. A., Eds.; ACS Symposium Series No. 143; American Chemical Society: Washington, DC, 1980; Chapter 6.
6. VELDHUIS, M. K.; SWIFT, L. J.; SCOTT, W. C. "Fully-Methoxylated Flavones in Florida Oranges Juices". *J. Agric. Food Chem.* 1970, 18, 590-592.
7. PELEG, H.; NAIM, M.; ROUSEFF, R. L.; ZEHAVI, U. "Distribution of Bound and Free Phenolic Acids in Oranges (*Citrus sinensis*) and Grapefruits (*Citrus paradisi*)". *J. Sci. Food Agric.* 1991, 57, 417-426.
8. NAIM, M.; STRIEM, B. J.; KANNER, J.; PELEG, H. "Potential of Ferulic Acid as a Precurser to Off-flavors in Stored Orange Juice". *J. Food Sci.* 1988, 53, 500-503 & 512.
9. SMITH, T. J.; YANG, S. "Effects of Food Phytochemicals on Xenobiotic Metabolism and Tumorigenisis". In *Food Phytochemicals for Cancer Prevention I: Fruits & Vegetables*; Haung, M. T.; Osawa, O., Ho, C. T.; Rosen, R., Eds.; ACS Symposium Series No. 546; American Chemical Society: Washington, DC, 1993; Chapter 2.
10. BRADDOCK, R. J.; CADWALLADER, K. R. "Citrus By-Products Manufacture for Food Use". *Food Technology* 1992, 46, 105-110.

11. FLORIDA DEPARTMENT OF AGRICULTURE AND CONSUMER SERVICES *1990-91 Annual Report* Florida Department of Agriculture Division of Fruit and Vegetable Inspection, Winter Haven, FL, 1991; p. 8.
12. KESTERSON, J. W.; HENDRICKSON, R.; BRADDOCK, R. J. *Florida Citrus Oils Bulletin 749* Institute of Food and Agricultural Sciences, University of Florida, 1971; p 38.
13. SINCLAIR, W. B. *The Grapefruit, Its Composition, Physiology and Products* Univ. Calif.: Riverside, CA 1972; p 225.
14. KUHNAU, J. "The Flavonoids, A Class of Semi-Essential Food Components: Their Role in Human Nutrition". *World Rev. Nutr. Dig.* 1976; 24, 117-119.
15. FISHER, K. D.; SENTI, F. R; ALLISON, R. G.; ANDERSON, S. A.; CHINN, H. I.; TALBOT, J. M. "Evaluation of the Health Aspects of Hesperidin, Naringin, and Citrus Bioflavonoid Extracts as Food Ingredients". FDA Report No. FDA/BF-82/62, Federation of American Societies for Experimental Biology, Bethesda, MD, 1982.
16. RUSZNYAK, S.; SZENT-GYORGYI, A. "Vitamin P: Flavonols as Vitamins". *Nature* 1936, 27, 138.
17. VICKERY, H.; NELSON, E.; ALMQUIST, H.; ELVEHJEM, C. "Joint Committee on Nomenclature—Term "Vitamin P" Recommendation to be Discontinued". *Science* 1950, 112, 628
18. VLIETINCK, A. 1990, Private Communication.
19. BOOTH, A. N.; JONES, F. T. AND DEEDS, F. "Metabolic Fate of Hesperidin, Eriodictyol, Homoeriodictyol, and Diosmin". *J. Biol. Chem.* 1958, 230, 661-668.
20. BOOTH, A. N.; JONES, F. T. AND DEEDS, F. "Metabolic and Glucosuria Studies on Naringin and Phloridzin". *J. Biol. Chem.* 1958, 233, 280-282.
21. WINTRAUB, R. A. "Determination of the Predominant Flavonoids of Citrus Fruit Present in Blood and Urine and Application in Human Oral Administration Experiments". Masters Thesis. The University of Florida at Gainesville, 1984.
22. KAUL, T. N.; MIDDLETON, E. JR.; OGRA, P. L. "Antiviral Effects of Flavonoids on Human Viruses". *J. Med. Virol.* 1985, 15, 71-74.
23. CARROLL, K. K. 1994, Private Communication.
24. ROBBINS, R. C. "Action of Flavonoids on Blood Cells: Trimodal Action of Flavonoids Elucidates Their Inconsistent Results". *Internal J. Vil. Nutr. Res.* 1974, 44, 203-216.
25. MIDDLETON, E. JR.; DZREWIECKI, G. "Effects of Flavonoids and Transitional Metal Cations On Antigen Induced Histamine Release From Human Basophils". *Biochem. Pharmacol.* 1982, 31, 1449-1453.
26. MIDDLETON, E. JR.; FUJIKI, H.; SAVLIWALA, M.; DZREWIECKI, G. "Tumor Promotor-Induced Basophil Histamine Release: Effect of Selected Flavonoids". *Biochem. Pharmacol.* 1987, 36, 29-48.
27. BRACKE, M. E.; VYNCKE, B.; OPDENAKKER, G; FOIDART, J. M.; DEPESTEL, G.; MAREEL, M. "Effect of Catechins and Citrus Flavonoids on Invasion in vitro". *Clin. Expl. Metastasis.* 1991, 9, 13-25.

28. KANDASWAMI, C.; PERKINS, E.; SOLONUIK, D. S.; DRZEWIECKI, G.; MIDDLETON, E. JR. "Antiproliferative Effects of Citrus Flavonoids on a Human Squamous Cell Carcinoma in vitro". *Cancer Letters* 1991, 56, 147-52.
29. LAM, L. K. T.; ZHANG, J.; HASEGAWA, S.; SCHUT, H. A. J. "Inhibition of Chemically Induced Carcinogenesis by Citrus Limonoids". In *Food Phytochemicals for Cancer Prevention I: Fruits & Vegetables*; Haung, M. T.; Osawa, O.; Ho, C. T.; Rosen, R., Eds. ACS Symposium Series No. 546; American Chemical Society: Washington, DC, 1993; Chapter 16.
30. MILLER, E. G.; GONZALES-SANDERS, A. P.; COUVILLON, A. M.; WRIGHT, J. M.; HASEGAWA, S.; LAM, L. K. T; SUNAHARA, G. I. "Inhibition of Oral Carcinogenesis by Green Coffee Beans and Limonoid Glucosides". In *Food Phytochemicals for Cancer Prevention I: Fruits & Vegetables*; Haung, M. T.; Osawa, O., Ho, C. T.; Rosen, R., Eds.; ACS Symposium Series No. 546; American Chemical Society: Washington, DC, 1993; Chapter 17.
31. FONG, C. H.; HASEGAWA, S.; HERMAN, Z.; OU, P. J. "Limonoid glucosides in commercial citrus juices". *J. Food Sci.* 1989, 54, 1505-6.
32. OZAKI, Y.; AYANO, S.; MIYAKE, M.; MAEDA, H.; IFUKU, Y.; HASEGAWA, S. "Limonoid glucosides in juices of satsuma mandarin (Citrus unshiu Marc.)". *Biosci. Biotech. Biochem.* 1992, 56, 836-837.
33. UNITED STATES DEPARTMENT OF AGRICULTURE. *United States Standards for Grades of Orange Juice.* Agr. Mark. Serv., Fruit Veg. Div., Processed Products Branch, Washington, D.C., 1982.
34. UNITED STATES DEPARTMENT OF AGRICULTURE. *United States Standards for Grades of Grapefruit Juice.* Agr. Mark. Serv., Fruit Veg. Div., Processed Products Branch, Washington, D.C., 1982.
35. STEWART, I. "Provitamin A and Carotenoid Content of Citrus Juices". *J. Agric. Food Chem.* 1977, 25, 1132-1137.
36. ROUSEFF, R. L.; SADLER, G. D.; PUTNAM, T. J.; DAVIS, J. E. "Determination of β-carotene and Other Hydrocarbon Carotenoids in Red Grapefruit Cultivars". *J. Agric. Food Chem.* 1992, 40, 47-51.
37. BYERS, T.; PERRY, G. "Dietary carotenes, vitamin C, and vitamin E as protective antioxidants in human cancers". *Ann. Rev. Nutr.* 1992, 12, 139-59.

6

Dietary Impact of Fat-Free Food Products

Judith S. Douglass
James T. Heimbach
Darin K. Waylett
Brooke E. Sever
Barbara J. Petersen

The contribution of different groups of foods to fat intake in the diets of U.S. adult males and adult females is examined. Using food consumption data from recent surveys by the U.S. Department of Agriculture, linked to databases of the nutrient content of foods, we identified the roll of different foods in providing total fat; saturated, monounsaturated, and polyunsaturated fatty acids; and fat soluble vitamins. This analysis provides a basis for projecting the impact of the introduction into the marketplace of reduced-fat or fat-free products and indicates the potential need for product reformulation or fortification.

The U.S. government and a variety of medical and public health associations and authorities have advised the American public to limit average fat intake to 30% of calories to decrease health risks, and to restrict energy intake to the level needed to achieve or maintain desirable body weight. These recommendations apply to healthy Americans two years of age and older, of all ethnic groups, male and female. Government programs emphasizing limitation of fat and energy intake include the Dietary Guidelines for Americans, the Food Guide Pyramid, the revised School Lunch Program, and the National Cholesterol Education Program's Step 1 Diet.

However, available data indicate that the average consumer is far from reaching the goal limiting fat intake to 30% of calories. In analyses conducted at TAS, Inc., percent calories from fat in diets of respondents in the 1989-90 and 1990-91 USDA Continuing Surveys of Food Intakes by Individuals (CSFII) (1,2) averaged 35%, and ranged from 33% to 39% in various age-sex subgroups of the population. Fat intake of CSFII respondents averaged 69 grams per day.

Consumers are generally aware that the fat content of their diets is often higher than is recommended. Surveys have shown that consumers are interested in lowering dietary fat and that they are willing to purchase foods with lower fat content. The 1990 survey conducted by the Food Marketing Institute (3), "Trends in the United States: Consumer Attitudes in the Supermarket," for example, showed that 54% of the population regards fats as "a serious health hazard"; the 1994 survey showed that 60% of the population takes this viewpoint. In surveys conducted by the American Dietetic Association and the International Food Information Council (4), the number of Americans reporting that they have changed their diets to reduce fat intake has risen from 42% in 1990 to 71% in the 1994 survey.

The food industry has responded to consumer concerns and the resulting market demand by reformulating products to remove fat. Although reduced-fat products have proliferated in recent years, their effectiveness in reducing fat intake of free-living populations has not been demonstrated. While some consumers may substitute low-fat products for the traditional high-fat versions and make no other dietary changes, it is possible that others may compensate for the reduction in fat by eating a greater volume of food or by adding high-fat foods not previously consumed. Caloric compensation for low-fat diets has been observed in some clinical studies (5,6), but not in others (7,8).

To examine the impact of low-fat or fat-free products on food and nutrient intakes of the U.S. population and population subgroups, we analyzed data from the 1989-90 and 1990-91 CSFIIs. Our goal was to answer the following questions:

What percent of the population consumes low-fat versions of traditionally high-fat foods?

Are low-fat foods and the high-fat versions of these foods eaten in similar quantities?

What are the potential fat savings if low-fat versions of traditionally high-fat foods are consumed?

Do consumers of low-fat foods retain the fat savings from these foods, or do they compensate by eating higher levels of fat from other sources?

Because intakes of fat-soluble vitamins would be expected to decrease with decreases in dietary fat, we also attempted to answer the following question:

Do consumers of low-fat foods have lower intakes of vitamin A or vitamin E than do consumers of the higher fat versions of these foods?

METHODS

The 1989-90 and 90-91 USDA CSFIIs were based on nationally representative samples of consumers, and provided information on all foods consumed, at home or away from home, over a three-day period, by 8,000 respondents of all ages living in U.S. households.

CSFII data on selected high-fat foods and low-fat counterparts were analyzed to determine user populations, amounts of foods consumed, and fat intakes from the foods. Foods investigated included whole, low-fat, and skim milk; regular and low-fat cheese; regular and low-fat table fat; and regular and low-fat salad dressings. Survey data were also analyzed to determine mean daily fat, vitamin A, and vitamin E intakes of users of each of the food products listed above.

Survey populations investigated for this study were the total U.S. population, females 20-54 and 55+ years of age, and males 20-54 and 55+ years of age.

RESULTS

A. Regular (full-fat) vs. low-fat versions of selected foods: user population, amounts consumed, and fat contributions to diets (Table 6.1).

Fluid Milks

Thirty-seven percent of the population reported consumption of whole milk, 39% reported consumption of low-fat milk (1 or 2%), and only 11% reported consumption of skim milk. About 20% of females age 55 and older were skim milk consumers.

Low-fat milk was consumed in higher quantities than were whole or skim milk; consumption amounts were 324, 374, and 318 g per day, respectively. Consumers of whole milk obtained 10.8 g of fat per day from milk, versus 6.4 g of fat per day from low-fat milk and 0.6 g of fat per day from skim milk.

Cheeses

About 47% of the survey population reported consumption of regular cheeses while only about 4% reported consumption of low-fat cheeses. When cheeses were consumed, the low-fat versions were consumed in much greater quantities—daily intake was 44 g for the regular cheeses and 78 g for the low-fat cheeses. Fat intake from the regular cheeses was 11.3 g, while the nearly-twice-as-large quantities of the low-fat versions provided only 2.2 g of fat.

Table Fats (Butter, Margarine, and Spreads)

About 57% of respondents reported consumption of regular table fats; 4% reported using "low-fat" table fats. Regular fats

TABLE 6.1. FULL-FAT FOODS AND LOW-FAT COUNTERPARTS: USER POPULATIONS, AMOUNT OF FOODS CONSUMED, AND FAT INTAKE FROM FOODS

	User Population %					Amt. Food Consumed g/user/day					Fat Intake From Food g/user/day				
	U.S.	Females		Males		U.S.	Females		Males		U.S.	Females		Males	
Foods		20-54	55+	20-54	55+		20-54	55+	20-54	55+		20-54	55+	20-54	55+
FLUID MILK															
Whole	37	31	30	32	28	324	212	235	320	264	10.8	7.1	7.9	10.7	8.8
Low-fat	39	37	34	36	36	374	306	251	423	277	6.4	5	4.3	7.4	4.8
Skim	11	13	20	10	18	318	305	261	414	289	0.6	0.5	0.5	0.7	0.5
CHEESES															
Regular	47	49	38	53	40	44	42	44	52	51	11.3	11	9.7	13.6	10.9
Low-fat	4	5	8	1	4	78	79	83	70	89	2.2	2.7	1.4	2.4	1.4
TABLE FATS															
Regular	57	58	63	59	61	15	13	13	18	17	11.5	10.3	10	14	13.3
Low-fat	4	4	9	3	5	12	11	10	12	12	4.7	4.4	3.8	4.5	4.5
SALAD DRESSINGS															
Regular	49	52	50	55	51	26	26	23	31	26	13.3	12.7	11.8	15.8	12.6
Low-fat	10	11	17	10	12	24	25	21	29	23	30	3.1	2.5	3.7	3.1

were consumed in somewhat higher quantities (15 g of regular table fats per day versus 12 g of low-fat products). Males age 20 to 54 consume an average of 18 g of regular table fat per day, 3 g/day more than the total population. Fat intake from table fat was 11.5 g/day for regular table fat and 4.7 g/day for low-fat table fat.

Salad Dressings

Forty-nine percent of the population reported consuming regular dressing, and 10% consumed low-fat dressing. Regular and low-fat salad dressings were consumed in approximately the same quantities, 26 g and 24 g per day, respectively. However, users of regular salad dressings consumed 13.3 g of fat per day from regular dressing while low-fat dressing users consumed only 3 g.

B. Nutrient intake of users of regular and low-fat foods: fat, vitamin A, and vitamin E

It should be noted in reviewing the following results that although data are presented for users of regular vs. low-fat foods, these groups are not mutually exclusive; for example, a consumer of whole milk might also be a consumer of skim milk.

Fat

Total daily fat intakes for consumers of whole milk, low-fat milk, skim milk, regular cheese, and low-fat cheese are shown in Fig. 6.1. Total daily fat intakes for consumers of regular and low-fat table fats and salad dressings are shown in Fig. 6.2.

On average, skim milk consumers consumed less fat on a daily basis than did whole milk or low-fat milk consumers. The mean daily fat intake was 62 g for skim milk drinkers, 72 g for whole milk drinkers and 69 g for low-fat milk drinkers.

Differences in total fat intake between consumers of regular cheese and consumers of low-fat cheese are more pronounced than differences seen with different types of milk choice. The average daily fat intake by low-fat cheese users was 55 g, while the average by regular cheese consumers was 75 g.

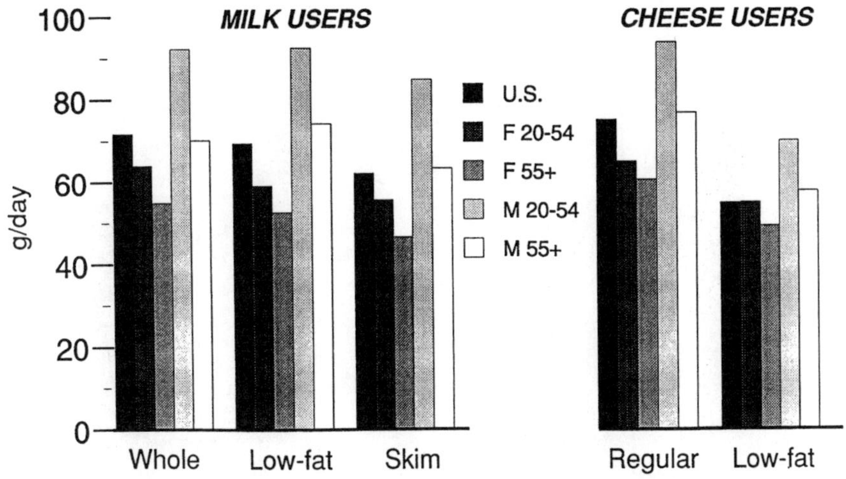

FIG. 6.1. MEAN DAILY FAT INTAKE OF FLUID MILK USERS AND CHEESE USERS.

The daily fat intake by users of regular table fats averaged 75 g for the total U.S. population. Daily fat intake by users of low-fat table fat averaged 57 g. Overall, daily fat intake was lower for users of low-fat table fat than for table-fat non-users (62 g/day); however, in several subpopulations this was not the case.

Consumers of regular salad dressings had higher daily fat intakes than did consumers of low-fat salad dressings. The daily fat intake by consumers of regular dressings was 75 g, while low-fat dressing users consumed 63 g—about the same as people who didn't use salad dressings at all.

Vitamin A

Daily vitamin A intake by users of skim milk and low-fat milk, cheese, table fat, and salad dressings was found to be higher than that by users of the regular versions of these foods in all cases. Intakes of vitamin A by users of whole, low-fat, and skim milk were 5414, 6399, and 7849 IU/day, respectively, by the total population. Mean daily vitamin A intake of regular cheese users was 6055 IU; that of low-fat cheese users was 7566 IU. Regular table fat users consumed a mean 6252 IU vitamin A

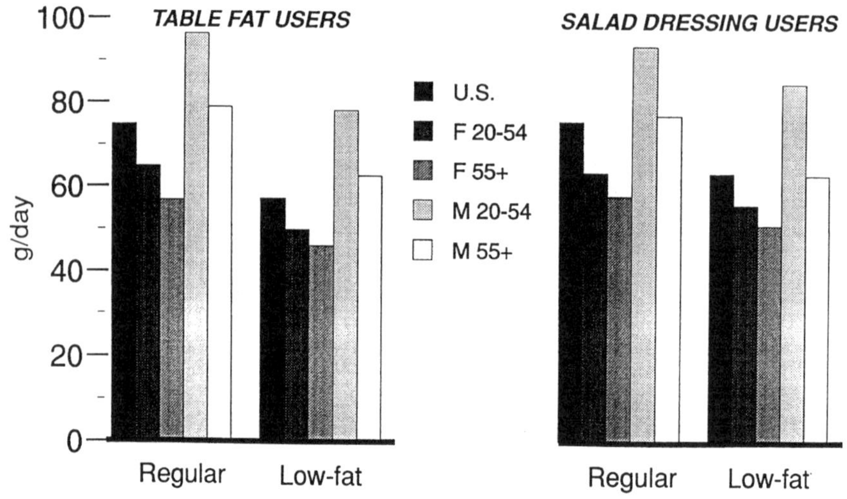

FIG. 6.2. MEAN DAILY FAT INTAKE OF TABLE FAT USERS AND SALAD DRESSING USERS.

per day, and low-fat table fat users consumed 7473 IU vitamin A per day. However, intake of vitamin A among salad dressing users was only slightly lower for regular dressing users (6544 IU/day) than for low-fat dressing users (6547 IU/day).

Vitamin E

The Recommended Dietary Allowances (RDA) for vitamin E are 8 mg alpha-tocopherol equivalents for nonpregnant, nonlactating adult females and 10 mg alpha-tocopherol equivalents for adult males (4). Mean daily vitamin E intake was below the RDA for most population groups, regardless of foods consumed (Fig. 6.3 and 6.4).

Vitamin E intake was about the same or perhaps slightly higher by skim milk drinkers than by people in the other groups. On the other hand, vitamin E intake does appear to be generally lower for those choosing low-fat cheese than for those consuming regular cheese. The latter pattern is also observed for consumers of low-fat table fats and salad dressings; consumers of low-fat versions tended to have lower daily intakes of vitamin E than do consumers of regular versions.

DISCUSSION

The goals of this study were to determine the percentage of the population consuming low-fat versions of traditionally high-fat foods, to compare the quantities consumed, and to estimate the potential fat savings if low-fat versions of traditionally high-fat foods are consumed. Most importantly, we wanted to determine if the fat savings from low-fat foods are retained in diets of consumers and to assess any impact of consuming low-fat food on intake of fat-soluble vitamins.

Results of this study show that low-fat foods are consumed by a much smaller segment of the population than are the high-fat foods they replace. However, these foods are generally consumed in similar quantities to the higher fat foods they might replace, and fat intakes from the low-fat versions are substantially less in each case.

Use of reduced-fat products resulted in lowered fat intake from the products themselves. Moreover, a key finding is that these fat reductions were not obviated by increased consumption or by fat increases elsewhere in the diet: consumers who

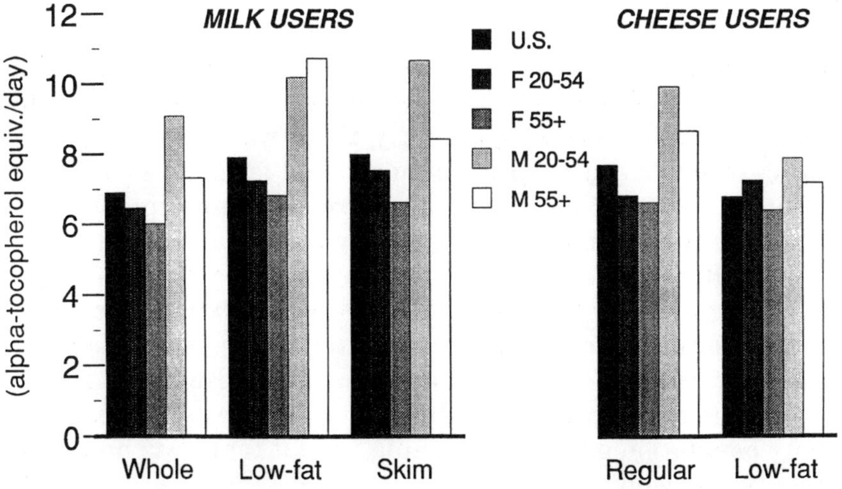

FIG. 6.3. MEAN DAILY VITAMIN E INTAKE OF FLUID MILK USERS AND CHEESE USERS.

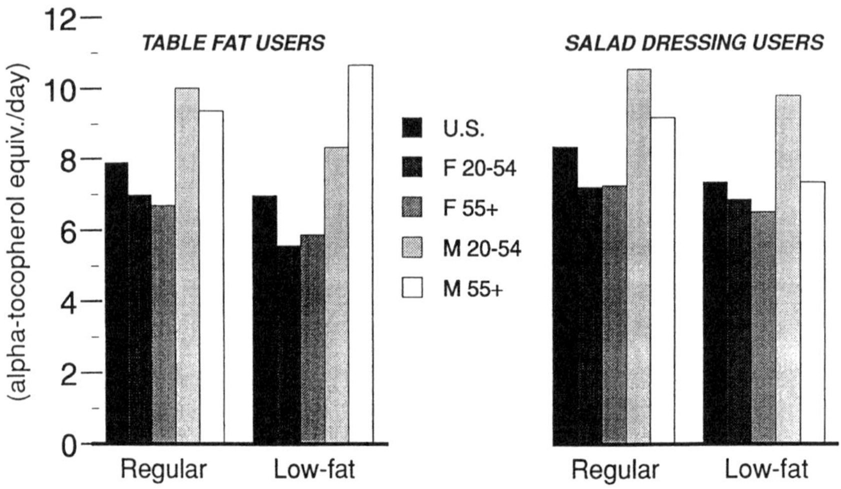

FIG. 6.4. MEAN DAILY VITAMIN E INTAKE OF TABLE FAT USERS AND SALAD DRESSING USERS.

used reduced-fat products consistently had lower total intakes of fat than did consumers who used their regular counterparts.

As previously noted, whole milk drinkers obtained about 11 g of fat from milk, while skim milk drinkers obtained less than 1 g. This 10-g difference in fat intake was retained and is indeed reflected in a 10-g difference in overall daily fat intake. On the other hand, low-fat milk drinkers obtained 6 g of fat from milk, but only 3 g of that 5-g savings (as compared to whole-milk drinkers) was retained. Apparently, there was some compensation in terms of consumption of additional fat in this case. This might be regarded as indicating a greater commitment to fat reduction by skim-milk as compared with low-fat-milk drinkers.

The difference in daily fat intake between consumers of regular cheese and low-fat cheese is much more than is accounted for by differences in fat intake from the cheeses alone and suggests that consumers who choose low-fat cheeses tend also to reduce their fat intake in other ways. This was the case for many population groups consuming low-fat table fats and salad dressings as well.

Might substitution of low-fat or fat-free foods for regular foods result in dangerously low intakes of fat-soluble vitamins?

Our results indicate that substitution of low-fat foods for regular foods does not necessarily have an adverse impact on vitamin A intake. In fact, daily vitamin A intake by users of skim milk and low-fat milk, cheese, table fat, and salad dressings was found to be higher than that by users of the regular versions of these foods in all cases. This is an interesting result for milk drinkers, because the milks are fortified with vitamin A at the same level, and the amounts of milk consumed by the two groups are approximately the same. It is clear that users of skim milk and other low-fat foods obtain more vitamin A from other sources, probably fruits and vegetables.

Choosing skim milk does not result in a reduction in vitamin E intake. On the other hand, vitamin E intake does appear to be generally lower for those choosing the other low-fat foods studied. This result was seen for users of low-fat cheese, who, as may be recalled, exhibit a pattern of low-fat eating that results in an overall fat reduction of more than 25% compared to consumers of regular cheeses. Consumers of low-fat table fat and low-fat salad dressings also generally had lower vitamin E intakes than did consumers of the regular versions of these foods.

There are many sources of vitamin A or its precursors, and it is clear that those people who are currently using reduced-fat foods are availing themselves of them. It remains to be seen whether this will continue to be the case. Vitamin E, however, is another story: the only real sources of vitamin E, absent fortification, are vegetable oils. As consumers reduce their consumption of these oils, we believe that even the limited data that we have seen today indicate that increased use of vitamin E fortification may be justified.

More research should be performed to further delineate the possible risks and benefits of expanded vitamin E fortification. For example, we examined nutrient intakes by groups that were not mutually exclusive; to further clarify differences between consumers of regular and low-fat items, we could contrast nutrient intake of people who consume regular items but not the low-fat versions and of people who consume low-fat items but not the regular versions.

Our overall conclusion is that reduced-fat foods can play a valuable part in helping consumers achieve dietary goals. We are actually somewhat surprised at this finding, because we expected that this would not be the case—that consumers of reduced-fat foods would simply get more fat elsewhere, thus ending up with no net change in their fat intake. It will be interesting to observe what happens as reduced-fat variations appear for more products. It is possible that those people who are choosing currently available reduced-fat foods are the more committed segments of the marketplace, who are really making serious efforts to change their diets. What will happen when more foods are available that may attract people with a more casual approach to achieving healthy diets?

Note: All consumption analyses were conducted using the TAS International Diet Research System® (TASDIET).

BIBLIOGRAPHY

1. Human Nutrition Information Service, USDA. Nationwide Food Consumption Survey: Continuing Survey of Food Intakes by Individuals 1989-90, 1992 Dataset.
2. Human Nutrition Information Service, USDA. Nationwide Food Consumption Survey: Continuing Survey of Food Intakes by Individuals 1990-91, 1993 Dataset.
3. Food Marketing Institute. "Trends in the United States: Consumer Attitudes in the Supermarket." Washington, D.C.: Food Marketing Institute, 1994.
4. Gallup Organization. "How are Americans Making Food Choices?" Survey Conducted for American Dietetic Association and International Food Information Council, April, 1994.
5. FOLTIN, R. W.; FISCHMAN, M. W.; EMURIAN, C. S.; et al. "Compensation for calorie dilution in humans given unrestricted access to food in a residential laboratory." *Appetite* 1988, 10, 13-24.
6. FOLTIN, R. W.; FISCHMAN, M. W.; MORAN, T. H.; et al. "Caloric compensation for lunches varying in fat and carbohydrate content by humans in a residential laboratory." *Am. J. Clin. Nutr.* 1990, 52, 969-980.
7. KENDALL-CASELLA, A.; LEVITSKY, D. A.; STRUPP, B. J.; LISSNER, L. "Weight loss on a low-fat diet: Consequence of the imprecision of the control of food intake in humans." *Am. J. Clin. Nutr.* 1991, 53, 1124-1129.
8. LISSNER, L.; LEVITSKY, D. A.; STRUPP, B. J.; KALKWARF, H. J.; ROE, D. A. "Dietary fat and the regulation of energy intake in human subjects". *Am. J. Clin. Nutr.* 1987, 46, 886-892.

7

Biological Basis for Dietary Modulation of Colon Carcinogenesis

Maurice R. Bennink

Studies of people with genetic predispositions to colon cancer (CC) have revealed that CC arises from mutations or gene deletions involving specific oncongenes and/or tumor suppressor genes. Other studies reveal these people have an upward shift in the proliferative compartment of the colon mucosa crypts and a hyperproliferative compartment of the colon mucosa crypts and a hyperproliferative state throughout the colon. Mitosis is tightly controlled by a complex sequence of protein phosphorylation/dephosphorylation of cellular proteins controlling cell division and differentation. Some of the known dietary influences on CC can be explained based on their impact on cell signals that alter phosphorylation states of cellular proteins that control the cell cycle.

During the past two decades, the relationship between diet and colon cancer (CC) was examined primarily through epidemiologic studies and by dietary manipulation of chemically induced CC in laboratory animals. These approaches demonstrated relationships between diet and CC, but very little could be learned about how diet modulates CC at a cellular level because of the limited understanding of tumorigenesis that existed 20 years ago. However, during the past few years, great progress has been made in our understanding of the genetic and molecular events involved in colon carcinogenesis. We now can study how diet influences molecular events involved in colon carcinogenesis.

The first section of this chapter will briefly review what has been learned about the relationship of diet and CC through epidemiologic studies and research with laboratory animals. The second section will focus on the relationship of colon epithelial cell proliferation to CC and on the molecular aspects of colon carcinogenesis. The last section will discuss how dietary calcium and genistein, caloric restriction, and sulindac can modulate colon cell proliferation and colon tumorigenesis.

DIETARY APPROACHES TO PREVENT COLON CANCER

Epidemiology provided clues as to dietary factors that increase CC incidence. Hypotheses based on epidemiologic studies were then tested in animal models of colon carcinogenesis. Approaches to reduce dietary enhanced colon carcinogenesis emerged from these studies and are discussed below.

Prevent Carcinogens From Contacting The Colon Mucosa

One approach to reduce dietary induced colon cancer is to prevent dietary carcinogens/mutagens from interacting with the colon mucosa and thus inhibit initiation of CC. Carcinogens/mutagens can be present in the diet because they occur naturally, because they are inadvertently added, or because they are produced during cooking or food processing. Potential genotoxic agents in the diet can be identified by *in vitro* mutagen assays such as the *Salmonella typhimurium* test (1) and the DNA repair test in hepatocytes (2). However, when dose, threshold effects, and *in vivo* detoxification mechanisms are considered, this line of research did not reveal that there are sufficient dietary genotoxins that occur naturally or that were inadvertently added to account for the higher incidence of CC in Western countries compared to Poland, Southern Europe, Japan or South America (3).

Potent mutagens can be formed during food preparation. Initial research focused on formation of polycyclic aromatic hydrocarbons produced by charcoal broiling of meat (4, 5). However, extensive research in this area has shown that polycyclic aromatic hydrocarbons do not significantly increase CC risk (6, 7). Later research has focused on the formation of heterocyclic aromatic amines during frying, broiling, and toasting. Some heterocyclic aromatic amines are extremely potent mutagens (8-10) and the presence of these compounds in food may be one cause for the increased incidence of CC in Western countries.

Reduce Contact Between Colon Mucosa and Carcinogens

Because the likelihood of identifying and removing all potential colon carcinogens/mutagens from the diet is remote, an alternative approach has been to reduce contact between a carcinogen and the colon mucosa. This can be achieved by diluting intestinal contents and/or by decreasing residence time of undigested food in the colon. Some types of dietary fiber can fulfill both roles. For example, fibers that are not fermented (i.e., lignin) or only partly fermented (i.e., cellulose and hemicellulose) adsorb and absorb water. These fibers plus related water dilute intestinal contents and any carcinogen that may be present. Also, dietary cellulose and hemicellulose speed passage of materials through the colon. However, pectins and gums (hydrocolloids) are often completely fermented by colonic microflora and, therefore, contribute very little to either minimizing contact between a colon carcinogen and the colon mucosa or to decreasing residence time of fecal material in the colon.

Epidemiologic studies suggest that dietary fiber is important in reducing CC incidence (11, 12). However, results from studies using dietary fiber to reduce chemical carcinogenesis in laboratory animals have been mixed—a decrease, no effect, or even enhancement of colon carcinogenesis has been reported (13). Considering all data, the preponderance of evidence suggests that dietary fiber decreases CC risk; however, the extent that dietary fiber can reduce CC incidence is uncertain.

Modify Colonic Microfloral Metabolism

Differences in CC incidence between countries with high and low incidence rates were hypothesized to be due to differences in colonic bacteria or to differences in bacterial metabolites (14). Careful studies enumerating facultative and strict anaerobes in colon contents failed to find major differences in number or type of bacteria in colons of people at high versus low risk for CC (15-17). Although type or number of colonic bacteria was not associated with CC incidence, populations that have a high incidence of CC have a greater concentration of mutagens in their stools (18, 19). Fecapentaenes are bacterial metabolites of unabsorbed fatty acids and they are mutagenic in bacterial mutation assays. However, fecapentaenes do not act as initiators of CC (20, 21) as originally hypothesized. A later study showed that fecapentaenes more likely function as promoters of CC (22). Because colonic concentrations of fecapentaenes are increased with high fat, low fiber diets, it is likely that fecapentaenes contribute to the increased incidence of CC seen in populations consuming that type of diet.

Prevent or Reduce Cellular Damage

Assuming that not all colon carcinogens—naturally occurring, formed during food preparation, food additives, or bacterial metabolites—can be eliminated from the diet or from reaching the colon, what measures can be taken to prevent or reduce their damage? Stimulating hepatic and intestinal "phase II" enzymes that detoxify xenobiotics can reduce chemically induced CC (23, 24). Phase II enzymes add glutathione, glucuronic acid, sulfate, or acetate to xenobiotics to reduce toxicity and to speed xenobiotic clearance via bile or urine. Epidemiologic studies often find an inverse relationship between CC and consumption of fruits, vegetables, and grains (12, 25, 26). This inverse relationship generally is attributed to increased consumption of antioxidants, fiber, and substances that enhance phase II enzymes (27). A variety of substances that induce phase II enzymes occur naturally in the diet in plant materials (28).

Oxidative damage to critical cellular macromolecules can both initiate and promote CC (28, 29, 30). Carotenoids, vitamins C and E, phenolics, and selenium—as part of glutathione peroxidase—act as general antioxidants at the cellular level. A deficiency of one or more of these antioxidants increases cancer at several sites (31); however, it is difficult to show that dietary intakes above minimum requirements offer a protective effect. For example, b-carotene, vitamin C plus vitamin E, or a combination of b-carotene with vitamins C and E did not reduce formation of colon polyps (a biomarker indicating initial stages of CC) in 864 patients (32).

Unabsorbed iron can catalyze peroxidation of unabsorbed polyunsaturated fatty acids to form lipid hydroperoxides that enhance chemically induced CC (33). Phytate may help prevent CC by reducing the amount of lipid hydroperoxides formed in the colon (33). However, since phytate inhibits cation absorption, the use of phytate as a cancer preventative agent should be considered with caution since phytate can cause trace mineral deficiencies.

Chemical carcinogens that are frequently used to induce CC are strong electrophiles that cause point mutations and ultimately result in CC. Organosulfur compounds in garlic (34) and vitamins C and E (28) can scavenge electrophiles, reduce point mutations, and reduce CC. Because the events initiating CC in humans are unknown, the general applicability of electrophile scavengers in preventing human CC is not known.

Inflammatory conditions stimulate oxidative damage to cells, production of growth factors, and cell proliferation (29); the net result is promotion of CC. The prostanoids—prostaglandin E_1, prostaglandin E_2, and leukotriene B_4—are potent proinflammatory agents. Inhibition of prostanoid synthesis can reduce the oxidative damage to cells and tissue, and thus inhibit colon carcinogenesis. Nonsteroidal anti-inflammatory drugs (NSAIDs) that inhibit prostanoid synthesis also inhibit chemically induced CC in rats (35) and lead to regression of colon polyps in humans (36).

Overall, research that has attempted to show that dietary constituents can prevent or reduce cellular damage and, in turn, prevent CC has been inconclusive. The most promising agents are the NSAIDs (aspirin, piroxicam, sulindac and indomethacin) (29, 30, 35) which are medicinals and not dietary constituents.

Reduce Fat Consumption

The amount of fat consumed has a strong bearing on CC risk. As the quantity of dietary fat increases, the quantity of fatty acids and bile acids passing through the colon also increases. Bile salts are strong detergents and are cytotoxic in high concentrations. The colonic concentrations of bile salts in individuals consuming high-fat, low-fiber diets are not cytotoxic. However, these concentrations of bile salts can irritate the colon mucosa, which in turn increases cell proliferation. Bile acids have been shown to promote CC in animal models (37). High-fat, low-fiber diets are consistently correlated with increased CC incidence in both epidemiologic and experimental CC studies (37), providing further indirect support that bile acids promote CC.

Reduce Caloric Intake

Diets rich in fat contribute to increased incidence of CC in another way—by increasing caloric intake. In general, high fat diets encourage greater caloric intakes. Western countries consume more calories per capita than countries with a low incidence of CC. It is clear from animal experiments that caloric restriction reduces CC incidence (38). Epidemiologic studies also support a positive correlation between caloric intake and CC incidence. The amount of fat in the diet and caloric intake appear to have independent roles in enhancing colon carcinogenesis (37).

BIOLOGY OF COLON CANCER

Identification of differences in the colon mucosa between individuals at high or low risk for CC has provided insights into the biology of CC. Histological studies identified aberrant growth patterns in colon mucosa of individuals with genetic predispositions to CC. Later studies, using molecular techniques, substantiated the early histologic studies and identified a number of genetic events that occur during the conversion of a normal colon epithelial cell to a fully transformed cell capable of developing into a malignant tumor.

Colon Mucosa Proliferation Characteristics

Increased cell proliferation and decreased cell differentiation are biomarkers considered indicative of an increased risk for developing colon cancer (39). In normal colon crypts, stem cells divide primarily in the bottom half of the crypt. As the cells travel toward the apex of the crypt (lumen surface), the cells mature, undergo terminal differentiation, and become incapable of further cell division. Because of cell differentiation, few mitotic cells are present in the top one third of normal crypts and essentially no dividing cells are present near the crypt mouths or in the flat mucosa (40). Differentiated cells in the flat mucosa undergo apoptosis and exfoliation. However, people with conditions associated with an increased risk for CC—familial adenomatous polyposis, Crohn's disease, ulcerative colitis, sporadic adenomas—typically have increased cell proliferation and decreased epithelial cell differentiation in their colon mucosa. Animals treated with colon carcinogens also have the characteristics of increased cell proliferation and decreased epithelial cell differentiation in the colon mucosa (41). As a result of decreased cell differentiation (in humans and animal models), there are more proliferative cells in the crypts and there are more mitotic cells in the top one third of crypts. In addition, a few mitotic cells appear at the mouth of crypts and in the flat mucosa. Hyperproliferation, along with abnormal differentiation and decreased apoptosis, leads to an accumulation of cells near the crypt mouths and in the flat mucosa. The accumulated cells eventually form small adenomas (hyperplastic polyps). With time, some polyps continue to grow and become adenomatous polyps that contain foci of transformed cells and, eventually, some of the polyps become malignant tumors (40). In general, a small but significant increase in the mitotic index is seen throughout crypts in early stages of colon carcinogenesis. However, a better criterion for distinguishing individuals at risk for CC is the mitotic frequency in the top 40% of the crypt. People predisposed to CC have increased cell proliferation in the top 40% of the crypt compared to individuals at low risk. Many clinical trials make use of this fact and assess treatment (dietary intervention or drug) effectiveness by measuring the mitotic frequency in the top 40% of colon mucosal crypts before and after treatment. A decrease in mitotic frequency either in the upper 40% of the crypts or in whole crypts is interpreted as lowering the risk for CC.

Inflammatory conditions, like Crohn's disease and ulcerative colitis, stimulate production of cytokines, such as transforming growth factor-a (TGF-a) and interleukins, which stimulate mucosal cell proliferation (42). Mucosal proliferation rates reflect the balance between cells in S, G_2, and M phases of the cell cycle on one hand and cells that have differentiated or are in the G_0 phase on the other hand. Cells appear to make the decision to differentiate, enter into G_0, or enter another round of cell division based on integration of signals derived from many interrelated pathways (43-45). Growth factors, cytokines, insulin, and insulin-like growth factor-1 are examples of extracellular signals. Internal signals reflect the energy state and adequacy of raw materials required for cell division and growth (43). Transduction of both extracellular and intracellular signals is done primarily via enzyme activation by phosphorylation and dephosphorylation of tyrosine, serine, or threonine residues on proteins. These proteins in turn regulate transcription or translation of proteins that ultimately control the cell cycle. Because there are many checks and balances, inappropriate control of one pathway usually does not produce cancer. However, if several pathways are inappropriately controlled, cancer can result.

Cellular Changes Associated With Colon Carcinogenesis

Some molecular events associated with initiation, promotion, and progression of colon carcinogenesis have been identified (46). Colon cancer results from a combination of activated oncogenes and inactivated tumor suppressor genes. The activation of oncogenes and/or inactivation of tumor suppressor genes can be caused by mutational events or by gene deletions (allelic loss of a gene).

In the genetic model of colon tumorigenesis presented by Fearon and Vogelstein (46), a hyperproliferative colon epithelium is the first identified abnormality. People that develope small mucosal adenomas (benign polyps) in the colon have increased mucosal cell proliferation throughout the colon (47). Progression from hyperproliferative normal crypts to small adenomas appears to require a gene mutation or deletion. Approximately two-thirds of colon adenomas and malignant tumors have a mutated or missing APC gene (48). Individuals with familial adenomatous polyposis inherit a mutated APC gene that acts in a dominant negative manner to allow mucosal adenomas to develop at a very young age, in some cases by nine years of age. A high percent of sporadic adenomatous polyps contain a mutated or deleted APC gene also.

The exact function of the protein encoded by the APC gene is not known (49). Expression of the APC protein increases gradually as the cells migrate up the crypt. This implies that the protein is involved in cell maturation and differentiation (49). Cleavage of the APC encoded protein by a proteolytic enzyme initiates loss of cell adhesion and apoptosis (50). Thus, when the APC gene is mutated or missing, the epithelial cell does not mature, differentiate, or proceed through apoptosis and exfoliation. Rather, the cell remains in the cell cycle, continues to proliferate, and ultimately leads to development of adenomas.

Mutation of the *ras* gene is frequently associated with the transformation of early adenomas to intermediate adenomas (46). Transformation to the cancerous state (adenocarcinoma) is frequently associated with loss of the DCC gene and/or a loss of the gene coding for p53. The specific order of mutational events/gene deletions is not as important as the total number of mutations (46). Several lines of evidence suggest that four to six mutations/gene deletions are required to transform a normal colon mucosal cell into a malignant cell.

An activating mutation of the *ras* oncogene occurs in approximately 50% of all colon carcinomas and adenomas greater than 1 cm, whereas less than 10% of small adenomas (< 1 cm) possess a mutated *ras* oncogene (46). The *ras* oncogene codes for a guanine-nucleotide-binding protein which acts as a "molecular switch" and whose activity is required to conduct many of the mitogenic signals (51). If *ras* is constitutively active because of mutations at critical sites, then mitogenic signals are sent to the nucleus in the absence of mitogens. Activating *ras* mutations confer a growth advantage to cells leading to the larger (intermediate) adenomas.

The DCC gene encodes a plasma membrane protein that is believed to function in cell-cell communication and/or cell-substrate interactions (52). As mucosal cells travel toward the apex of the crypt, the DCC encoded protein may pass signals from the submucosa directing cells to undergo terminal differentiation. There is a strong relationship between lack of DCC expression, lack of cell differentiation, and tumorigenesis (53). Approximately 75% of colorectal tumors and 40% of adenomas with foci of carcinomatous transformation have a mutated or missing DCC gene (54).

The p53 gene encodes a protein that can block cells with DNA damage from passing from G_1 to S in the cell cycle (55). Mutated p53 protein binds to and inactivates wild type p53 protein. This allows the cell to pass into S and provides a proliferative advantage to the cell (56). A mutated or deleted p53 gene plus a *ras* mutation is sufficient to transform a normal cell to a cancer cell. Approximately 60 to 85% of colon tumors have mutated p53 genes (56, 57).

NORMALIZATION OF THE HYPER-PROLIFERATIVE COLON MUCOSA

Is there any evidence that hyperproliferation in the colon mucosa can be reversed to reduce the risk of CC? The next section discusses data that suggest that dietary calcium (Ca) and genistein, caloric restriction, and the NSAID sulindac can reduce colon mucosa hyperproliferation and, presumably, CC risk.

Effects of Dietary Calcium On Cell Proliferation and Colon Cancer

Hints that Ca intake may affect the incidence of CC were provided by Reddy et al. (18). Finnish populations that consume a diet high in fat and high in Ca have a CC incidence comparable to populations consuming a low fat diet. The low incidence of CC despite consuming a high fat diet was partly attributed to the high intake of calcium (37). Another indirect piece of evidence was provided by studies with colon tissue explants and with primary colonic epithelial cell cultures (58). Culture medium containing 2.2 mM Ca (the Ca level in blood) inhibited cell division and caused terminal cell differentiation. Conversely, colonocytes cultured in 0.1 mM Ca continued to proliferate and did not differentiate.

Dietary Ca levels also can affect cell proliferation and cell differentiation *in vivo*. Several clinical trials have shown that supplemental Ca decreases cell proliferation in the upper 40% of colon crypts in people at intermediate or high risk of CC (59-62). In two other studies (63, 64), supplemental Ca did not reduce colon mucosa proliferation rates. The reason for the negative results is not clear. It should be noted that the mitotic index for the entire crypt may not change with Ca supplementation. However, the frequency of proliferating cells in the top 40% of the crypt decreases (normalizes) in response to Ca supplementation. As noted previously, the proliferative pattern is a better discriminator for CC risk than the overall mitotic frequency in the crypt.

Research with animals strongly suggests that Ca inhibits CC biomarkers and tumor incidence. High Ca diets normalize the distribution of proliferating colon cells in rats treated with N-methyl-N'-nitro-N-nitrosoguanidine, a direct-acting carcinogen (65). Also, high Ca diets reduce aberrant crypt formation (precancerous lesions) (66) and chemically induced CC in rats (67, 68). Epidemiologic data, animal studies, and five of seven clinical trials all suggest that Ca consumed above normal metabolic needs will normalize colon mucosal cell proliferation in people at increased risk for CC.

The precise mechanism by which Ca reduces CC is not known, although there are at least two possibilities. First, Ca forms less toxic salts of bile acids and second Ca could act directly on the epithelial cells to reduce cell proliferation and to induce terminal cell differentiation. Typically, 40 to 90% of ingested Ca is not absorbed in the small intestine and can form Ca salts with bile acids. Ca salts of bile acids may be less irritating to the colon mucosa than bile salts formed with sodium or potassium (69). Therefore, when high-fat diets are consumed and there are more bile acids passing through the colon, increasing dietary Ca provides more Ca to complex with bile acids. Since Ca salts of bile acids are less irritating, mucosal cell proliferation is reduced. Thus, Ca could act in a nonspecific, noncellular manner to reduce CC incidence by reducing cell proliferation.

Conversely, increasing the intraluminal concentrations of Ca in the colon may produce results similar to those observed when colon tissue explants and cells were cultured in medium containing 2.2 mM Ca; i.e., increased intraluminal Ca concentrations may decrease cell proliferation and increase cell differentiation by acting directly on mucosal cells (58). It is noteworthy that addition of the Ca ionophore A23187 to cell cultures stimulates proteolysis of the APC protein and induces apoptosis (50).

Administration of azoxymethane, a colon carcinogen, increases colon mucosal cell proliferation and tyrosine kinase activity (70). However, high levels of dietary Ca attenuate the increased cell proliferation and tyrosine kinase activity caused by azoxymethane injections (70). These observations suggest that intraluminal Ca is directly affecting mucosal cells in a manner entirely independent of bile salts.

Effect of Genistein On Colon Carcinogenesis

Another possible chemopreventive agent in the diet is genistein. Soybeans are a rich source of the isoflavone genistein and populations that regularly consume soy foods have a lower incidence of CC (71). Genistein is a specific, irreversible inhibitor of tyrosine kinases (72-74) and can inhibit colon epithelial cell proliferation. Gastrin stimulates colonic mucosal cell proliferation (75) and induces colon tumor growth (76, 77). Also, gastrin stimulates increases in tyrosine kinase activity and phosphorylation of a 57 kda membrane protein in rat colon mucosa explants (78). Addition of genistein abolished the increased tyrosine kinase activity and tyrosine phosphorylation induced by gastrin (78). Genistein fed at 75 and 150 ppm to rats injected with a colon carcinogen reduced formation of aberrant crypts by 29 and 34%, respectively (66). Taken together, these observations suggest that genistein inhibits tyrosine phosphorylation, which slows cell division in colon mucosa and, ultimately reduces formation of precancerous lesions (aberrant crypts). A clinical trial to determine if consuming genistein in soy protein will reduce the mitotic index and cause a downward shift in the proliferative zone of colonic crypts of individuals at increased risk of CC is in progress.

Caloric Restriction and Colon Epithelium

Rodents treated with a colon carcinogen and undergoing 10 to 40% caloric restriction exhibit a lower mitotic index and a downward shift in the proliferative zone in their colon mucosa and have fewer tumors compared to controls fed ad libitum (79). Steinbach et al. (80) reported data from obese subjects who had reduced their caloric intake by 34% for 12 weeks. The caloric restriction lead to a 39% reduction in whole-crypt mitotic index and a 57% reduction in cell proliferation in the top 40% of the crypts. These results imply that caloric restriction may lead to reduced CC in humans also. However, is the reduced risk of CC associated only with a caloric intake that causes a negative energy balance, or would the reduced risk persist during weight maintenance at a reduced or normal body weight? It would be interesting to determine colon mucosa proliferation patterns in obese subjects before and after weight reduction and then again several months after maintaining a reduced weight. Epidemiologic studies show a weak, inconsistent association between body mass index and CC incidence (81). One interpretation of the epidemiologic data is that overconsumption of energy leading to obesity causes only slight increases in CC risk compared to normal weight individuals. Animal research suggests that cancer is reduced only when caloric intake is restricted sufficiently to slow growth and to produce very lean animals. Similar caloric restriction with humans would produce a leaner person than what is currently considered “normal weight”.

Inhibition of Colon Carcinogenesis by Suppressing Prostanoid Metabolism

Non-steroidal anti-inflammatory drugs have been used to inhibit chemically induced CC in animals. Reduction of colon carcinogenesis by NSAIDs is generally attributed to inhibition of arachidonic acid metabolism and suppression of prostaglandin synthesis (82). The NSAID sulindac is particularly effective as a chemopreventive agent against CC. Two trials with patients that have familial polyposis showed that polyps either disappear or become smaller when patients consumed sulindac (36, 83). These results suggest that chemopreventive agents can effectively inhibit or reverse colon carcinogenesis at an intermediate stage of cancer development even when mutation of a tumor suppressor gene (APC gene) is the cause of colon carcinogenesis. As described earlier, arachidonic acid metabolism and prostaglandin synthesis can be modulated by dietary agents. Organosulfur compounds, such as those found in garlic and onion, and eicosopentaenoic acid are potential chemopreventive agents because they can suppress prostanoid synthesis.

CONCLUSIONS

Diet can inhibit colon carcinogenesis through a variety of mechanisms as described in the beginning of this chapter. Diet can also potentially inhibit CC by suppressing cell proliferation and by stimulating colon epithelial cell differentiation. Preliminary observations suggest that dietary components can inhibit mitogenic signals from being transmitted to the nucleus, which results in decreased cell proliferation. The mechanisms by which diet may stimulate colon cell differentiation are less clear. The daunting task that lies ahead is the identification of precise biochemical steps that slow cell proliferation and/or enhance cell differentiation in response to dietary manipulation.

BIBLIOGRAPHY

1. MARON, D. M.; AMES, B. N. "Revised methods for the *Salmonella* mutagenicity test." *Mutat Res.* 1983, 113, 173-215.
2. WILLIAMS, G. M.; LASPIA, M. F.; DUNKEL, V. C. "Reliability of the hepatocyte primary culture/DNA repair test in testing of coded carcinogens and noncarcinogens." *Mutat. Res.* 1982, 97, 359-370.
3. HENDERSON, B. E. "Summary report of the sixth symposium on cancer registries and epidemiology in the Pacific basin." *J. Natl. Cancer Inst.* 1990, 82, 1186-1190.
4. LIJINSKY, W.; ROSS, A. E. "Production of carcinogenic polynuclear hydrocarbons in the cooking of food." *Food Cosmet. Toxicol.* 1967, 5, 343-347.
5. BARNETT, D. "Polycyclic aromatic hydrocarbons and foods." *Food Res Q.* 1976, 36, 8-12.
6. WEISBURGER, J. H. "Chemical carcinogens and their mode of action in colonic neoplasia." *Dis. Colon Rectum* 1973, 16, 431-437.
7. TOTH, B. "Tumorigenesis by benzo(a)pyrene administered intracolonically." *Oncology* 1980, 37, 77-82.
8. FELTON, J. S.; KNIZE, M. "New mutagens from cooked foods." In: *Mutagens and Carcinogens in the Diet*; Felton, J. S. and Sato, S., Eds.; Wiley-Liss Inc.: New York, 1990, pp. 19-38.
9. SUGIMURA, T. "Multistep carcinogenesis:" A 1992 perspective. *Science* 1992, 258, 603-607.
10. WEISBURGER, J. H.; RIVENSON, A.; REINHARDT, J.; et al. "Genotoxicity and carcinogenicity in rats and mice of 2-amino-3,6-dihydro-3-methyl-7H-imidazolo[4,5-f]quinolin-7-one: An intestinal bacterial metabolite of 2-amino-3-methyl-3H-imidazo[4,5-f]quinoline." *J Natl. Cancer Inst.* 1994, 86, 25-30.

11. GREENWALD, P.; LANZA, E.; EDDY, G. A. "Dietary fiber in the reduction of colon cancer risk." *J Am Diet Assoc.* 1987, 87, 1178-1188.
12. TROCK, B.; LANZA, E.; GREENWALD, P. "Dietary fiber, vegetables, and colon cancer: Critical review and meta-analyses of the epidemiologic evidence." *J. Natl. Cancer Inst.* 1990, 82, 650-661.
13. GLAUERT, H. P; BENNINK, M. R.; SANDER, C. H. "Enhancement of 1,2-dimethylhydrazine-induced colon carcinogenesis in mice by dietary agar." *Fd. Cosmet. Toxicol.* 1981, 19, 281-286.
14. HILL, M. J.; CROWTHER, J. S.; DRASAR, B. S.; et al. "Bacteria and aetiology of cancer of large bowel." *Lancet.* 1971, 1, 95-100.
15. FINEGOLD, S. M.; ATTEBERY, H. R.; SUTTER, V. L. "Effect of diet on human fecal flora: Comparison of Japanese and American diets." *Am. J. Clin. Nutr.* 1974, 27, 1456-1469.
16. MOORE, W. E. C.; HOLDEMAN, L. V. "Discussion of current bacteriological investigations of the relationship between intestinal flora, diet, and colon cancer." *Cancer Res.* 1975, 35, 3418-3420.
17. GOLDBERG, M. J.; SMITH, J. W.; NICHOLS, R. L. "Comparison of the fecal microflora of seventh-day adventists with individuals consuming a general diet." *Ann. Surgery* 1977, 186, 97-100.
18. REDDY, B.; ENGLE, A.; KATSIFIS, S.; et al. "Biochemical epidemiology of colon cancer: Effects of types of dietary fiber on fecal mutagens, acid, and neutral sterols in healthy subjects." *Cancer Res.* 1989, 49, 4629-4635.
19. VAN TASSLEE, R. L.; KINGSTON, D. G. I.; WILKINS, T. D. "Metabolism of dietary genotoxins by the human colonic microflora; the fecapentaenes and hetrocyclic amines." *Mutat.Res.* 1990, 238, 209-221.
20. WARD, J. M.; ANJO, T.; OHANNESIAN, L.; et al. "Inactivity of fecapentaene-12 as a rodent carcinogen or tumor initiator." *Cancer Letters* 1988, 42, 49-59.
21. WEISBURGER, J. H.; JONES, R. C.; WANG, C-X.; et al. "Carcinogenicity tests of fecapentaene-12 in mice and rats." *Cancer Letters* 1990, 49, 89-98.
22. ZARKOVIC, M.; QIN, X.; NAKATSURU, Y.; et al. "Tumor promotion by fecapentaene-12 in a rat colon carcinogenesis model." *Carcinogenesis* 1993, 14, 1261-1264.
23. DESCHNER, E. E.; RUPERTO, J.; WONG, G.; MEWMARK, H. L. "Quercetin and rutin as inhibitors of axozymethanol-induced colonic neoplasia." *Carcinogenesis* 1991, 12, 1193-1196.
24. YOSHIMI, N.; WANG, A.; MORISHITA, Y.; et al. "Modifying effects of fungal and herb metabolites on azoxymethane-induced intestinal carcinogenesis in rats." *Jpn. J. Cancer Res.* 1992, 83, 1273-1278.
25. STEINMETZ, K. A.; POTTER, J. D. "Vegetables, fruit, and cancer. I. Epidemiology." *Cancer Causes, Occurrence and Control* 1991, 2, 325-357.
26. BLOCK, G.; PATTERSON, B.; SUBAR, A. "Fruit, vegetables, and cancer prevention: A review of the epidemiological evidence." *Nutr. Cancer* 1992, 18, 1-29.

27. STEINMETZ, K. A.; POTTER, J. D. "Vegetables, fruit and cancer. II. Mechanisms." *Cancer Causes, Occurrence and Control* 1991, 2, 427-442.
28. WATTENBERG, L. W. "Prevention-therapy-basic science and the resolution of the cancer problem: Presidential address." *Cancer Res.* 1993, 53, 5890-5896.
29. CERUTTI, PETER A.; TRUMP, B. F. "Inflammation and oxidative stress in carcinogenesis." *Cancer Cells* 1981, 3, 1-7.
30. LIPPMAN, S. M.; BENNER, S. E.; HONG, W. K. "Cancer chemoprevention." *J. Clin. Oncol.* 1994, 12, 851-873.
31. BLOT, W. J.; LI, J-Y.; TAYLOR, P. R.; et al. "Nutrition intervention trials in Linxian, China: Supplementation with specific vitamin/mineral combinations, cancer incidence, and disease-specific mortality in the general population." *J. Natl. Cancer Inst.* 1993, 85, 1483-1492.
32. GREENBERG, E. R.; BARON, J. A.; TOSTESON, T. D.; et al. "A clinical trial of antioxidant vitamins to prevent colorectal adenoma." *N. Engl. J. Med.* 1994, 331, 141-147.
33. GRAF, E.; EATON, J. W. "Antoxidant functions of phytic acid." *Free Radical's & Medicine* 1990, 8, 61-69.
34. SUMIYOSHI, H.; WARGOVICH, M. J. "Chemoprevention of 1,2-dimethylhydrazine-induced colon cancer in mice by naturally occurring organosulfur compounds." *Cancer Res.* 1990, 50, 5084-5087.
35. REDDY, B. S.; RAO, C. V.; RIVENSON, A.; KELLOFF, G. "Inhibitory effect of aspirin on azoxymethane-induced colon carcinogenesis in F344 rats." *Carcinogenesis* (Lond.) 1993, 14, 1493-1497.
36. LABAYLE, D.; FISCHER, D.; VIELH, P.; et al. "Sulindac causes regression of rectal polyps in familial adenomatous polyposis." *Gastroenterology* 1991, 101, 635-639.
37. WEISBURGER, J. H. "Causes, relevant mechanisms, and prevention of large bowel cancer." *Sem. Oncol.* 1991, 18, 316-336.
38. KUMAR, S. P.; ROY, S. J.; TOKUMO, K.; et al. "Effect of different levels of calorie restriction on azoxymethane-induced colon carcinogenesis in male F344 rats." *Cancer Res.* 1990, 50, 5761-5766.
39. LIPKIN, M. "Biomarkers of increased susceptibility to gastrointestinal cancer: New applications to studies of cancer prevention in human subjects." *Cancer Res.* 1988, 48, 235-245.
40. LIPKIN, M. "Phase I and Phase 2 proliferative lesions of colonic epithelial cells in diseases leading to colon cancer." *Cancer* 1974, Suppl. 34, 878-888.
41. DESCHNER, E. E.; MASKENS, A. P. "Significance of the labeling index and labeling distribution as kinetic parameters in colorectal mucosa of cancer patients and DMH treated animals." *Cancer* 1982, 50, 1136-1141.
42. STADNYK, A. W. "Cytokine production by epithelial cells." *FASEB J.* 1994, 8, 1041-1047.
43. NORBURY, C.; NURSE, P. "Animal cell cycles and their control." *Annu. Rev. Biochem.* 1992, 61, 441-470.

44. DOREE, M.; GALAS, S. "The cyclin-dependent protein kinases and the control of cell division." *FASEB J.* 1994, 8, 1114-1121.
45. LEWIN, B. "Cell cycle and growth regulation." In: *Genes V*, Oxford University Press: New York, 1994, pp. 349-373.
46. FEARON, E. R.; VOGELSTEIN, B. "A genetic model for colorectal tumorigenesis." *Cell* 1990, 61, 759-767.
47. TERPSTRA, O. T.; VAN VLANKENSTEIN, M.; DEES, J.; EILERS, G. A. M. "Abnormal pattern of cell proliferation in the entire colonic mucosa of patients with colon adenoma or cancer." *Gastroenterol.* 1987, 92, 704-715
48. MIYOSHI, Y.; MAGASE, H.; ANDO, H.; et al. "Somatic mutations of the *APC* gene in colorectal tumors: Mutation cluster region in the *APC* gene." *Hum. Molec. Genet.* 1992, 1, 229-233.
49. SMITH, K. J.; JOHNSON, K. A.; BRYAN, T. M.; et al. "The *APC* gene product in normal and tumor cells." *Proc. Natl. Acad. Sci. USA* 1993, 90, 2846-2850.
50. BROWNE, S. J.; WILLIAMS, A. C.; HAGUE, A.; et al. "Loss of APC protein expressed by human colonic epithelial cells and the appearance of a specific low-molecular-weight form is associated with apoptosis *in vitro.*" *Int. J. Cancer* 1994, 59, 56-64.
51. KHOSRAVI-FAR, R.; DER, C. J. "The ras signal transduction pathway." *Cancer and Metastasis Reviews* 1994, 13, 67-89.
52. CHO, K. R.; OLINER, J. D.; SIMONS, J. W.; et al. "The DCC gene: Structural analysis and mutations in colorectal carcinomas." *Genomics* 1994, 19, 525-531.
53. HEDRICK, L.; CHO, K. R.; FEARON, E. R; et al. "The DCC gene product in cellular differentiation and colorectal tumorigenesis." *Genes & Development* 1994, 8, 1174-1183.
54. FEARON, E. R.; CHO, K. R.; NIGRO, J. M.; et al. "Identification of a chromosome 18q gene that is altered in colorectal cancers." *Science* 1990, 247, 49-56.
55. HUNTER, T.; PINES, J. "Cyclins and Cancer II: Cyclin D and CDK inhibitors come of age." *Cell* 1994, 79, 573-582.
56. YAMAGUCHI, A.; MAKIMOTO, K.; GOI, T.; et al. "Overexpression of p53 protein and proliferative activity in colorectal adenoma." *Oncology* 1994, 51, 224-227.
57. BAKER, S. J.; PREISINGER, A. C.; MESSUP, J. M.; et al. "p53 gene mutations occur in combination with 17p allelic deletions as late events in colorectal tumorigenesis." *Cancer Res.* 1990, 50, 7717-7722.
58. BUSET, M.; LIPKIN, M.; WINAWER, S.; et al. "Inhibition of human colonic epithelial cell proliferation in vivo and in vitro by calcium." *Cancer Res.* 1987, 46, 5426-5430.
59. LIPKIN, M.; NEWMARK, H. "Effects of dietary calcium on colonic epithelial cell proliferation in subjects at high risk for familial colonic cancer." *N. Engl. J. Med.* 1985, 313, 1381-1384.

60. LIPKIN, M.; FRIEDMAN, E.; WINAWER, S. J. "Colonic epithelial cell proliferation in responders and non-responders to supplemental dietary calcium." *Cancer Res.* 1989, 49, 248-254.
61. ROZEN, P.; FIREMAN, A.; FINE, N.; et al. "Oral calcium suppresses increased rectal epithelial proliferation of persons at risk of colorectal cancer." *Gut* 1989, 30, 650-655.
62. WARGOVICH, M. J.; ISBELL, G.; SHABOT, M.; et al. "Calcium supplementation decreases rectal epithelial cell proliferation in subjects with sporadic adenoma." *Gastroenterology* 1992, 103, 92-97.
63. GREGOIRE, R. C.; STERN, H. S.; YEUNG, K. S.; et al. "Effect of calcium supplementation on mucosal call proliferation in high risk patients for colon cancer." *Gut* 1989, 30, 376-382.
64. STERN, H. S.; GREGORIE, R. C.; KOSHTAN, H. "Long-term effects of dietary calcium on risk markers for colon cancer in patients with familial polyposis." *Surgery* 1990, 108, 528-533.
65. RESHEF, R.; ROZEN, P.; FIREMAN, Z.; et al. "Effect of a calcium-enriched diet on the colonic epithelial hyperproliferation induced by N-methyl-N'-nitro-N-nitrosoguanidine in rats on a low calcium and fat diet." *Cancer Res.* 1990, 50, 1764-1767.
66. PEREIRA, M. A.; BARNES, L. H.; RASSMAN, V. L.; et al. "Use of azoxymethane-induced foci of aberrant crypts in rat colon to identify potential cancer chemopreventive agents." *Carcinogenesis* 1994, 15, 1049-1054.
67. APPLETON, G. V. N.; DAVIES, P. W.; BRISTOL, J. B.; et al. "Inhibition of intestinal carcinogenesis by dietary supplementation with calcium." *Br. J. Surg.* 1987, 74, 523-525.
68. HU, P. J.; BAER, A. R.; WARGOVICH, M. J. "Calcium and phosphate: Effect of two dietary confounders on colonic epithelial cellular proliferation." *Nutr. Res.* 1989, 9, 545-553.
69. WARGOVICH, M. J.; ENG, V. W. S.; NEWMARK, H. L.; et al. "Calcium ameliorates the toxic effect of deoxycholic acid on colonic epithelium." *Carcinogenesis* 1983, 4, 1205-1207.
70. ARLOW, F. L.; WALCZAK, S. M.; LUK, G. D,; MAJUMDAR, A. P. N. "Attenuation of azoxymethane-induced colonic mucosal ornithine decarboxylase and tyrosine kinase by calcium in rats." *Cancer Res.* 1989, 49, 5884-5888.
71. MESSINA, M.; PERSKY, V.; SETCHELL, K.; BARNES, S. "Soy intake and cancer risk: A review of the in vitro and in vivo data." *Nutr. Cancer* 21, 113-131.
72. AKIYAMA, T.; ISHIDA, J.; NAKAGAWA, S.; et. al. "Genistein, a specific inhibitor of tyrosine-specific protein kinases." *J. Biol. Chem.* 1987, 262, 5592-5595.
73. OGAWARA, H.; AKIYAMA, T.; WATANABE, S.; et. al. "Inhibition of tyrosine protein kinase activity by synthetic isoflavones and flavones." *J. Antibiot.* 1989, XLI, 340-343.

74. TERAOKA, H.; OHMURA, Y.; TSUKADA, K. "The nuclear matrix from rat liver is capable of phosphorylating exogenous tyrosine-containing substrates." *Biochem. Intern.* 1989, 18, 1203-1210.
75. JOHNSON, L. R. "Regulation of gastrointestinal growth." In: *Physiology of the Gastrointestinal Tract,* Johnson, L.R., Ed.; Raven Press: New York, 1987, pp. 301-333.
76. MCGREGOR, D. B.; JONES, R. D.; KARLIN, D.; ROMSDAHL, M. M. "Trophic effects of gastrin on colorectal neoplasms in the rat." *Ann. Surg.* 1982, 195, 219-223.
77. BEAUCHAMP, R. D.; TOWNSEND JR., C. M.; SINGH, P.; GLASS, E. J.; THOMPSON, J. C. "Proglumide, a gastrin receptor antagonist, inhibits growth of colon cancer and enhances survival in mice." *Ann. Surg.* 1985, 202, 303-309.
78. MAJUMDAR, A. P. N. "Role of tyrosine kinases in gastrin induction of ornithine decarboxylase in colonic mucosa." *Am. J. Physiol.* 1990, 259 (Gastrointest Liver Physiol 22), G626-630.
79. STEINBACH, G.; HEYMSFIELD, S.; OLANSEN, N. E.; et al. "Effect of caloric restriction on colonic proliferation in obese persons: implications for colon cancer prevention." *Cancer Res.* 1994, 54, 1194-1197.
80. STEINBACH, G.; KUMAR, S. P.; REDDY, B. S.; et al. "Effects of caloric restriction and dietary fat on epithelial cell proliferation in the rat colon." *Cancer Res.* 1993, 53, 2745-2749.
81. KUNE, G. A.; KUNE, S.; WATSON, L. F. "Body weight and physical activity as predictors of colorectal cancer risk." *Nutr. Cancer* 1990, 13, 9-17.
82. KELLOFF, G. J.; BOONE, C. W.; CROWELL, J. A.; et al. "Chemopreventive drug development: Perspectives and progress." *Cancer Epidem. Biomark. Prev.* 1994, 3, 85-98.
83. GIARDIELLO, F. M.; HAMILTON, S. R.; KRUSH, A. J.; et al. "Treatment of colonic and rectal adenomas with sulindac in familial adenomatous polyposis." *N. Engl. J. Med.* 1993, 328, 1313-1316.

8

Cancer Chemoprevention by Constituents of Plant Essential Oils

Luke K. T. Lam
Guo-Qiang Zheng
Jilun Zhang
Patrick M. Kenney

Plant essential oils are commonly used in food flavorings and cosmetics. Many oils and their processing by-products were found to have high activity as inducers of the detoxifying enzyme glutathione S-transferase (GST). Since the ability of a compound to increase GST activity has been positively correlated with its capacity to inhibit carcinogenesis, the essential oils that showed high enzyme inducing activity in at least two tissues were further fractionated. Pure compounds from seven essential oils were found to induce increased GST activity in the liver and small bowel of mice. Two of the monoterpenes, carvone and limonene, have been previously determined to inhibit chemically induced carcinogenesis in several animal tumor models. The active components, myristicin isolated from

> parsley leaf oil, and sedanolide and 3-n-butyl phthalide isolated from celery seed oil, were found to inhibit forestomach and lung tumors in mice. In addition, sedanolide from celery seed was determined to inhibit the promotional stage of carcinogenesis in the skin tumor model system.

Essential oils are volatile components of plants, spices, and herbs. Commercial use of essentials oils includes soft drinks, food flavoring, cosmetics, detergents, and many other products that are ingested by or come in contact with the general population. Recent research findings from several laboratories have indicated that some compounds present in essential oil may have chemoprevention properties for different types of cancer. Garlic and onion oils are sources of sulfur-containing compounds, which have anticarcinogenic action against many forms of cancer in animal models (1-5). Orange peel oil contains mainly d-limonene which is known to inhibit forestomach, lung, and mammary tumors (5-8). Caraway oil and dillweed oil have the main ingredient d-carvone that is an inhibitor of nitrosamine-induced tumors in mice (5). In our laboratories, we have screened a large number of essential oils and their processing by-products for potential chemopreventive agents (9).

A total of 46 commercially available oils and by-products have been tested using a biochemical assay. Twenty-six of these were judged to have high inducing activity of the detoxifying enzyme system, glutathione S-transferase (GST). Those that induced increased GST activity in at least two tissues were chosen for further fractionation (Table 8.1). In this chapter, the active constituents of seven essentials oils will be presented. The anticarcinogenic potential of the active compounds from celery seed oil and parsley leaf oil were investigated using *in vivo* tumor models.

INDUCTION OF GLUTATHIONE S-TRANSFERASE

A biochemical method developed as a rapid screening assay for potential inhibitors of chemical carcinogenesis has been

TABLE 8.1. LIST OF ESSENTIAL OILS AND BY-PRODUCTS THAT ARE ACTIVE AS GST INDUCERS IN AT LEAST TWO TISSUES IN MICE

Ambrette musk residues	Fennel oil
Angelica root	Fennel terpenes
Camomile oil	Galanga root oil
Caraway oil	Hops oil
Celery seed oil	Lemongrass oil
Clove terpenes	Lime oil tails
Dillweed oil	Origanum oil
Dillweed terpenes	Parsley leaf oil
Eucalyptus terpenes	Spearmint residues

used successfully in our laboratories to study the essential oils. This screening technique is based on the induction of the detoxifying enzyme system, GST (10). The rationale for using GST is that it is the major detoxifying enzyme system (11). An enhancement of the activity of this powerful enzyme system signifies an increase in the host's ability to detoxify xenobiotics, including carcinogens. The essential oil that showed significant inducing activity was fractionated by normal phase preparative liquid chromatography. The fractions or pure compounds thus obtained were tested for their GST-inducing activity. Structure determination and purity check of the active constituents were performed using spectroscopic methods and chromatographic techniques.

The induction of GST was performed with a standardized protocol where 30 mg doses of the essential oil or 20 mg doses of the fractions were administered to mice by gavage every other day for a total of 3 doses (9). In the case of pure compounds the dosages may be as low as 5 mg. Twenty-four hours after the last dose, the mice were sacrificed and the cytosolic fractions of the liver, small bowel mucosa, and other tissues of interest were prepared. The cytosolic GST activity was measured according to the method of Habig *et al.* using 1-chloro-2,4-dinitrobenzene as the substrate (10).

Clove Terpenes

Clove terpenes are the high boiling fraction of clove oil, which can be obtained by steam distillation of the dried flower buds of *Eugenia caryophyllata* Thunberg (12). This tropical tree, originated in the Moluccas, is cultivated in many tropical countries. Clove oil is frequently used in perfumery, medicine and flavorings. Five active compounds, β-caryophyllene, β-caryophyllene oxide, α-humulene, α-humulene epoxide and eugenol, were isolated from clove terpenes that elicit GST activity (13). They were found to stimulate GST activity in both the small bowel and liver of mice (Fig. 8.1). β-Caryophyllene oxide was determined to have the highest activity and eugenol the lowest. The former compound induced GST activity 2.88 and 4.80 times over the control levels (T/C=Test/Control) in the liver and small bowel, respectively.

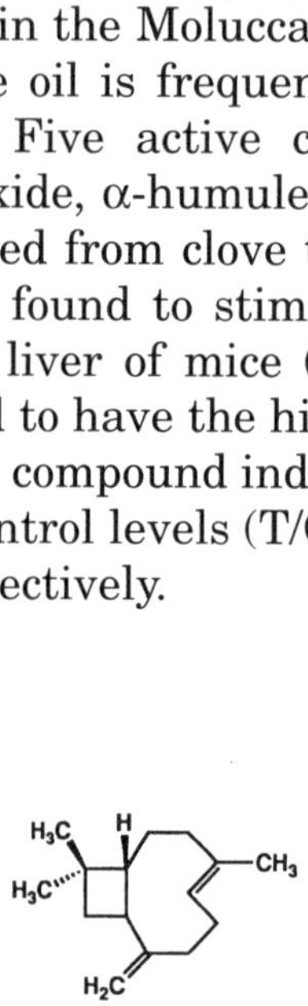

β-Caryophyllene

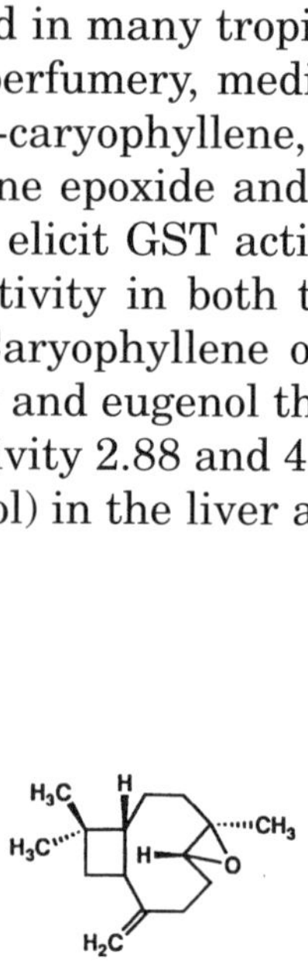

β-Caryophyllene oxide

	β-Caryophyllene T/C	β-Caryophyllene oxide T/C
Liver	2.59	2.88
Small bowel	3.00	4.80

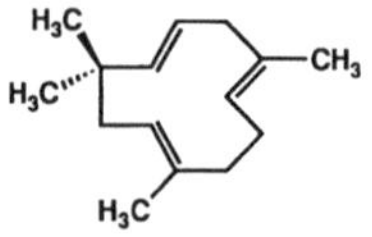

α-Humulene

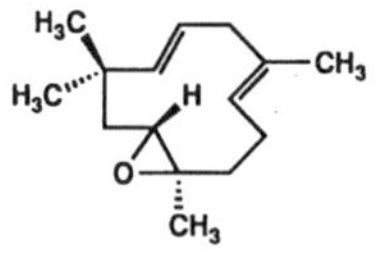

α-Humulene oxide

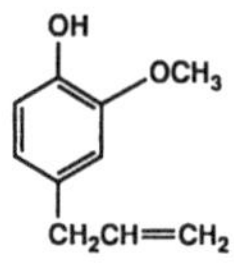

Eugenol

	α-Humulene T/C	α-Humulene oxide T/C	Eugenol T/C
Liver	1.99	2.08	1.26
Small bowel	2.52	3.24	2.36

FIG. 8.1. THE GST-INDUCING ACTIVITY OF ACTIVE CONSTITUENTS FROM CLOVE TERPENES. T/C = TEST/CONTROL.

Caraway and Dillweed Oils

Caraway oil is obtained by steam distillation of the crushed mature seeds of the plant *Carvum carvi* L. which is cultivated in northern and central Europe and central Asia (14). The oil is used mainly in cosmetics, food favoring and to a lesser extent, medicine. Dillweed oil is the steam distillation product of the flowering dill plant, *Anethum graveloens* L. (15). Dill, a native plant of southern Europe, is cultivated in England, Hungary, Germany and the United States. Dillweed oil is mainly used for seasoning and flavoring in food. The main active ingredient in caraway and dillweed oils is carvone which had been determined to have GST-inducing activity and chemopreventive property (5,16). In our study, carvone was found to enhance GST activity in both the liver (T/C= 2.69) and the small bowel (T/C=3.83). In addition to carvone, other active constituents identified in these oils were anethofuran from dillweed and limonene from caraway. Both compounds were found to have GST-inducing activity greater than the control level (Fig. 8.2).

Lemongrass and Galanga Root Oils

Lemongrass oil is produced by steam distilling the leaves of *Anclropogon citratus* DC. or *Cymbopogon citratus* Stapf. (17). *C. citrancs*, native to Sri Lanka and India, is now cultivated in

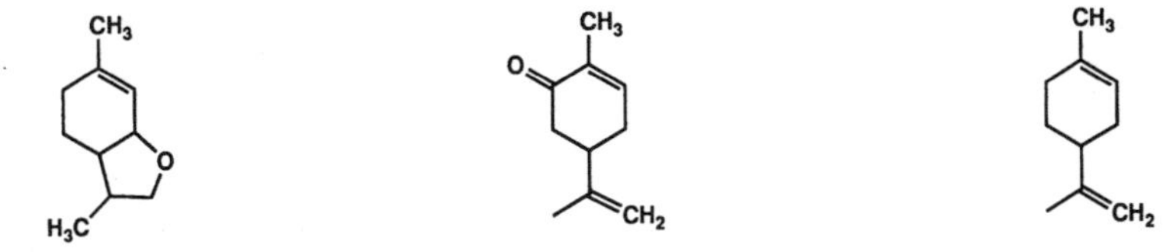

	Anethofuran	Carvone	Limonene
	T/C	T/C	T/C
Liver	2.44	2.69	2.03
Small Bowel	2.68	3.83	1.33

FIG. 8.2. THE GST-INDUCING ACTIVITY OF ACTIVE CONSTITUENTS FROM CARAWAY OIL (CARVONE AND LIMONENE) AND DILL WEED OIL (ANETHOFURAN AND CARVONE). T/C = TEST/CONTROL.

India, Africa, Philippines, Madagascar, Central and South America, the West Indies and Southeast Asia. Galanga root oil is obtained from the fresh and dried rhizomes of *Alpinia galanga* Wild, or *Languas pyramidata* (Blume) Merr. (18). This plant is cultivated throughout Malaysia and the Philippines and is used as a common spice. The rhizomes are used for flavoring foods. Both lemongrass oil and galanga root oil are used mainly in food flavorings, and to a lesser extent in cosmetics and perfumery. Four compounds were identified to be responsible for the high activity of the oils as GST inducers (10). d-Limonene (5%) and geraniol (5.5%) were obtained from lemongrass oil. Ethyl *trans*-cinnamate (13%) and ethyl 4-methoxy-*trans*-cinnamate (4%) were fractionated from galanga root oil (Fig. 8.3).

Parsley Leaf Oil

Parsley (*Petroselinum sativum* Hoffm.) is a small biennial flowering plant 2 to 3 ft high. It has greatly divided pinnately-compound leaves. Parsley is used extensively as a culinary herb for garnishing and seasoning. The essential oil that is present in all parts of the plant, including the seed, is responsible for the pronounced odor and flavor of parsley. Two types of oil, the parsley leaf or herb oil and parsley seed oil are steam-distilled from the fresh leaves and the seeds, respectively (20). Typical yield for the leaf oil is about 500 grams of oil per ton of the plant material. Parsley leaf oil has a superior taste and aroma of the plant than parsley seed oil. The former is used primarily in the food industry as flavorings and seasonings. It is used to a lesser extent in perfumery. The main active ingredient from parsley was identified to be myristicin which is present in greater than 14%. Some preparation may have myristicin present in greater than 70%.

The GST-inducing activity of myristicin was found to be very high (21). At 10 mg per dose, which was half the normal dose for active constituents from other oils, myristicin was able to induce four times the control level of GST activity in the liver (T/C=4.27) and more than three times the control level in the small bowel (T/C=3.25) (Fig. 8.4). Because of this unusually

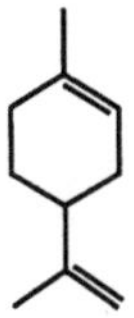

d-Limonene

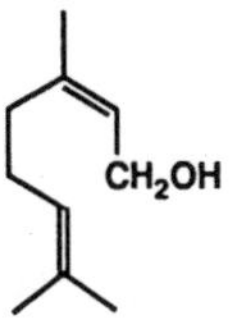

Geraniol

	d-Limonene T/C	Geraniol T/C
Liver	3.02	1.22
Small Bowel	2.36	2.62

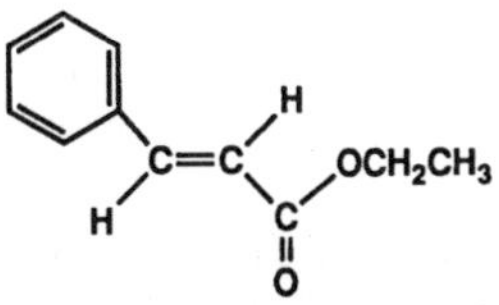

Ethyl *trans*-cinnamate

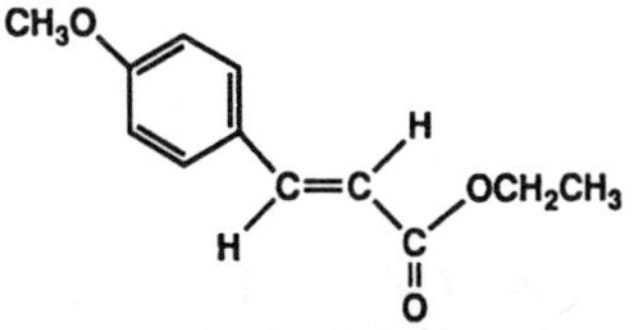

Ethyl 4-methoxy-*trans*-cinnamate

	Ethyl *trans*-cinnamate T/C	Ethyl 4-methoxy-*trans*-cinnamate T/C
Liver	1.30	1.68
Small Bowel	1.43	2.16

FIG. 8.3. THE GST-INDUCING ACTIVITY OF ACTIVE CONSTITUENTS FROM GALANGA ROOT OIL (ETHYL TRANS-CINNAMATE AND ETHYL 4-METHOXY-TRANS-CINNAMATE) AND LEMONGRASS OIL (D-LIMONENE AND GENEROIL). T/C = TEST/CONTROL.

high activity an experiment was carried out to test the anticarcinogenic activity of this compound.

The chemical structure of myristicin differs from that of safrole by an extra methoxy group at the 6 position of the benzene ring. Safrole is carcinogenic in some animal test systems and the mechanism of action is believed to involve oxidation of the benzylic carbon at the propenyl side chain (22, 23). Hydrogenation of the double bond in safrole to give dihydrosafrole resulted in total elimination of the carcinogenicity. To eradicate the potential carcinogenic property of myristicin, hydrogenation was carried out to obtain dihydromyristicin. With the saturation of the double bond the site of oxidation is greatly deactivated, thus the carcinogenic moiety, is expected to be

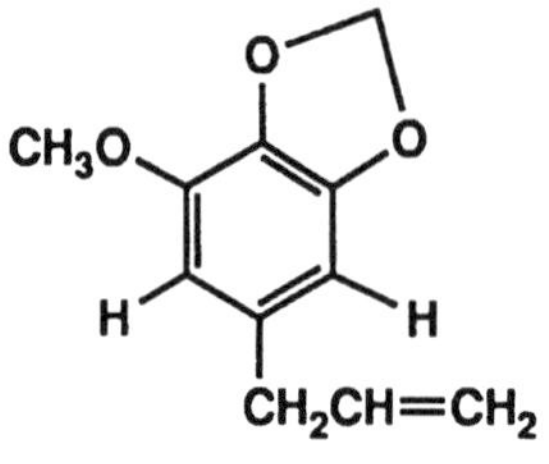

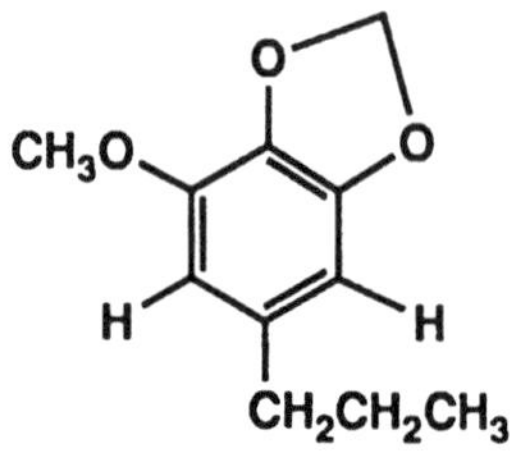

	Myristicin T/C	Dihydromyristicin T/C
Liver	4.27	3.40
Small bowel	3.25	2.21

FIG. 8.4. THE GST-INDUCING ACTIVITY OF THE ACTIVE CONSTITUENT FROM PARSLEY LEAF OIL (MYRISTICIN) AND ITS HYDROGENATED PRODUCT (DIHYDROMYRISTICIN). T/C = TEST/CONTROL.

eliminated. The dihydromyristicin from hydrogenation retained a high percentage of the GST-inducing activity of the parent compound (Fig. 8.4) (21).

Celery Seed Oil

Celery is a common vegetable that is regularly consumed by humans almost all over the world. Celery seed oil is used frequently in food flavorings and seasonings, in cosmetics and perfumery, and in pharmaceutical preparation. The volatile oil is obtained by steam distillation from the ripe fruits of wild or cultivated celery, *Apium graveolens* L.(17). Five compounds that are major components of celery seed oil appeared to be responsible for the high GST-inducing activity of the oils observed in the preliminary screening. They can be divided into two groups, limonene-type monoterpenes (d-limonene, p-mentha-2,8-dien- 1-ol, and p-mentha-8(9)-en-1,2-diol) and butyl phthalides (3-n-butyl phthalide and sedanolide) (25, 26). The GST assay data showed that the phthalide compounds are more active than the limonene-type monoterpenes (Fig. 8.5) (24). The most active compound in the latter group is p-mentha-2,8-dien-l-ol with T/C=3.72 and 3.74 in the liver and small bowel, respectively. For the phthalates, the five-membered lactone ring appeared to be important for the high enzyme-inducing activity, while the aromatic ring may not be required for the maintenance of such high activity. This conclusion is consistent with the observation that sedanolide is only slightly less active than 3-n-butyl phthalide as GST inducers.

INHIBITION OF TUMORIGENESIS

Induction of the major detoxifying enzyme system, GST, signifies an increased response to eliminate xenobiotics including carcinogens. Many GST inducers have been found to inhibit chemically induced carcinogens in various tumor models. The widely used antioxidant, butylated hydroxyanisole, is a potent

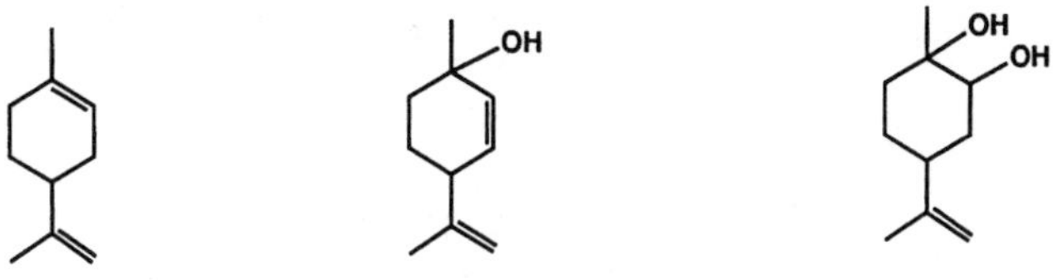

	d-Limonene	*p*-Mentha-2,8-dien-1-ol	*p*-Mentha-8(9)-en-1,2-diol
	T/C	T/C	T/C
Liver	2.78	3.72	1.73
Small Bowel	1.64	3.74	2.73

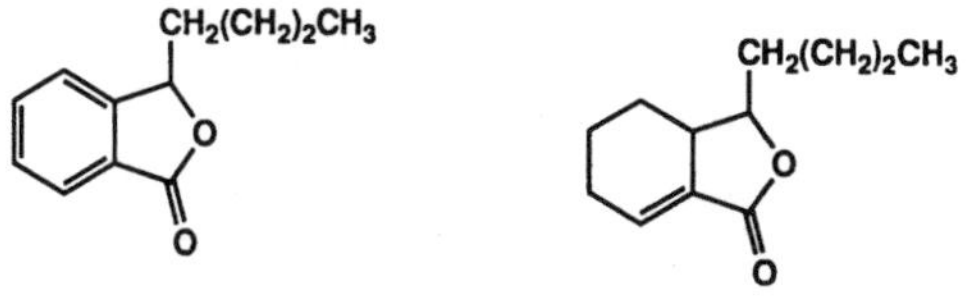

3-*n*-Butyl phthalide	Sedanolide
T/C	T/C
5.29	4.72
5.18	4.50

FIG. 8.5. THE GST-INDUCING ACTIVITY OF ACTIVE CONSTITUENTS FROM CELERY SEED OIL. T/C = TEST/CONTROL.

GST inducer and inhibitor of carcinogenesis (27, 28). The synthetic dithiothione, oltipraz, is an inducer of phase 2 enzymes including GST (29). Its inhibitory effect in carcinogenesis covers many tissues that are relevant to human cancer (30). Phase I clinical trials have been conducted to test its efficacy as a chemopreventive agent (31). Naturally occurring compounds such as citrus limonoids in citrus fruits (32, 33, 34), diterpenes in coffee beans (35, 36), furans, and thiophenes in cooked meat (37) have been determined to possess GST-inducing property and tumor inhibition quality. The active constituents isolated from essential oils using the GST induction assay have been found to follow the same trend.

D-Carvone

The characteristic smell of caraway oil is due to the presence of the main ingredient, D-carvone (38). Both the oil and D-carvone have been found to inhibit N-nitrosodiethylamine (NDEA)-induced tumorigenesis in the forestomach and lung of mice (5).

D-Limonene

Citrus fruit oils such as lemon oil and orange oil have been found to have anticarcinogenic properties. They inhibit both forestomach and lung tumor formation induced by the tobacco specific nitrosamine 4-(methylnitrosamino)-1-(3-pyridyl)-1-butanone (NNK) in mice (7). The monoterpene, D-limonene, is the major constituent of citrus fruit oils. It has been found to inhibit tumorigenesis in mice induced by the carcinogens NDEA and NNK (5, 7). It was also found effective in rats as an inhibitor of mammary tumor formation induced by 7,12-dimethylbenz[a]anthracene and nitrosomethylurea (6, 8). More interestingly, D-limonene and its metabolites were found to cause significant regression of mammary tumors (39, 40). These findings appear to pave the way for further research into the therapeutic effects of the constituents of essential oils.

Myristicin

Myristicin, the major constituent of parsley oil is the most active GST inducer found in all of the essential oils tested thus far. In mice, the benzo[a]pyrene-induced lung and forestomach tumors were reduced by the administration of myristicin at 10 mg per dose for a total of 12 doses. The number of tumors per mouse was reduced by 65% and 31% in the lung and forestomach, respectively (Table 8.2) (41). The hydrogenated product, dihydromyristicin, though it retains most of the GST-inducing property, was not able to inhibit tumor formation in this system. It is possible that the dosage applied in the experiment was too low to effectively inhibit carcinogenesis by this semi-synthetic compound.

Inhibitors of carcinogenesis discovered by the GST induction assay are often effective antipromoters. For this reason, an experiment to test the inhibition of two-stage skin carcinogenesis by myristicin was carried out. High and low doses of myristicin were applied to the skin of mice initiated with 7,12-dimethylbenz[a]anthracene and promoted with phorbol ester. The results showed a slight enhancement of tumor formation by myristicin when the compound was given both at the initiation and promotion stages (Fig. 8.6). The enhancement was more pronounced at the promotion phase. It is not clear at this time what the relative ratio of risk versus benefit may be.

3-n-Butyl Phthalide and Sedanolide

The two most active enzyme inducers of celery seed oil were tested as potential chemopreventive agents. The tumor inhibi-

TABLE 8.2. EFFECTS OF MYRISTICIN AND DIHYDROMYRISTICIN ON BENZO[A]PYRENE-INDUCED FORESTOMACH AND LUNG TUMORS IN A/J MICE

	Lung		Forestomach	
	% Mice with tumors	No. of tumors per mouse	% Mice with tumors	No. of tumors per mouse
BP Control	100	9.9±1.8	70.6	1.9±0.5
Myristicin	100	3.4±0.5	72.3	1.3±0.5
Dihydromyristicin	100	7.4±1.0	63.3	1.4±0.3

tion data indicated that 3-n-butyl phthalide and sedanolide significantly inhibit carcinogenesis in the mouse forestomach when given 1 week prior to and during carcinogen administration (24). The inhibition was manifested by a reduction in both the percentage of mice with tumors and the number of tumors

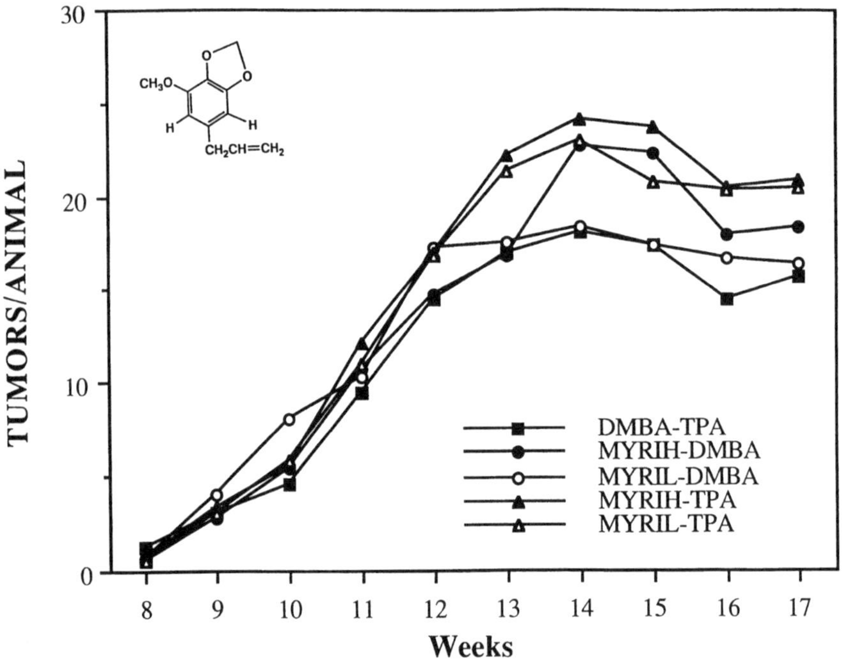

FIG. 8.6. THE EFFECTS OF MYRISTICIN ON THE TWO-STAGE SKIN TUMORIGENESIS IN SENCAR MICE WAS MEASURED FOR 17 WEEKS. ALL 5 GROUPS WERE TREATED WITH A SINGLE DOSE OF THE INITIATOR, 7,12-DIMETHYLBENZ[A]ANTHRACENE (DMBA, 50 NMOL/200μL ACETONE) FOLLOWED 1 WEEK LATER BY THE PROMOTER, 12-O-TETRADECANOYLPHORBOL-13-ACETATE (TPA, 5μG/200μL ACETONE) APPLIED TWICE WEEKLY FOR 17 WEEKS. DMBA-TPA WAS THE CONTROL GROUP WITHOUT INHIBITOR TREATMENT. MYRIH-DMBA AND MYRIL-DMBA WERE TREATED WITH 8 μMOL/DAY OR 2 μMOL/DAY OF MYRISTICIN BEFORE AND DURING INITIATOR APPLICATION. MYRIH-TPA AND MYRIL-TPA WERE TREATED WITH 8 μMOL/DAY OR 2 μMOL/DAY OF MYRISTICIN DURING THE PROMOTION PERIOD.

per mouse (Table 8.3). The results represented a greater than 55 and 83% reduction of tumor incidence for the two compounds, respectively.

Sedanolide was also tested as inhibitor of two-stage carcinogenesis in the skin tumor model. In contrast to myristicin it did not cause any appreciable change in the number of tumors per animal when it was applied during initiation. When the compound was given during the promotional period, however, almost 50% inhibition was observed (Fig. 8.7). Both the number of tumors and the percentage of malignancy values indicated that sedanolide was an effective inhibitor of carcinogenesis at the promotional phase.

SUMMARY

The essential oils and other natural products that provide most of the raw materials for seasoning and flavoring needs are being produced in huge quantities. Other commercial use of these materials in medicine and cosmetics is wide spread. The total consumption of and exposure to any one oil by an individual on a daily basis, however, are estimated to be quite low. The discovery that many essential oils contain large number of compounds that induce detoxifying enzymes and inhibit chemically induced tumorigenesis suggests that ultra-nutritious components of food may be potentially useful to combat cancer.

TABLE 8.3. EFFECTS OF CELERY SEED OIL CONSTITUENTS ON BENZO[A]PYRENE-INDUCED FORESTOMACH TUMORS IN MICE

	Forestomach	
	% Mice with tumors	No. of tumors per mouse
BP control	68.4	1.16±0.23
p-Mentha-2,8-dien-1-ol	50.0	0.64±0.19
3-n-Butylphthalide	33.3	0.40±0.16
Sedanolide	11.1	0.17±0.12

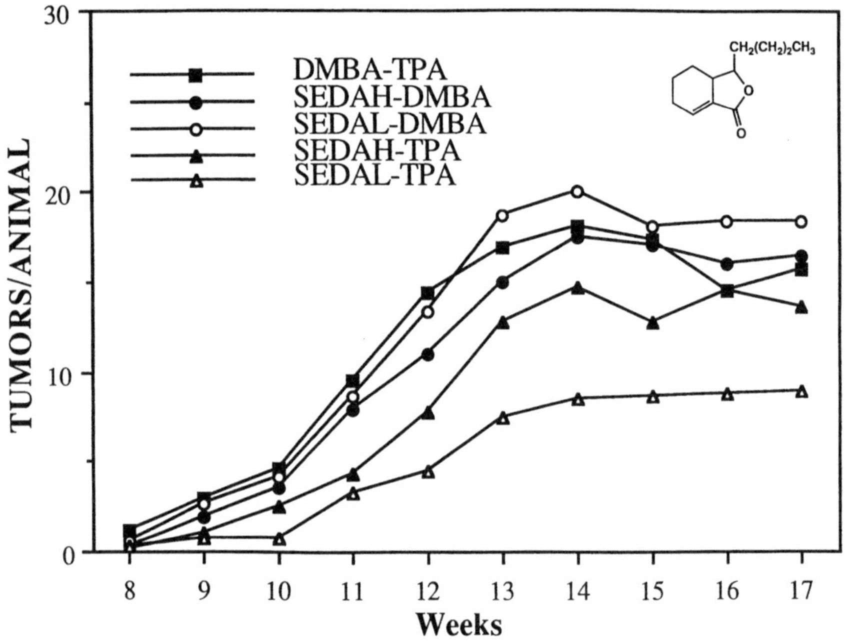

FIG. 8.7. THE EFFECTS OF SEDANOLIDE ON THE TWO-STAGE SKIN TUMORIGENESIS IN SENCAR MICE WAS MEASURED FOR 17 WEEKS. ALL 5 GROUPS WERE TREATED WITH A SINGLE DOSE OF THE INITIATOR, 7,12-DIMETHYLBENZ[A]ANTHRACENE (DMBA, 50 NMOL/200 μL ACETONE) FOLLOWED 1 WEEK LATER BY THE PROMOTER, 12-O-TETRADECANOYLPHORBOL-13-ACETATE (TPA, 5 μG/200μL ACETONE) APPLIED TWICE WEEKLY FOR 17 WEEDS. DMBA-TPA WAS THE CONTROL GROUP WITHOUT INHIBITOR TREATMENT. SEDAH-DMBA AND SEDAL-DMBA WERE TREATED WITH 8 μMOL/DAY OR 2 μMOL/DAY OF SEDANOLIDE BEFORE AND DURING INITIATOR APPLICATION. SEDAH-TPA AND SEDAL-TPA WERE TREATED WITH 8 μMOL/DAY OR 2 μMOL/DAY OF SEDANOLIDE DURING THE PROMOTION PERIOD.

BIBLIOGRAPHY

1. BELMAN, S. "Onion and garlic oils inhibit tumour promotion". *Carcinogenesis (Lond.)* 1983, 4, 1063-1065.
2. WARGOVICH, M. J. "Diallyl sulfides, a flavor component of garlic (Allium sativum) inhibits dimethylhydrazine-induced colon cancer". *Carcinogenesis (Lond.)* 1987, 8, 487-489.

3. SPAMINS, V. L.; BARANY, G.; WATTENBERG, L. W. "Effects of organosulfur compounds from garlic and onions on benzo(a)pyrene-induced neoplasia and glutathione S-transferase activity". *Carcinogenesis (Lond.)* 1988, 9, 131-134.
4. WARGOVICH, M. J.; WOODS, C.; ENG, V. W. S.; STEPHENS, L. C.; GRAY, K. "Chemoprevention of N-nitrosomethylbenzylamine-induced esophageal cancer in rats by the naturally occurring thioether, diallyl sulfide". *Cancer Res.* 1988, 48, 6872-6875.
5. WATTENBERG, L. W.; SPARNINS, V. L.; BARANY, G. "Inhibition of N-nitrosodiethylamine carcinogenesis in mice by naturally occurring organosulfur compounds and monoterpenes". *Cancer Res.* 1989, 49, 2689-2692.
6. ELSON, C. E.; MALTZMAN, T. H.; BOSTON, J. L.; TABBER, M. A.; GOULD, M. N. "Anti-carcinogenic activity of D-limonene during initiation and promotion/progression stages of DMBA-induced mammary carcinogenesis". *Carcinogenesis (Lond.)* 1988, 9, 331-332.
7. WATTENBERG, L. W.; COCCIA, J. B. "Inhibition of 4-(methylnitrosamino)-1-(3-pyridyl)-1-butanone carcinogenesis in mice by D-limonene and citrus fruit oils". *Carcinogenesis (Lond.)* 1991, 12, 115-117.
8. MALTZMAN, T. H.; HURT, L. M.; ELSON, C. E.; TANNER, M. A.; GOULD, M. N. "The prevention of nitrosomethylurea-induced mammary tumors by d-limonene and orange oil". *Carcinogenesis (Lond.)* 1989, 10, 781-783.
9. LAM, L. K. T.; ZHENG, B.-L. "Effects of essential oils on glutathione S - transferase activity in mice". *J. Agric. Food Chem.* 1991, 39, 660-662.
10. HABIG, W. H.; PABST, M. J.; JAKOBY, W. B. "Glutathione S-transferase". *J. Biol. Chem.* 1974, 249, 7130-7139.
11. JAKOBY, W. B.; HABIG, W. H. "Glutathione S-transferase". In *Enzymatic Basis of Detoxification*; Academic Press: New York, 1980; Vol. 2, pp. 63-94.
12. FORMACEK, V.; KUBCEZKA, K.-H. "Celery seed oil". In *Essential Oil Analysis by Capillary Gas Chromatography and Carbon-l3 NMR Spectroscopy*; Wiley and Sons: New York, 1982; pp. 37-39.
13. ZHENG, G.-Q.; KENNEY, P. M.; LAM, L. K. T. "Sesquiterpenes from clove (Eugenia caryophyllata) as potential anticarcinogenic agents". *J. Nat. Prod.* 1992, 55, 999-1003.
14. IKEDA, R. M.; STANLEY, W. L.; VARMIER, S. H.; SPITLER, E. M. "The monoterpene hydrocarbon composition of some essential oils". *J. Food Sci.* 1962, 27, 445-458.
15. HUOPALAHTI, R; LINKO, R. R. "Composition content of aroma compounds in dill,*Anethum graveolens* L. at three different growth stages". *J. Agric. Food Chem.* 1983, 31, 331-333.
16. ZHENG, G.-Q.; KENNEY, P. M.; LAM, L. K. T. "Anethofuran, carvone, and limonene: potential cancer chemopreventive agents from dill weed oil and caraway oil". *Planta Med.* 992, 58, 338-341.

17. FORMACEK, V.; KUBCEZKA, K.-H. *Essential oil analysis by capillary gas chromatography and carbon-l3 NMR spectroscopy.* Wiley: New York, 1982; pp. 155-157.
18. DE POOTER, H. L.; OMAR, M, N.; COOLSAET, B. A.; SCHAMP, N. M. "The essential oil of greater galanga (*Alpinia galanga*) from Malaysia". *Phytochemistry* 1985, 24, 93-96.
19. ZHENG, G.-Q.; KENNEY, P. M.; AND LAM, L. K. T. "Potential anticarcinogenic natural products isolated from lemongrass oil and galanga root oil". *J. Agric. Food Chem.* 1993, 41, 153-156,
20. SHAATH, N. A.; GRIFFIN, P.; DEDEIAN, S.; PALOYMPIS, L. "The chemical composition of Egyptian parsley seed, absolute and herb oil". In *Flavors and Fragrances: A World Perspective*, Lawrence, B. M.; Mookherjee, B. D., Willis, B. J., Eds.; Proceedings of the 10th International Congress of Essential Oils, Fragrances and Flavors: Washington, DC, 1986; pp. 715-729.
21. ZHENG, G.-Q.; KENNEY, P. M.; LAM, L. K. T. "Myristicin: a potential cancer chemopreventive agent from parsley leaf oil". J. *Agric and Fd Chem.* 1992, 40, 107-110.
22. BORCHERT, P.; MILLER, J. A.; MILLER E. C. "The metabolism of the naturally-occurring hepatocarcinogen safrole to 1'-hydroxy-safrole and electrophilic reactivity of 1'-acetoxysafrole". *Cancer Res.* 1973, 33, 575-589.
23. WISLOCKI, P G.; BORCHERT, P.; MILLER, J. A.; MILLER, E. C. "The metabolic activation of the carcinogen 1'-hydroxysafrole in vivo and in vitro and the electrophilic reactivities of possible ultimate carcinogens". *Cancer Res.* 1976, 36, 1686-1695.
24. ZHENG, G.-Q.; KENNEY, P. M.; ZHANG, J.; LAM, L. K. T. "Chemoprevention of benzo[a]pyrene-induced forestomach cancer in mice by natural phthalides from celery seed oil". *Nutr. Cancer.* 1993, 19, 77-86.
25. BJELDANES, L. F.; KIM, I. S. "Phthalide components of celery essential oil". *J. Org. Chem.* 1977, 42, 2333-2335.
26. MACLEOD, A. J.; MACLEOD, G.; SUBRAMANIAN, G. "Volatile aroma constituents of celery". *Phytochemistry* 1988, 27, 373-375.
27. LAM, L. K. T.; SPARNINS, V. L.; HOCHALTER, J, B.; WATTENBERG, L. W. "Effects of 2- and 3-tert-butyl-4-hydroxyanisole on glutathione S-transferase and epoxide hydrolase activities and sulfhydryl levels in liver and forestomach of mice". *Cancer Res.* 1981, 41, 3940-3943.
28. WATTENBERG, L. W.; LAM, L. K. T. "Phenolic antioxidants as chemical carcinogenesis". In *Radioprotectors and Anticarcinogens Inc.*; Nygaard, O. F., Simic, M. G., Eds.; Academic Press: New York, 1983; pp 461-469.
29. EGNER, P. A.; KENSLER, T. W.; PRESTERA, T.; TALALAY, P.; LIBBY, A. H.; JOYNER, H. H.; CURPHEY, T. J. "Regulation of phase 2 enzyme induction by oltipraz and other dithiolethiones". *Carcinogenesis (Lond.)* 1994, 15, 177-181.
30. KENSLER, T. W.; GROOPMAN, J, D.; ROEBUCK, B. D. "Chemoprevention by oltipraz and other dithiolethiones". In *Cancer Chemoprevention;*

Wattenberg, L. W., Lipkin, M., Boone, C. and Kelloff, G. Eds.; CRC Press; Boca Raton, FL, 1992; pp. 205-225.

31. DIMITROV, N. V.; BENNETT, J. L.; MACMILLAN, J.; PERLOFF, M.; LEECE, C. M.; MALONE W. "Clinical pharmacology studies of oltipraz-a potential chemopreventive agent". *Invest. New Drugs* 1992, 10, 289-298.
32. LAM, L. K. T.; LI, Y.; HASEGAWA, S. "Effects of citrus limonoids on glutathione S-transferase activity in mice". *J. Agric. Food Chem.* 1989, 37, 878-880.
33. MILLER, E. G.; FANOUS, R.; RIVERA-HIDALGO, F.; BINNIE, W, H,; HASEGAWA, S.; LAM, L. K. T. "The effect of citrus limonoids on hamster buccal pouch carcinogenesis". *Carcinogenesis (Lond.)* 1989, 10, 1535-1537.
34. LAM, L. K. T.; HASAGAWA, S. "Inhibition of benzo[a]pyrene-induced forestomach neoplasia in mice by citrus limonoids". *Nutr. Cancer* 1989, 12, 43-47.
35. LAM, L. K. T.; SPARNINS, V. L.; WATTENBERG, L. W. "Effects of derivatives of kahweol and cafestol on the activity of glutathione S-transferase in mice". *J. Med. Chem.* 1987, 30, 1399-1403.
36. WATTENBERG, L. W.; LAM, L. K. T, "Protective effects of coffee constituents on carcinogenesis in experimental animals". *Banbury Rep.* 1984, 17, 137-145.
37. LAM, L. K. T.; ZHENG, B.-L. "Inhibitory effects of 2-n-heptylfuran and 2-n-butylthiophene on benzo[a]pyrene-induced lung and forestomach tumorigenesis in A/J mice". *Nutr. Cancer* 1992, 17, 19-25.
38. JUSAIN, A.; VIRMANI, O. P.; SHARMA, A.; KUMAR, A.; MISRA, L. N. "Major essential oil-bearing plants of India". In *Central Institute of Medicinal and Aromatic Plants*; 1988, pp. 17-22.
39. ELEGBEDE, J. A.; ELSON, C. E.; TANNER, M. A.; QURESHI, A.; GOULD, M. N. "Regression of rat primary mammary tumors following dietary d-limonene". *J. Nat. Cancer Inst.* 1986, 76, 323-325.
40. CROWELL, P. L.; KENNAN, W. S.; HAAG, J. D.; AHMAD, S.; VEDEJS, E.; GOULD, M. N. "Chemoprevention of mammary carcinogenesis by hydroxylated derivatives of d-limonene". *Carcinogenesis (Lond.)* 1992, 13, 1261-1264.
41. ZHENG, G.-Q.; KENNEY, P. M.; ZHANG, J.; LAM, L. K. T. "Inhibition of benzo[a]pyrene-induced tumorigenesis by myristicin, a volatile aroma constituent of parsley leaf oil". *Carcinogenesis (Lond.)* 1992, 13, 1921-1923.

9

The Isoflavone Genistein: A Good Reason for Eating Soy

Stephen Barnes
Lori Coward
Marion Kirk

A reduction in the risk of certain cancers and of cardiovascular disease is associated with the increased consumption of soy. Soy contains high levels (1-3 mg/g) of the isoflavone genistein (5,7,4'-trihydroxyisoflavone) which has been shown to inhibit cell growth and the biochemical events involved with this action (receptor signalling pathways, DNA replication and expression of immediate early response genes such as c-fos). In unprocessed soybeans and unheated soy flours, genistein is found principally as its 6”-O-malonylglucoside conjugate. However, the use of heat in the preparation of soy flours and isolated soy protein leads to decarboxylation of genistein 6”-O-malonylglucoside to its 6”-O-acetylglucoside. Soy foods, such as full fat soy milk and tofu, which are prepared using a hot aqueous leaching step contain mostly the ß-glucoside, genistin, a result of de-esterification of the 6OMalGlc conjugate.

This chemical reaction can also occur during extraction of isoflavones with aqueous organic solvents from soy matrices prior to reversed-phase HPLC analysis. Thus, not all forms of soy foods are necessarily equivalent, since the glycosidic conjugate forms may have quite different bioavailabilities and hence degree of physiologic effects. Recent improvements in analytical methodology will allow for selection of the most appropriate form of soy for clinical experiments.

Diet is widely believed to be an important factor for the international variation in the incidence of several chronic diseases, such as cancer (1) and cardiovascular disease (2). Most of the investigative efforts to establish which parts of the diet account for this variation have concentrated on the macronutrients. Such research led to the recommendation that Americans should decrease their consumption of fats and increase consumption of fruits and vegetables to five servings or more a day (3). More recently, greater interest has been placed on the minor dietary components, particularly the non-nutritive substances.

Breast cancer, prostate cancer and heart disease are characterized by involvement of estrogens. Exposure to estrogens increases the risk of breast cancer, whereas the antiestrogen tamoxifen is effective in the treatment of estrogen-dependent breast cancer (4). Tamoxifen is also under trial as a chemopreventive agent in women at high risk of breast cancer (5). Synthetic estrogens such as diethylstilbestrol have been used in the treatment of prostate cancer in its early stages (6). The risk of heart disease in premenopausal women is substantially below that in men (7). However, following menopause and cessation of ovarian estrogen synthesis, heart disease risk in women rises rapidly (8). Intense investigations to determine the optimum form of estrogen-replacement therapy are underway. However, they have been complicated by the increased risk of endometrial cancer (9). This can be overcome by including a progestin in the therapy, but at the cost of an increased risk of breast cancer (10).

In addition to the physiological estrogens (the steroids estradiol and estrone), we are exposed to other sources of estrogen-like activities. These may occur from foods and nonfood environmental sources (11). The principal food sources of estrogens arise from compounds in edible plants (phytoestrogens) or from microbial contamination (moulds and yeasts). In general, these nonphysiological estrogens are less potent than their steroid counterparts. Nonetheless, exposure to them can often be substantial.

Soy, a food eaten widely in Southeast Asia, contains mg/g quantities of two phytoestrogens, the isoflavones daidzein and genistein (12-14). On average, 25-100 mg/day of each of these compounds is consumed each day by Southeast Asians (15). In contrast, Americans eat less than 2 mg/day (15). It has been speculated that this increased exposure to phytoestrogens in Southeast Asians is a large factor in their lower risk of breast and prostate cancer and of cardiovascular disease (16-18). Experiments using animal models of breast cancer have confirmed that soy reduces the risk of cancer (17, 19, 20) - indeed, the most recent experiments have shown that genistein alone is capable of this effect (21).

The mechanism by which genistein exerts its anticancer effects is unknown. However, since it was discovered in 1987 that genistein is a potent and specific inhibitor of protein tyrosine kinases (22), it has been assumed that genistein interferes with signal transduction pathways stimulated by growth factors. These pathways are abnormally activated in many cancers. However, several other critical biochemical events are also regulated by genistein and at this time it is not known which one is the most relevant to the cancer disease process (23, 24). In a fascinating recent study, Uckun et al. (25) reported that genistein conjugated to an antibody to the CD19 receptor on human leukemia cells, was highly effective as an immunotherapy agent in a nude mouse model of pre-B precursor cell leukemia, the most common form of childhood leukemia and the second most common form of acute leukemia in adults. In this study genistein was chosen as a broad spectrum inhibitor of Src tyrosine kinases.

A role for the isoflavones in preventing cardiovascular disease is just emerging. It has been long known that when soy protein is used to replace animal protein in the diet that there is a marked improvement in the blood lipid profiles, particularly causing a lowering of the serum cholesterol concentration. This effect has also been observed in men on a soy-containing diet (26, 27). In a recent study in rhesus monkeys, it was found that depletion of the isoflavones from soy protein used in diets results in the loss of the hypocholesterolemic effect of soy (28). Genistein also inhibits the activity of osteoclasts (29) which are responsible for the bone reabsorption leading to osteoporosis that occurs in the postmenopausal period.

In soy foods daidzein and genistein occur as several glucoside conjugates (30) (Fig. 9.1), as well as the free aglucone (mostly in fermented foods) (12). In soybeans, the principal conjugate is the 6"-O-malonate ester of the ß-glucoside (6OMalGlc) (Fig. 9.1) (31). This conjugate can undergo chemical alterations during extraction of soy proteins from soybeans and during processing to form second generation foods such as soy protein concentrates and isolated soy proteins (12, 32). The rapidly increasing market for soy foods, particularly those low in fat, is leading to many new products which may have quite different isoflavone composition from the traditional soy foods.

In this chapter we examine the isoflavone conjugate profile of several soy foods in order to understand the chemical changes which occur in their preparation. In addition, we consider the implications for the bioavailability of the isoflavones from different soy foods.

MATERIALS & METHODS

Materials

Soybeans and soy milks (full fat and lite) were obtained from a national food store chain specializing in vegetable products. Defatted soy flour and an isolated soy protein (Supro*) were kindly donated by Protein Technologies International, St. Louis, MO. Several grades of soy flour were provided by the Archer

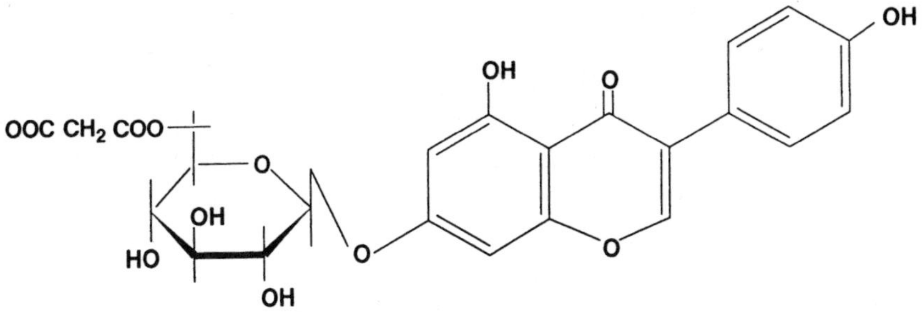

MALONYLGLUCOSIDE

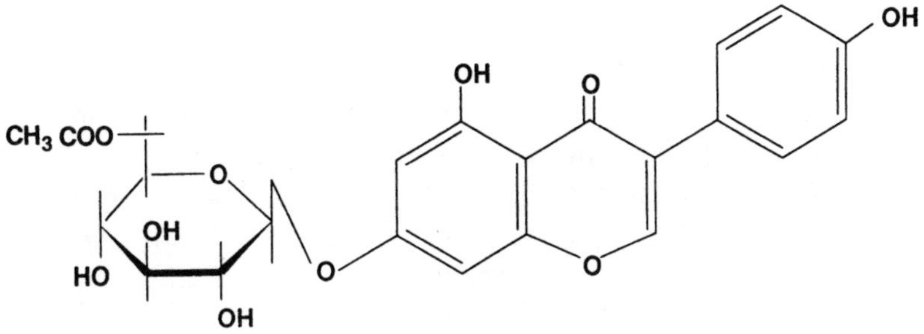

ACETYLGLUCOSIDE

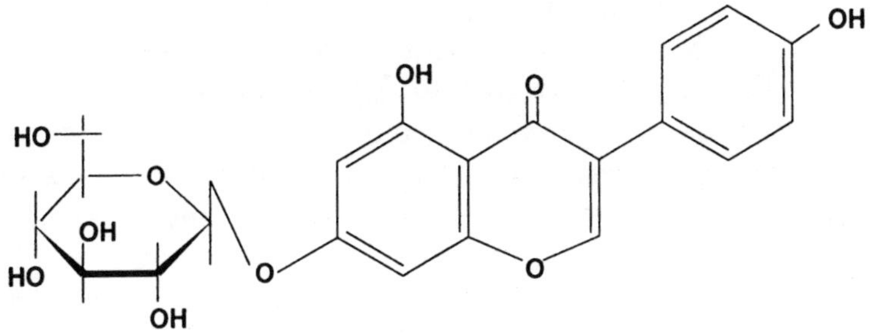

β-GLUCOSIDE

FIG. 9.1. CHEMICAL STRUCTURE OF THE 6"-O-MALONYLGLUCOSIDE, 6"-O-ACETYLGLUCOSIDE AND ß-GLUCOSIDE OF GENISTEIN.

Daniels Midland Co., Decatur, IL. Full fat and lite tofu were donated by Morinaga Nutritional Foods, Inc., Torrance, CA. Miso was a gift of Westbrae, Carson, CA.

HPLC grade methanol and acetonitrile and the disodium salt of fluorescein were used without further purification. Double distilled water was filtered through a 0.45 μm pore size Superpore nylon membrane.

Daidzein and genistein and their ß-glucoside conjugates were isolated and purified as described elsewhere (12, 33).

Extraction of Isoflavones From Soy Foods

Portions of soy material (500 mg) were mixed with 4 ml of 80% aqueous methanol containing the internal standard fluorescein (1 mg). The mixtures were then placed in a tumbling mixer for 2 h at room temperature (22°C). Aliquots of each mixture were clarified by centrifugation at 14,000 × g in an Eppendorf centrifuge prior to reversed-phase HPLC analysis.

Isoflavone Analysis

Reversed-phase HPLC analysis of isoflavones was carried out on a 25 cm × 4.6 mm Aquapore C_8 column (Applied Biosystems, Foster City, CA) as recently described (30).

HPLC mass spectrometry experiments were performed on an API III triple quadrupole mass spectrometer (PE-Sciex, Thornhill, Ontario, Canada) controlled by two MacIntosh Quadra 950 computers, one of which was used for data analysis. The isoflavones in the soy extracts were separated by reversed-phase HPLC on a 10 cm × 4.6 mm Aquapore C_8 column at a flow rate of 1.0 ml/min using a linear 0-50% gradient of acetonitrile (5% per min) in 10 mM ammonium acetate. Positive ions from eluted solutes were introduced into the mass spectrometer following their generation by atmospheric pressure chemical ionization caused by a corona discharge needle in the heated nebulizer interface of this instrument.

Theoretical Plasma Concentration-time Curves

The pharmacokinetic parameters governing intestinal absorption, distribution and excretion for the isoflavones have yet to be defined. However, the different chemical forms should be expected to behave in a manner analogous to many therapeutic drugs. Intestinal uptake was defined as obeying a gamma function,

$$p_t(t) = 1/\Gamma(\alpha + 1)\beta^{\alpha + 1^{t^{\alpha} \cdot e^{-t/\beta}}}$$

where α and β were set to (20, 3), (20, 6) and (20,16) for duodenal, jejunal and colonic sites of absorption, respectively, and t was the time in min. The disappearance of genistein from the blood compartment was modeled as following first order kinetics with a $T_{1/2}$ of 30 min. Thus the loss of genistein for each 10 min period was,

[initial blood concentration] . 10 . (ln 2)/30

This was subtracted from the accumulating genistein in the blood compartment by the function in equation 1. A multiplying factor F for the gamma function was set at 20,000. This value was chosen to satisfy the average plasma genistein concentration of 300 nM observed in four subjects 6.5 hours after taking an isolated soy protein beverage (containing 70% malonyl- and acetylglucosides, 20% ß-glucosides and 5% aglucone) studied over a 14-day period (Barnes and co-workers, unpublished observations).

RESULTS

Full-fat soy milks prepared by boiling water extraction of crushed soybeans contain only the ß-glucosides, with just traces of the 6OMalGlc conjugates (Fig. 9.2). A similar distribution was observed for full fat tofu (Fig. 9.3) and "lite" soy milk (Fig. 9.4). The "lite" soy milk contained a two-fold lower concentration of isoflavones than full-fat soy milk.

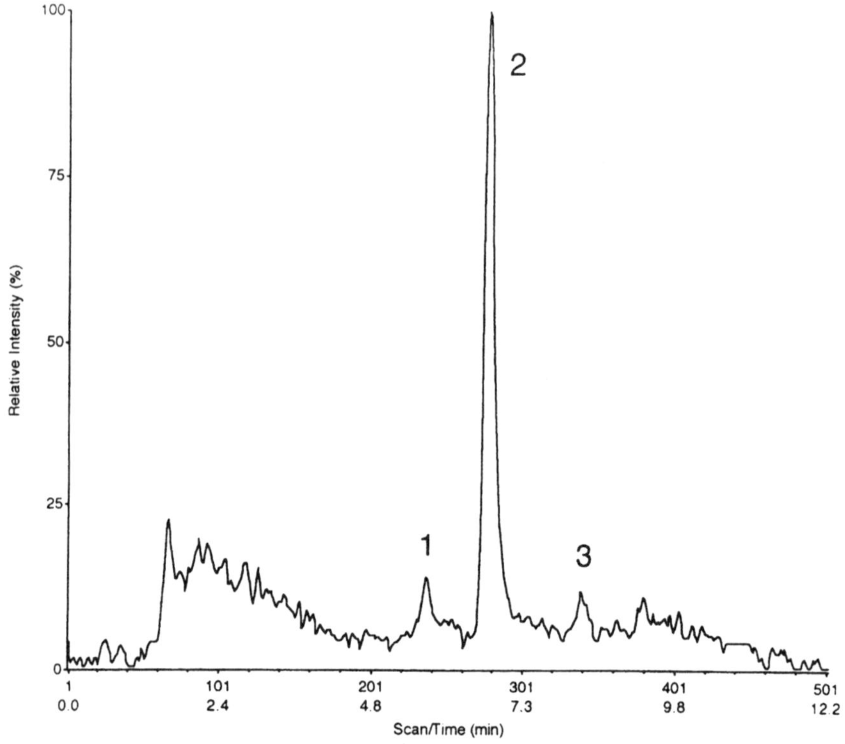

FIG. 9.2. RECONSTRUCTED ION CHROMATOGRAM OF DAIDZEIN CONJUGATES FOLLOWING HPLC-MASS SPECTROMETRY OF AN EXTRACT OF FULL-FAT SOY MILK. THE CHROMATOGRAM IS THE SUM OF THE $[M+H]^+$, $[M+H-COOH]^-$, $[M+H-MALONATE]^+$ AND $[AGLUCONE+H]^+$ IONS. PEAK IDENTIFICATION: 1 = 6"-O-MALONYLGLUCOSYLDAIDZEIN, 2 = DAIDZIN, 3 = DAIDZEIN. THE FULL SCALE ION COUNT IS 253,708.

"Lite" versions of tofu from different manufacturers contained two patterns of isoflavone conjugates. In one, the 6OMalGlc conjugates predominated, with significant amounts of both the ß-glucosides and the 6OAcGlc conjugates. This pattern was very similar to that observed for isolated soy protein, the soy material used in these products (30). In the other type of "lite" tofu, the ß-glucosides predominated (Fig. 9.5). The concentrations of isoflavones in this "lite" tofu were 4 to 5 times lower than in the full-fat tofu.

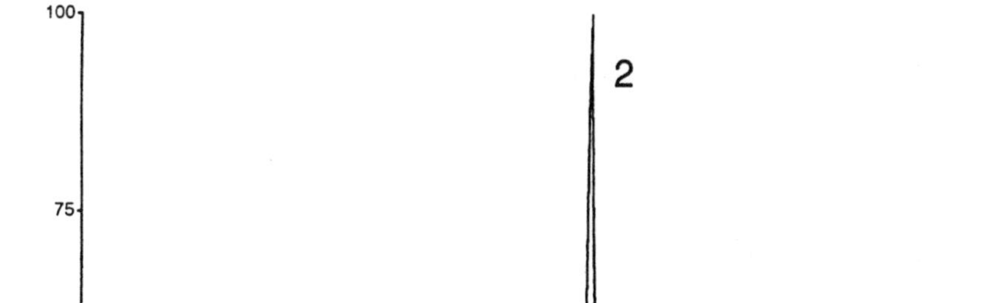

FIG. 9.3. RECONSTRUCTED ION CHROMATOGRAM OF DAIDZEIN CONJUGATES FOLLOWING HPLC-MASS SPECTROMETRY OF AN EXTRACT OF FULL-FAT TOFU. PEAK IDENTIFICATION AS IN FIG. 9.2. THE FULL SCALE ION COUNT IS 457,876.

Miso, a fermented soy food, contains a large proportion of the isoflavones as their aglucones (13). In the sample analyzed in this study, only the aglucones were detected (Fig. 9.6).

Predicted serum genistein concentrations based on simulation of intestinal uptake and a plasma disappearance $T_{1/2}$ of 30 min showed that aglucones (absorbed in the upper small intestine) produce a three-fold higher peak concentration than the 6OMalGlc and 6OAcGlc conjugates (absorbed in the colon) (Fig. 9.7). The area under the plasma concentration-time curve was the same for each type of compound. The use of a $T_{1/2}$ of 500 min as determined for ^{125}I-labeled genistein (25) led to a highly

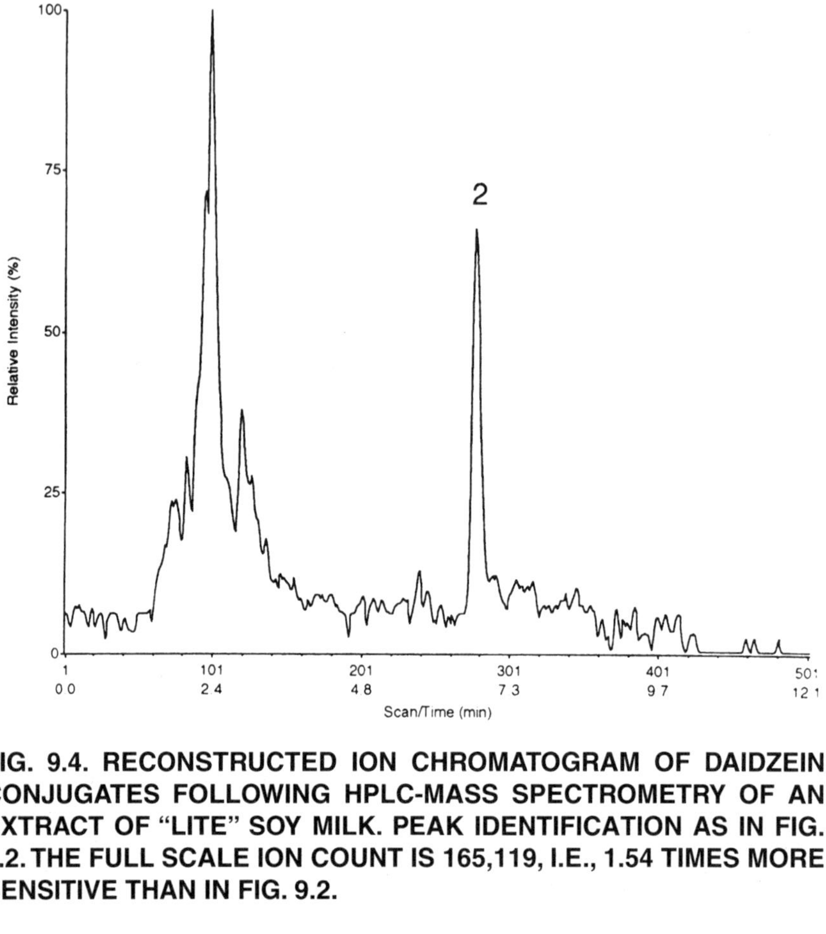

FIG. 9.4. RECONSTRUCTED ION CHROMATOGRAM OF DAIDZEIN CONJUGATES FOLLOWING HPLC-MASS SPECTROMETRY OF AN EXTRACT OF "LITE" SOY MILK. PEAK IDENTIFICATION AS IN FIG. 9.2. THE FULL SCALE ION COUNT IS 165,119, I.E., 1.54 TIMES MORE SENSITIVE THAN IN FIG. 9.2.

skewed plasma concentration-time curve which did not match experimentally observed data.

A soy product composed of both simple and complex glucosides would be expected to produce an elevated plasma genistein concentration for a greater period of time, and perhaps cause the appearance of two peaks of concentration (Fig. 9.8).

DISCUSSION

In the past year there has been a marked increase in the interest in plant estrogens, particularly the isoflavones in soy,

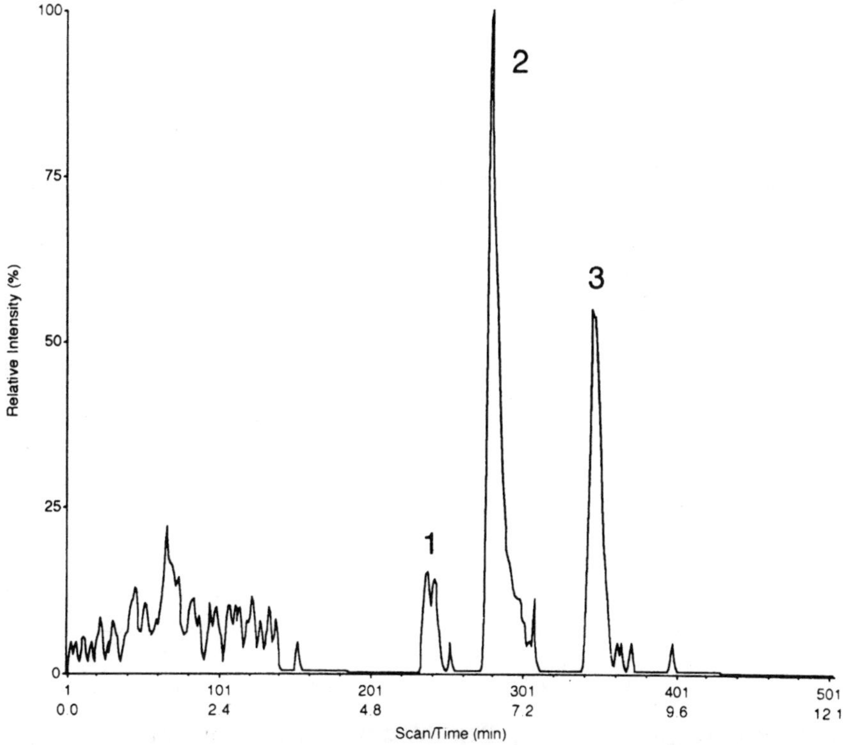

FIG. 9.5. RECONSTRUCTED ION CHROMATOGRAM OF DAIDZEIN CONJUGATES FOLLOWING HPLC-MASS SPECTROMETRY OF AN EXTRACT OF "LITE" TOFU. PEAK IDENTIFICATION AS IN FIG. 9.2. THE FULL SCALE ION COUNT IS 110,00, I.E., 4.16 TIMES MORE SENSITIVE THAN IN FIG. 9.3.

daidzein and genistein. This has arisen because of the apparent association between soy consumption and a lower risk of certain cancers (15) and of cardiovascular disease (26, 27).

There are advantages in the use of a food matrix to deliver a chemopreventive substance. In particular, the dose of the substance lies in a range that does not cause untoward or toxic effects. Soy foods have been eaten on a regular basis by nearly a third of the world's population for several hundred years. In the United States, the soybean is a major crop, but instead of being consumed here it is either exported or used in animal feeds. It is

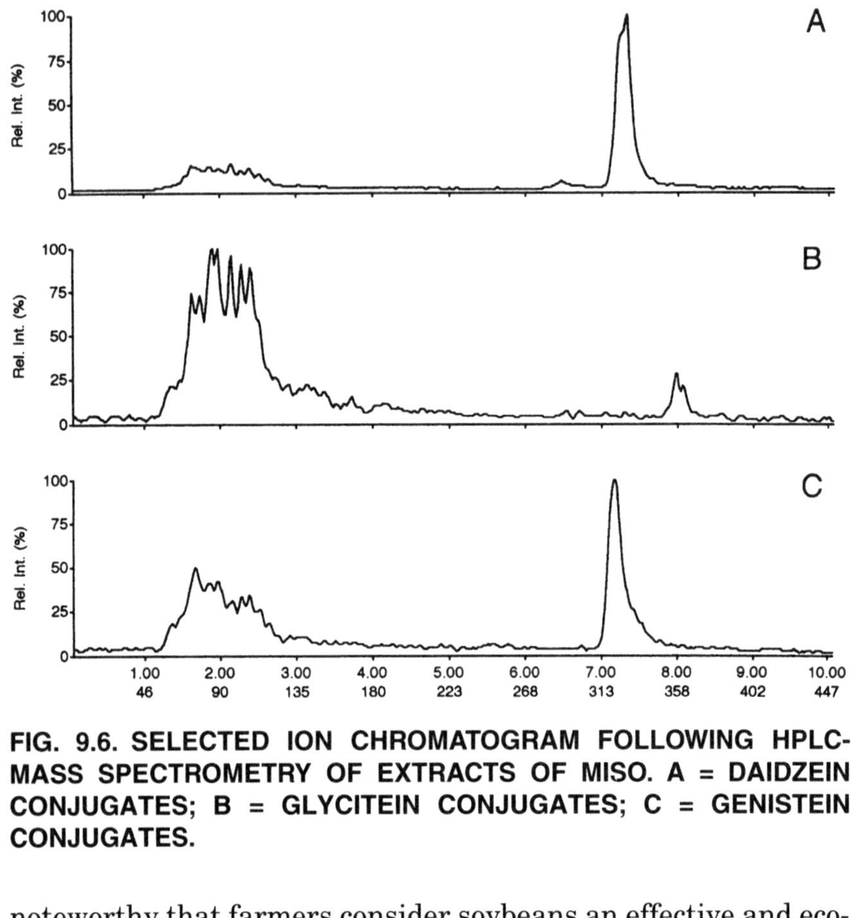

FIG. 9.6. SELECTED ION CHROMATOGRAM FOLLOWING HPLC-MASS SPECTROMETRY OF EXTRACTS OF MISO. A = DAIDZEIN CONJUGATES; B = GLYCITEIN CONJUGATES; C = GENISTEIN CONJUGATES.

noteworthy that farmers consider soybeans an effective and economic source of protein for their livestock. Nonetheless, the cadre of soy users is on the increase in the United States, including those who have gastrointestinal disturbances due to lactase deficiency, and those who are alert to the need to reduce the intake of animal fats. The latter include a large group of serious athletes.

In order for the isoflavones in foods to reach the tissues of the body, they have to conform to the same pharmacological principles that govern the absorption and distribution of orally administered, conventional pharmaceutical drugs. In general, drugs are absorbed by passive absorption, with hydrophobic compounds passing through the intestinal mucosal membranes

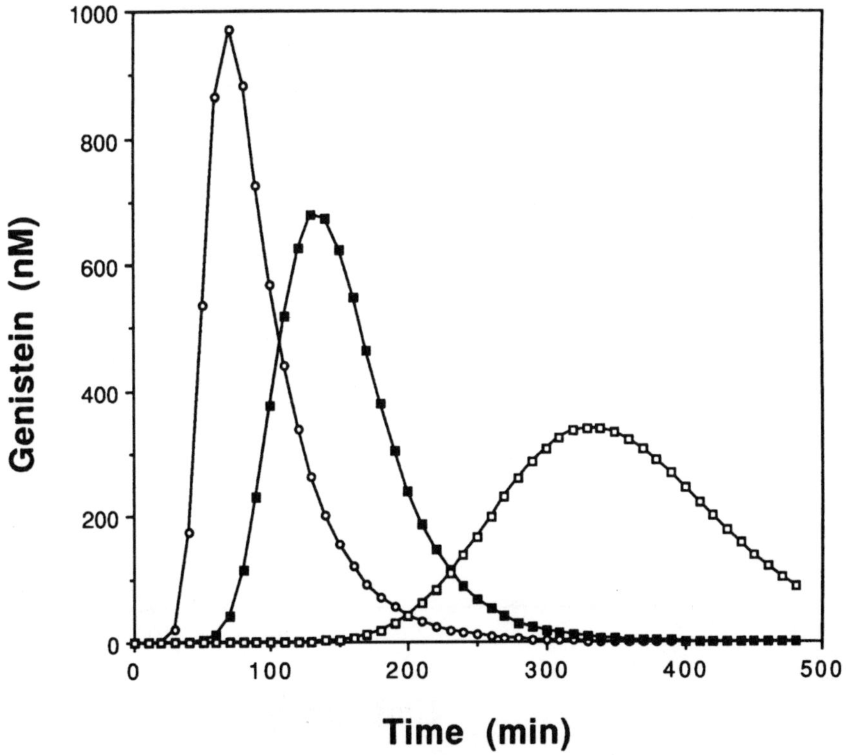

FIG. 9.7. THEORETICAL PLASMA CONCENTRATION-TIME CURVES FOLLOWING THE INGESTION OF ISOFLAVONES IN MISO (O; UNCONJUGATED), FULL-FAT SOY MILK (N;ß-GLUCOSIDES), AND SOY BEVERAGES BASED ON DEFATTED SOY FLOUR (P; MALONYLGLYCOSIDES).

more rapidly. Indeed, in recent experiments using rats with in dwelling biliary cannulas we have shown that unconjugated genistein is rapidly absorbed in the upper small intestine (34). Since the isoflavone glucosidic conjugates are hydrophilic, it is unlikely that they will be absorbed intact. Instead, the absorption of these isoflavones will depend on the ability of intestinal ß-glucosidases to hydrolyze them to the unconjugated isoflavones. It should be expected that the more complex 6OAcGlc and 6OMalGlc isoflavone conjugates would be hydrolyzed with

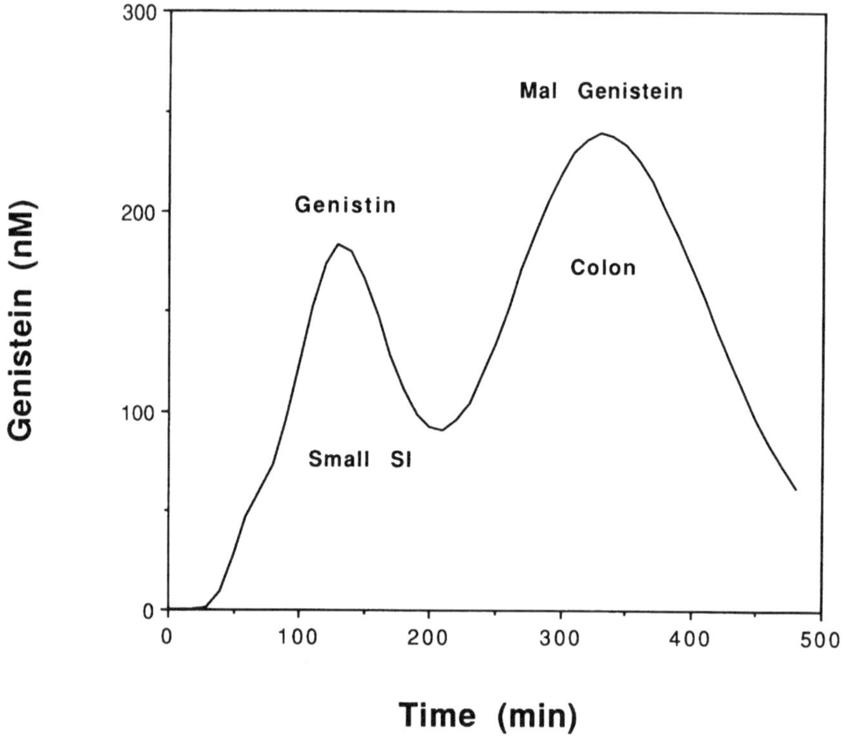

FIG. 9.8. THEORETICAL PLASMA CONCENTRATION-TIME CURVES FOLLOWING THE INGESTION OF ISOFLAVONES IN ISOLATED SOY PROTEIN BEVERAGES (A MIXTURE OF 75% ACETYL- AND MALONYLGLUCOSIDES, 20% ß-GLUCOSIDE AND 5% AGLUCONE).

greater difficulty than the ß-glucosides (35), possibly not until they reach the large bowel (Fig. 9.8).

The range of pH throughout the intestine is such that the unconjugated isoflavones should be always non-ionized and hence easily absorbed. However, as the effective surface area of the intestine decreases from the duodenum onwards, this may lead to slower rates of absorption in the more distal regions of the intestine.

Bearing in mind these pharmacological considerations, the various forms of soy foods may not be necessarily equivalent in their biological effect because of differences in total absorption, the shape of the plasma concentration-time curve, and the extent to which bacterial metabolism contributes to their pharmacokinetics. This is a very important consideration for those investigators embarking on clinical trials involving the use of a soy food product. There is the risk that they may select a soy food that because of processing has a low concentration of isoflavones. The "lite" versions of soy milks and tofu tested in this study had substantially lower concentrations of isoflavones than their full-fat counterparts. Further, "non-fat" versions of soy milk appear to be made from alcohol extracted soy protein concentrates which have little or any isoflavones (12).

Miso, since it mostly consists of the isoflavone aglucones, provides the most easily absorbable form. However, if all the isoflavones are absorbed rapidly from miso, then a large peak will occur in their plasma concentration which would be followed by a trough (Fig. 9.7). This is not ideal from the perspective of maintaining a steady plasma concentration. In contrast, the glucosidic forms of the isoflavones will have a delayed absorption. The ß-glucosides would be expected to give rise to a peak in the plasma isoflavone concentration at 1 to 2 h after ingestion (Fig. 9.7), a result of hydrolysis by ß-glucosidases in the small bowel. The 6OMalGlc and 6OAcGlc conjugates are more resistant to ß-glucosidases (35) and therefore would not be hydrolyzed until they entered the large bowel. This would result in a delayed plasma concentration peak 4 to 6 h after ingestion (Fig. 9.7).

Selection of the soy food for a clinical trial may also depend on the nature of the disease under examination. Clearly, miso might be a poor choice (because it is rapidly absorbed) for diseases of the large bowel (colonic and rectal cancer, or ulcerative colitis). Similarly, the non-fermented foods are unlikely to have a luminal effect on stomach ulcers or stomach cancer. On the other hand, foods rich in the 6OMalGlc and 6OAcGlc conjugates will target the delivery of the isoflavones to large bowel—this is analogous to the recent use of N,N'-diazosalicylic acid to deliver 5-aminosalicylic acid to the colonic lumen (the diazo bond is cleaved only by the bacteria in the large bowel).

From these various considerations, the ideal form of soy would contain the aglucones, the ß-glucosides and the 6OMalGlc and 6OAcGlc conjugates, which together would provide a steady plasma concentration (Fig. 9.8). This is the case for many of the non-fermented soy foods, particularly those containing the complex glucosidic conjugates; this has recently been demonstrated by capillary HPLC-electrospray ionization MS-MS in volunteers consuming an isolated soy protein beverage which contained ß-glucosides and the 6OMalGlc and 60AcGlc conjugates (36). Further studies are urgently called for to address these issues by direct experimentation.

Acknowledgments

Research on soy and a reduction in cancer risk has been supported by grants from the American Cancer Society (BC-599), the American Institute for Cancer Research (91B58, MG92A42), the United Soybean Board, the Nebraska Soybean Board, the National Cancer Institute (1R01 CA61668) and Protein Technologies International of St. Louis, MO. The UAB Comprehensive Center Mass Spectrometry Shared Facility is supported in part by a Core Support Grant (5P30 CA-13148) from the National Cancer Institute and by a Shared Instrumentation grant (S10RR06487) from the NIH.

BIBLIOGRAPHY

1. GRAY, G. E.; PIKE, M. C.; HENDERSON, B. E. "Breast cancer incidence and mortality rates in different countries in relation to known factors and dietary practice." *Br. J. Cancer* 1979, 39, 1-7.
2. KATO, H.; TILLOTSON, J.; NICHAMEN, M. Z.; RHOADS, G. G.; HAMILTON, H. B. "Epidemiologic studies of coronary heart disease and stroke in Japanese men living in Japan, Hawaii and California: serum lipids, and diet." *Am. J. Epidemiol.* 1973, 97, 372-385.
3. NESTLE, M. "Dietary recommendations for cancer prevention: public policy implementation." *Monogr. NCI* 1992, 12, 153-157.
4. LIPMANN, M. E. "The NIH Consensus Development Conference for Breast Cancer." *NCI Monogr.* 1986, 1.
5. NAYFIELD, S. G.; KARP, J. E.; FORD, L. G.; DORR, F. A.; KRAMER, B. S. "Potential role of tamoxifen in prevention of breast cancer." *J. Nat. Cancer Inst.* 1991, 83, 1450-1459.

6. HERBST, W. P. "Effects of estradiol dipropionate and diethylstilbestrol on malignant prostatic tissue." *Trans. Am. Assoc. Genitourin. Surg.* 1941, 34, 195-202.
7. JOHANSSON, S.; VEDIN, A.; WILHELMSSON, C. "Myocardial infarction in women." *Epidemiol. Rev.* 1983, 5, 67-95.
8. ROSENBERG, L.; HENNEKENS, C. H.; ROSNER, B.; BELANGER, C.; ROTHMAN, K. J.; SPEIZER, F. E. "Early menopause and the risk of myocardial infarction." *Am. J. Obst. Gynecol.* 1981, 139, 47-51.
9. SHAPIRO, S.; KELLY, J. P.; ROSENBERG, L.; KAUFMAN, D. W.; HELMRICH, S. P.; ROSENSHEIN, N. B.; LEWIS, J. L.; KNAPP, R. C.; STOLLEY, P. D., SCHOTTENFIELD, D. "Risk of localized and widespread endometrial cancer in relation to current and discontinued use of oral contraceptives." *N. Engl. J. Med.* 1985, 313, 969-972.
10. COLDITZ, G. A.; EGAN, K. M; STAMPFER, M. J. "Hormone replacement therapy and risk of breast cancer: Results from epidemiologic studies." *Am. J. Obstet. Gynecol.* 1993, 168, 1473-1480.
11. PRICE, K. R.; FENWICK, G. R. "Naturally occurring oestrogens in foods - a review." *Food Addit. Contam.* 1985, 2, 73-106.
12. COWARD, L.; BARNES, N. C.; SETCHELL, K. D. R.; BARNES, S. "Genistein and daidzein, and their -glycoside conjugates: anti-tumor isoflavones in soybean foods from American and Asian diets." *J. Agric. Food Chem.* 1993, 41, 1961-1967.
13. WANG, H-J.; MURPHY, P. A. "Isoflavone content in commercial soybean foods." *J. Agric. Food Chem.* 1994, 42, 1666-1673.
14. FRANKE, A. A.; CUSTER, L. J.; CERNA, C. C.; NARALA, K. K. "Rapid HPLC analysis of dietary phytoestrogens from legumes and from human urine." *Proc. Soc. Exp. Biol. Med.* 1995, 208, 18-26.
15. MESSINA, M.; PERSKY, V.; SETCHELL, K. D. R.; BARNES, S. "Soy intake and cancer risk: A review of the *in vitro* and *in vivo* data." *Nutr. Cancer* 1994, 21, 113-131.
16. SETCHELL, K. D. R.; BORRIELLO, S. P.; HULME, P.; KIRK, D. N.; AXELSON, M. "Non-steroidal estrogens of dietary origin: possible roles in hormone-dependent disease." *Am. J. Clin. Nutr.* 1984, 40, 569-578.
17. BARNES, S.; GRUBBS, C.; SETCHELL, K. D. R.; CARLSON, J. "Soybeans inhibit mammary tumors in models of breast cancer." In *Mutagens and Carcinogens in the Diet*; Pariza, M., Ed.; Wiley-Liss, Inc.: New York, 1990, 239-253.
18. ADLERCREUTZ, H. "Western diet and Western diseases: some hormonal and biochemical mechanisms and associations." *Scand. J. Clin. Lab. Invest.* 1990, 50 (suppl 201), 3-23.
19. TROLL, W.; WIESNER, R.; SHELLABARGER, C. J.; HOLTZMAN, S.; STONE, J. P. "Soybean diet lowers breast tumor incidence in irradiated rats." *Carcinogenesis* 1980, 1, 469-472.
20. BARNES, S.; PETERSON, T. G.; GRUBBS, C.; SETCHELL, K. D. R. "Potential Role of Dietary Isoflavones in the Prevention of Cancer." In

Diet and Cancer: Markers, Prevention and Treatment, Jacobs, M., Ed.; Plenum Press: New York, 1994, 135-148.

21. LAMARTINIERE, C. A.; MOORE, J.; HOLLAND, M. B.; BARNES, S. "Neonatal genistein chemoprevents mammary carcinogenesis." *Proc. Soc. Exptl. Biol. Med.* 1995, 208, 120-123.
22. AKIYAMA, T.; ISHIDA, J.; NAKAGAWA, S.; OGAWARA, H.; WATANABE, S.; ITOH, N. M.; SHIBUYA, M.; FUKAMI, Y. "Genistein, a specific inhibitor of tyrosine-specific protein kinases." *J. Biol. Chem.* 1987, 262, 5592-5595.
23. BARNES, S.; PETERSON, T. G. "Biochemical targets of the isoflavone genistein in tumor cell lines." *Proc. Soc. Exp. Biol. Med.* 1995, 208, 103-108.
24. PETERSON, T. G. "Evaluation of the biochemical targets of genistein in tumor cells." *J. Nutr.* 1995, 125, 784S-789S.
25. UCKUN, F. M.; EVANS, W. E.; FORSYTH, C. J.; WADDICK, K. G.; AHLGREN, L. T.; CHELSTROM, L. M.; BURKHARDT, A.; BOLEN, J.; MYERS, D. E. "Biotherapy of B-cell precursor leukemia by targeting genistein to CD19-associated tyrosine kinases." *Science* 1995, 267, 886-891.
26. POTTER, S. M.; BAKHIT, R. M.; ESSEX-SORLIE, D.; WEINGARTNER, K.; CHAPMAN, K.; NELSON, R.; PARBHUESAI, M.; SAVAGE, W.; NELSON, A. I.; WINTER, L.; ERDMAN, J. W. "Depression of plasma cholesterol in men by consumption of baked products containing soy protein." *Am. J. Clin. Nutr.* 1993, 58, 501-506.
27. BAKHIT, R. M.; KLEIN, B. P.; ESSEX-SORLIE, D.; HAM, J. O.; ERDMAN, J. W.; POTTER, S. M. "Intake of 25 g soy protein reduces plasma cholesterol in men with elevated cholesterol concentrations." *J. Nutr.* 1994, 124, 213-222.
28. ANTHONY, M.; BURKE, G. L.; HUGHES, JR., C. L.; CLARKSON, T. B. "Does soy supplementation improve coronary heart disease (CHD) risk?" *Circulation* 1995, 91, 925.
29. BLAIR, H.; WILLIAMS, J.; BARNES, S. "Response of osteoclastic acid transport to tyrosine kinase inhibitors." *J. Bone Mineral Res.* 1994, 9 (S1), S133.
30. BARNES, S.; KIRK, M.; COWARD, L. "Isoflavones and their conjugates in Soy Foods: Extraction and Analysis by HPLC-Mass Spectrometry." *J. Agric. Food Chem.* 1994, 42, 2466-2474.
31. KUDOU, S.; FLEURY, Y.; WELTI, D.; MAGNOLATO, D.; UCHIDA, T.; KITAMURA, K.; OKUBO, K. "Malonyl isoflavone glycosides in soybean seeds (*Glycine max* MERRILL)." *Agric Biol. Chem.* 1991, 55, 2227-2233.
32. BARNES, S.; COWARD, L.; KIRK, M. "Isoflavonoids in soy - all is not what it seems." In: *Physiologically Functional Foods*, Caragay, A. and Orthoefer, F., Eds.; AOCS Press: Champaign, IL, in press.
33. WALTER, E. D. "Genistin (an isoflavone glucoside) and its aglucone, genistein from soybean." *J. Am. Oil Chem. Soc.* 1941, 63, 3273-3276.

34. SFAKIANOS, J.; BARNES, S. "The isoflavone genistein undergoes an enterohepatic circulation." *Hepatology* 1995, 22, 247A.
35. FARMAKALIDIS, E.; MURPHY, P. A. "Isolation of 6"-O-acetyldaidzein and 6"-O-acetylgenistein from toasted defatted soy flakes." *J. Agric. Food Chem.* 1985, 33, 385-389.
36. BARNES, S.; COWARD, L.; WILSON, L.; KIRK, M. "Serum conjugated and unconjugated isoflavones by capillary reversed-phase hplc-electrospray ionization-mass spectrometry." Presented at the NCI Workshop on *"Dietary Phytoestrogens: Cancer Cause or Cure?"*, Washington, DC, 1994.

10

The Role of Pectin in Cholesterol Regulation

James J. Cerda

Our laboratory has had a particular interest in the role of grapefruit pectin (GFP) in health and disease. We have developed *in vitro* and *in vivo* techniques to systematically study dietary pectin in lowering plasma cholesterol in several animal models and in human studies. Results have demonstrated that GFP consistently lowers plasma cholesterol and LDL cholesterol with no significant effect on HDL cholesterol or triglycerides. We have recently assessed the effect of GFP in microswine with established hypercholesterolemia. There was a significant reduction in atherosclerosis observed in the coronary vessels and the aorta. This strongly suggests that GFP may also inhibit the development of atherosclerosis even in animals with established hypercholesterolemia either by promoting regression or interfering with lesion progression. The implications of these findings will be discussed.

For the past two decades my colleagues and I at the University of Florida have been systematically evaluating the role of citrus fruits and their products in human nutrition. Our initial interest was in establishing the role of citrus in providing certain vitamins, particularly vitamin C and folacin, in replenishing loss to electrolytes, and possibly inhibiting viral infections (1). We next focused on the study of the chemistry and the biological role of dietary grapefruit pectin, as a model soluble dietary fiber. A comprehensive review of dietary fibers has recently been published (2).

We chose to study pectin because of its abundance in citrus fruits. Pectin is a heterogenous mixture of a number of pectic polysaccharides. Pectin appears early during plant cell wall biogenesis. It is obtained by aqueous extraction of appropriate edible plant material, usually oranges, grapefruit and apples. All land and plants contain pectic substances, which in combination with cellulose, are responsible for the structural properties of fruits and vegetables. Pectin has been evaluated and cleared toxicologically by the Joint World Health Organization Expert Committee on food additives. This organization deemed it unnecessary to establish an acceptable daily uptake. National and international food regulations recognized that pectin is a valuable food additive. Pectin is included in the list of permitted additives of standardized foods when a technological need can be proven.

We, and others (2, 3), in early studies found that pectin, when supplemented in the diet of laboratory animals and/or human volunteers, caused a significant reduction in serum cholesterol levels. This is an important observation, as it has been shown that the etiology of atherosclerosis and coronary artery disease is associated with elevated serum cholesterol levels. If one could develop pectin so that it could be ingested in therapeutic quantities and in a palatable form, it would hold great promise for the treatment and/or prevention of these important diseases.

Our initial studies focused on the role of dietary grapefruit pectin (GFP) with an emphasis into examining its complex nature and possible biochemical basis by which it might cause lowering of serum and/or liver cholesterol. We initially developed techniques which incorporated radioactivity into GFP (4, 5). We achieved this by supplying radioactive myoinositol to a ripening grapefruit or by treating isolated dietary pectic polysaccharides with galactose-oxidase, followed by a reduction with tritiated sodium borohydride. Having achieved this, we prepared radiolabeled pectin which was then fed to mice (6). The radiolabel was prepared by supplying radioactive methionine to germinating lily pollen tubes. Following ingestion the radiolabeled pectin was monitored in the serum, liver and gastrointestinal tract of those mice. Our results suggest that some metabolism and degradation products of pectin does occur in mice.

We then studied the comparative effectiveness of cholestyramine and GFP as hypocholesterolemic agents (7). Circulating levels of serum cholesterol and lipoprotein-associated cholesterol were measured in rats with high cholesterol diets supplemented with either cholestyramine or pectin. In this study we demonstrated that both cholestyramine and pectin were comparable and effective hypocholesterolemic agents. In addition, the observed hypocholesterolemic effect appeared to be mediated through the lowering of the cholesterol-associated low density lipoprotein (LDLC). We then demonstrated that the feeding of pectin (as does feeding of cholestyramine), results in an increase in the activity of hepatic HMGCoA reductase (8). As an extension to those studies we also studied the effect of dietary GFP on cholesterol and hepatic 7α-hydroxy cholesterol (C7H) formation. We concluded that dietary cholesterol in the presence of GFP results in a significant decrease in C7H formation (9). These initial observations need further study.

We were concerned that if high concentrations of pectin were supplemented in the diet, it would be possible for colonic bacteria to degrade pectin, causing a significant amount of methanol to be released from the galacturonic residues. In a study evaluating normal human fecal flora against known pectinolytic bacteria, we demonstrated that colonic microflora present in fecal material degrade pectin and release free methanol, but the amount of methanol release is trivial (10).

There is usually a layer of relatively unstirred water next to the human intestinal brush border through which some molecules must move in order to be transported. Obviously, changes in the unstirred water layer might affect nutrient absorption. We estimated the change in the unstirred water layer in rabbit small intestine with both pectin and guar gum. Our studies demonstrated that both pectin and guar gum significantly increased the thickness of the unstirred water layer in rabbit intestine, explaining in part, the reduction in the rate of absorption of certain substances such as cholesterol (11, 12).

We then examined the effect of GFP on the absorption and/or turnover of minerals such as iron, zinc and calcium. We studied rats maintained on a low iron diet with 59 Fe and compared them to the group of rats maintained on normal iron levels. GFP had no influence on iron uptake and/or turnover in rats (13). Furthermore, we studied the effect of GFP on zinc and calcium balance (14). The hypocholesterolemic effect of GFP has been thought to be due, in part, to binding of bile salts. We studied the *in vitro* interaction of pectin with bile salts by the utilization of centrifugation and equilibrium dialysis techniques. We were unable to find any binding (15).

Miniature swine are excellent animals to study hypercholesterolemia and atherosclerosis. They are considered superior to rabbits and rats. Because of this, we studied the effectiveness of GFP in lowering plasma cholesterol in miniature swine (16). In this study the effect of GFP on total cholesterol, LDLC, and LDLC:HDLC ratio was investigated. The pigs were randomized to either (1) a control diet (hog chow), (2) an atherogenic diet with 3% cellulose, or (3) an atherogenic diet with 3% GFP. The results demonstrated that GFP significantly lowered plasma cholesterol by nearly 30%, and improved the LDLC:HDLC by 31% as compared to the atherogenic cellulose diet with no effect on serum triglycerides. Upon completion of the feeding experiments, the animals were sacrificed and the effect of GFP on the development of atherosclerosis was examined. Thoracic and abdominal aorta, the arches and main branches of the coronary arteries were removed and examined grossly by histology. Surface area of plaques was measured by planimetry and computer graphic techniques. Despite variability, the affected pigs on the pectin supplemented atherogenic diet demonstrated up to an 85% decrease in plaque formation in the surface area of the aorta and 88% decrease in the narrowing of the coronary arteries. These studies strongly suggested that not only does GFP lower plasma cholesterol but might reduce formation of atheromatous plaque in the aorta and coronary vessels. We, therefore, extended these studies to determine if GFP would affect cholesterol levels and atherogenesis in animals with established hypercholesterolemia. Yucatan microswine were fed the aforementioned atherogenic diet with cellulose to establish hypercholesterolemia. The plasma cholesterols rose rapidly and were sustained at a level at least 12 times higher than baseline. One of the animals was sacrificed to establish atherosclerosis and the remaining animals were randomized to an atherogenic diet of 3% GFP or continued on the 3% atherogenic cellulose diet. The animals were sacrificed 270 days later and the extent of atherosclerosis was determined as previously described. Although cholesterol levels decreased, they did not decrease to a level of significance. However, GFP reduced the extent of atherosclerosis in both the aorta and coronary arteries. The mean surface area covered by atherosclerosis in the aorta was 13% in the group that did not receive the pectin compared to 5.3% in the group that did receive pectin. The mean coronary artery narrowing was 45% without pectin and 24% with pectin. These observations strongly suggest that GFP may have a direct beneficial effect on atherosclerosis by a mechanism independent of cholesterol levels (17).

A major problem in treating subjects with hypercholesterolemia is compliance. Because of this, we studied the effect of GFP on plasma cholesterol, triglycerides, and the lipoprotein fractions in a group of subjects with hypercholesterolemia who were unable or unwilling to alter their lifestyle. There were 27 subjects (nine males, 18 females, whose mean baseline plasma cholesterols were 273 mg/dl (range 208-420 mg/dl). All subjects were healthy volunteers who were not on steroids, hormones or medications that could alter or affect cholesterol levels. A four week equilibration period was followed by a four week treatment (placebo or pectin), followed by a four week period of no treatment, and then a four week treatment in which patients were crossed over with each subject acting as his/her own control. Because it is difficult to blind the mouthfeel of pectin, the GFP was given in capsule form, 0.5 gm GFP/capsule, 9- for three meals. This totaled 27 capsules per day, calculated so that patients would receive 15 gm/day. If the subjects did not eat three meals a day, they were still required to take the 15 gm in three-5 gm doses at the "normal" meal time. Placebo (starch) and pectin were encapsulated by our Pharmacy Service. At no time during the study was the code broken. Dietary records were kept and supervised by a dietician on the nutrition service. Since all subjects lived in the Gainesville area, this was an easy task. Compliance by the subjects was outstanding (98.4%). There was a 7.6% decrease in the mean plasma cholesterol level with 88.9% of the subjects demonstrating decreases. When the subjects were given placebo, cholesterol levels did not vary from the normal baseline of 275 mg/dl. No deviation from baseline occurred and only 44.4% of the subjects showed any decrease in plasma cholesterol. There was no significant change in the HDLC and TG. The LDLC decreased but was not significant (18). Our next effort was to develop a pectin product which was palatable and could allow ingestion of 15 gm of water-soluble daily fiber (WSF). Therefore, a dietary supplement made from a combination of GFP and eggwhite protein was developed. We initially tested this product in guinea pigs using our standard atherogenic diet protocol (19). We compared a chow diet versus an atherogenic cellulose diet, atherogenic eggwhite protein-pectin diet, and an atherogenic eggwhite-pectin cellulose diet. Only with the eggwhite pectin diet were we able to achieve significantly lower plasma cholesterol levels. We have recently reported that supplementing flax meal results in an even further lowering of the LDLC (20). We have extended these early observations on animals to a field study on 7 patients who were placed on a WSF product containing pectin, guar gum and eggwhite protein (Pro-Fibe™)diet.

All patients were instructed to take one serving of the product containing 5 gm of soluble fiber three times a day, preferably

TABLE 10.1. EFFECT OF PROFIBE™ ON SERUM LIPIDS

	Baseline				Day 30				% Decrease		
Patient	TC	LDLC	HDLC	Ratio	TC	LDLC	HDLC	Ratio	TC	LDLC	Ratio
C.S.	241	154	41	3.8	202	125	36	3.5	16	19	8
M.V.	244	172	39	4.4	205	141	38	3.7	16	18	16
C.C.	293	161	29	5.5	243	114	27	4.2	17	29	24
S.E.	291	219	36	6.1	255	176	43	4.1	12	20	33
F.R.	263	124	24	5.2	219	76	27	2.8	17	39	46
C.B.	233	166	28	5.9	172	117	27	4.3	26	29	27
J.S.	276	183	33	5.5	229	139	32	4.3	17	24	22
Average	263	168	33	5.2	218[1]	127[2]	33	3.8[3]	17	25	25

TC = Total Cholesterol
LDLC = Low Density Lipoprotein Cholesterol
HDLC = High Density Lipoprotein Cholesterol
[1] $p < 0.009$
[2] $p = 0.008$
[3] $p = 0.003$

at mealtime. ProFibe™ was mixed in the beverage of their choice. Patients were encouraged to follow a diet low in fat as recommended by the American Heart Association and exercise as prescribed by their physician. Gastrointestinal symptoms were determined by patient responses to a questionnaire which included items regarding stool frequency and stool consistency. In addition, patients were asked to maintain detailed records on frequency of cramping, bloating and dyspepsia.

Table 10.1 demonstrates the average cholesterol and cholesterol fraction changes. After 30 days cholesterol dropped from an average of 263 to 218. The LDLC had dropped from 168 to 127 and the LDLC/HDLC ratio had dropped from 5.2 to 3.8. No differences were noted in the HDLC estimation. This pilot study is very encouraging and verifies the benefit of following a reasonable diet and exercise program along with soluble fiber consumption. The finding of a 17% drop in total cholesterol, 25% drop in LDLC and 25% drop in LDLC/HDLC ratio is gratifying. Patient acceptance of the product has been enthusiastic and compliance has been excellent. We conclude, therefore, that these initial results demonstrate that dietary supplementation with 15 gm of water-soluble fiber is extremely useful in significantly lowering plasma cholesterol and improving the LDLC as well as improving the ratio of the LDLC/HDLC in patients with moderate hypercholesterolemia.

Recent evidence shows that one in four Americans has a cholesterol level which imparts an increased risk for premature coronary heart disease. A broader application in the form of dietary recommendations which include pectin-rich foods, and water-soluble fiber products such as the one we have developed, incorporated into a prudent diet aimed at the primary prevention of atherosclerosis and hypercholesterolemia in the general public seems justifiable.

ACKNOWLEDGEMENTS

Supported by grant No. 4910290562112 from the Florida Citrus Commission and No. RR-0082 from the General Clinical Research Grants, Division of Research Resources, National Institutes of Health.

I am grateful to my collaborators who contributed so much to these studies: Drs. A. W. Nelson, M. M. Baig, R. T. Guild, T. G. Baumgartner, R. Siragusa, and Messrs. C. W. Burgin, F. L. Robbins and R. W. Rice. The expert technical assistance of Patricia R. Vance and Ms. Elizabeth Patrick is also gratefully acknowledged.

BIBLIOGRAPHY

1. BAIG, M. M.; CERDA, J. J. "Studies on the role of citrus in health and disease." In *Citrus Nutrition and Quality.* Nagy, S.; Attaway, J. A.; Eds.; American Chemical Society: Washington, D.C., 1980, pp. 25-41.
2. BENNET, W. G.; CERDA, J. J. "Dietary fiber: fact and fiction." *Dig. Dis.* 1995, 14, 43-58.
3. KAY, R. N.; TRUSWELL, A. S. "Effect of citrus pectin on blood lipid and fecal steroid secretion in man." *Am. J. Clin. Nutr.* 1977, 30, 171.
4. BAIG, M. M.; CERDA, J. J. "Use of galactose oxidase tritiated-potassium borohydride method for labeling pectin polysaccharides." *Anal. Biochem.* 1979, 98, 429.
5. BAIG, M. M.; BURGIN, C. W.; CERDA, J. J. "Labeling and chemistry of grapefruit pectin substance." *Phytochemistry* 1980, 19, 1425.
6. GUILD, R. T.; BAIG, M. M.; BURGIN, C. W.; et al. "Absorption and distribution of orally administered radiolabeled pectin in the mouse." *Gastroenterology* 1981, 80, 1165.
7. BAIG, M. M.; BURGIN, C. W.; CERDA, J. J. "A comparison of the relative effectiveness of cholestyramine and pectin in rats." *Drug Nutr. Interac.* 1985, 5, 100.
8. BAIG, M. M.; BURGIN, C. W.; CERDA, J. J. "Influence of dietary pectin and cholestyramine on the activity of hepatic 3-hydroxyl 3-methylglutaryl coenzyme: a reductase in the rat." Med. Proc. 1983, 42, 171-187.
9. CERDA, J. J.; ROBBINS, F. L.; RICE, R. W.; BURGIN, C. W. "The effect of dietary grapefruit pectin and cholesterol on hepatic 7-hydroxy-cholesterol formation in the rat." *Clin. Res.* 1988, 36(3), 355A.
10. SIRAGUSA, R. J.; CERDA, J. J. "Methanol production from the degradation of pectin by human colonic bacteria." *Am. J. Clin. Nutr.* 1988, 47, 848-851.
11. GERENCSER, G. H.; CERDA, J. J.; BURGIN, C. W.; et al. "Unstirred water layers in rabbit intestine: effects of pectin." Proc. Soc. Exp. Biol. Med. 1984, 176, 183.
12. CERDA, J. J.; ROBBINS, F. L.; BURGIN, C. W.; et al. "Unstirred water layers in rabbit intestine: effects of guar gum." *J. PENN.* 1980, 11, 63.
13. BAIG, M. M.; BURGIN, C. W.; CERDA, J. J. "Effect of dietary pectin on iron absorption and turnover in rat." *J. Nutr.* 1983, 113, 2385.
14. BAEKEY, P. A.; BAIG, M. M.; BURGIN, C. W.; et al. "The effect of pectin on zinc and calcium absorption and turnover in rat." *Nutr. Int.* 1986, 2(2), 108.

15. CERDA, J. J.; BURGIN, C. W. "Non-binding of pectin to bile salts." *Dig. Dis. Sci.* 1986, 31(10), 1435.
16. BAEKEY, P. A.; CERDA, J. J.; BURGIN, C. W.; ROBBINS, F. L.; et al. "Grapefruit pectin inhibits hypercholesterolemia and atherosclerosis in miniature swine." *Clin. Cardiol.* 1988, 11, 595-600.
17. CERDA, J. J.; NORMANN, S. F.; SULLIVAN, M. P.; BURGIN, C. W.; et al. "Inhibition of atherosclerosis by dietary pectin in microswine with sustained hypercholesterolemia." *Circulation* 1994, 89, 1247-1253.
18. CERDA, J. J.; ROBBINS, F. L.; BURGIN, C. W.; BAUMGARTNER, T. G.; et al. "The effects of grapefruit pectin on patients at risk for coronary heart disease without altering diet or lifestyle." *Clin. Cardiol.* 1988, 11, 589-594.
19. CERDA, J. J.; ROBBINS, F. L.; BURGIN, C. W.; VATHUDA, S.; SULLIVAN, M. P. "Effectiveness of a grapefruit pectin product in lowering plasma cholesterol in guinea pigs." *Clin. Res.* 1991, 39, 80A.
20. CERDA, J. J.; ROBBINS, F. L.; SIRAGUSA, R. J.; BURGIN, C. W. "The effects of a protein-fiber product (PFP) supplemented with flax meal in total cholesterol and lipoprotein in rats." *Fed. Am. Soc. Exp. Biol. J.* 1994, 8, 5A162.

11

Folic Acid and Provitamin A Contents of Citrus Fruits and Their Products

Steven Nagy
Russell L. Rouseff

Citrus fruits and their juice products are considered important dietary sources for many health-promoting phytochemicals. Two vitamins found at noticeable levels in citrus are folic acid and provitamin A precursors (carotenoids). Recent evidence from our laboratories has indicated that the methodology to determine folic acid (folates) in citrus products considerably underestimated its true value. Recently developed HPLC methods coupled with a pretreatment utilizing conjugase enzymes included polyglutamate forms of folic acid that had previously been overlooked by standard microbiological methods. In an 8-fluid ounce glass of orange juice, folic acid values were noted to range from 10.8% to 24.0% RDI. With respect to vitamin A, the provitamin A contents of most citrus cultivars are primarily derived from ß-cryptoxanthin, ß-carotene and α-carotene. Tangerines, tangerine hybrids, and pigmented grapefruit are excellent sources of provitamin A, whereas oranges, white grapefruit, lemons and limes are poor sources. The edible portion of the following pigmented grapefruit contained the following amounts of ß-carotene: Ruby Red (4.2 μg/g), Ray Ruby (7.0 μg/g), Flame (8.6 μg/g) and Star Ruby (9.6 μg/g).

A large body of information has accumulated within the past two decades that strongly suggests individuals who regularly consume higher amounts of fruits and vegetables have a lower risk of developing diverse types of disease (1). Because of these findings, the National Academy of Sciences, the American Cancer Society and the National Cancer Institute have proposed modifications to our diets. Perhaps one of the most important is that individuals increase their consumption of fresh fruits and vegetables, especially citrus fruits and yellow/green vegetables.

Citrus fruits and their juice products have been historically recognized as an excellent dietary source of vitamin C, but more recently have been recognized as good sources for folic acid and provitamin A precursors. This chapter will focus on the composition, and potential health and nutritional benefits of folic acid and provitamin A precursors (carotenoids) in citrus.

FOLIC ACID

Folic acid (also known as folacin or folate) is a water-soluble B vitamin. The basic structure is represented by tetrahydrofolate and this molecule is a versatile carrier of activated one-carbon units. The one-carbon group carried by tetrahydrofolate is bonded to the N-5 or N-10 nitrogen atoms or to both. The one-carbon group may exist in three oxidation states, namely, most reduced (methyl), intermediate (methylene) or most oxidized (formyl, formimino or methenyl). The principal form of folate in citrus is found in the most reduced state, i.e., N^5-methyl tetrahydrofolate. Other polyglutamate forms have also been reported (2,3) and all are found in the reduced methyl state in citrus.

Folacin coenzymes play important metabolic roles in the transfer of single carbon units from one compound to another in amino acid metabolism and nucleic acid synthesis. These coenzymes are needed for the synthesis of purine, methionine and thymidylate, for the conversion of serine to glycine, and for the catabolism of histidine. The metabolism of folacin and vitamin B_{12} is linked as noted by the fact that the coenzyme, 5'-deoxyadenosyl, and methyl forms of vitamin B_{12} (cobalamins) catalyze a transmethylation from a folic acid cofactor to homocysteine to form methionine.

Determination and Content

Currently, the most common methods utilized for determination of folic acid are by microbiological assay. These assay systems generally employ either *Streptococcus faecalis* (4) or *Lactobacillus casei* (5). The microbiological method used for folate analysis in citrus juices is the method of Herbert (5) as modified by Strieff (6) utilizing *L. casei*. The AOAC method (4) utilizing *S. faecalis* is not used for citrus folate determination because Herbert (5) noted that *S. faecalis* can grow in a medium containing folic acid (pteroylglutamic acid) but does not grow in a medium containing N^5-methyltetrahydrofolate (a methylated form of folic acid), which is the predominant form in citrus.

Pretreatment of a food sample with folate polyglutamate hydrolase (conjugase) enzyme prior to assay by *L. casei* was reported as early as 1972 (7). Essentially, Tamura (7) noted that the response of *L. casei* alone to folates was dependent on the polyglutamyl chain; poor responses were elicited for folate compounds with greater than three glutamic acid residues. The use of a conjugase enzyme to digest polyglutamated forms of folate prior to assay by *L. casei* resulted in higher and more accurate values for total folates in food.

Recognizing the limitations of an assay system for citrus that relies only on *L. casei*, many investigators (2,3,8) now pretreat citrus samples with conjugase enzyme. Engelhardt and Gregory (8) examined the types of conjugase and found that hog kidney conjugase was appropriate and resulted in complete deconjugation of extracted polyglutamly folates in orange juice. Those investigators, however, raised some concerns regarding the use of chicken pancreas as a conjugase for foods containing citrate.

Additionally, in recent years, folate analyses has departed from the traditional use of microbiological assay (*L. casei*) to more sophisticated analytical techniques using reversed-phase HPLC methods and differing detection methods. Rouseff (9) and Gregory et al. (2) noted that fluorometric detection methods underestimate the amount of folate in orange juice. The method developed by White et al. (3) using selective amperometric detection on a glassy carbon electrode accurately quantifies 5-methyl tetrahydrofolate. However, White's method only detects the monglutamate form and must use conjugase pretreatment to deconjugate polyglutamate forms to the monoglutamate form. Nevertheless, the White method (3) is one of the more accurate methods to evaluate the total folate contents of citrus products.

Comparative examination of 5-methyl tetrahydrofolate in orange and grapefruit juices by the standard *L. casei* assay (no conjugase pretreatment) and by the HPLC/EC method of White et al. (3) is noted in Fig. 11.1. This figure shows that the HPLC/EC method yields folic acid values abut 16-63% higher than the *L. casei* assay. An 8-fl. oz. serving juice would yield about 7 to 10% of the RDI. Two salient features of the White et. al. (3) study were that: (A) conjugase enzyme pretreatment is required for a reasonably accurate determination of total folate and, (B) the response of *L. casei* to 5-methyl tetrahydrofolate is lower than when calibrated with oxidized folic acid monoglutamate. *L. casei* assay that does not include conjugase pretreatment and uses oxidized folic acid as the calibration standard will undoubtedly yield low folate values for citrus juice.

Table 11.1 lists orange juice folate values compiled from four recent studies. The studies of White et al. (3) and Bailey (10) used hog kidney conjugase for pretreatment of samples, whereas the study by Fellers et al (11) did not include conjugase pretreatment. Treatment conditions for orange juice were not reported by Souci et al. (12). Clay (13) evaluated several studies dating back to 1971 and reported that the average RDI value

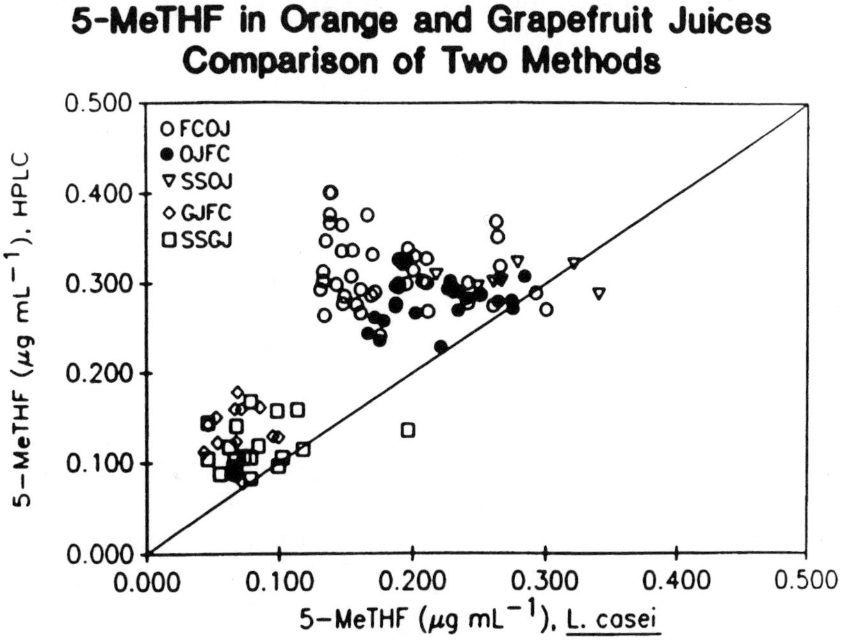

FIG. 11.1. 5-METHF IN ORANGE AND GRAPEFRUIT JUICES. HPLC METHOD VERSUS MICROBIOLOGICAL ASSAY (*L. CASEL*). FROM WHITE ET AL. (3)

for folate in 240 ml of orange juice ranged from 17.2% to 31.6% with a mean of 27.7%. The values compiled by Clay (13) show higher range and mean value than reported in Table 11.1, and may be due to less sophisticated methodologies used for folate determination during the 1970s and 80s.

Bioavailability

The bioavailability of folate from citrus juice is high (14-16). Only the monoglutamate form of folic acid is directly absorbed from the upper part of the small intestine. Polyglutamate forms in citrus are not absorbed and must be converted to the monoglutamate form by folypolyglutamate hydrolase enzymes associated with the intestinal mucosa. Coleman et al. (17) noted that 90% of folate monoglutamate and 50 to 90% of folate poly-

TABLE 11.1. ORANGE JUICE FOLATE VALUES (SELECTED STUDIES)

	240 ml at 11.8 BRIX		
Investigator	Low RDI	High RDI	Mean
White et al. (1991)	13.7%	24.0%	—
Fellers et al. (1991)	10.8%	21.6%	16.2%
Bailey (1994)	15.3%	19.3%	17.2%
Souci et al. (1989)	15.5%	24.0%	—

glutamate ingested from food is absorbed. The bioavailability of folate (mono- and polyglutamate forms) in citrus juice (18) approximates the absorption values of folate noted by Coleman et al. (17). The folate in orange juices is 50 to 60 percent monoglutamate, whereas 40 to 50 percent is di-, tri-, tetra-, penta-, hexa- and heptaglutamate (19, unpublished results).

Disease Conditions

Cancer Risk.—Folate deficiency has been shown to cause chromosomal damage. Extensive cellular changes in thymidylate activities and deoxynucleotide levels during folate deficiency may impede DNA repair and may lead to mutations and chromosomal damage (20). Butterworth et al. (21) administered oral folic acid to women with cervical cancer; there results suggested that folic acid may prevent progressions of cervical dysplasia or promote regression to normalcy. Patients with cervical dysplasia manifested low serum folate levels and Potischman (22) suggested that folate may have a role in protecting women from these dysplastic lesions.

In humans, hypomethylation of DNA has been observed in colorectal cancers and in their adenomatous polyp precursors. Giovannucci et al. (23) showed that high dietary folate intakes were inversely associated with the risk of colorectal adenoma in women. The apparent protective effect of fresh fruits and vegetables, major folate sources, on colorectal cancer incidence suggests that a methyl-deficient diet contributes to occurrence of this type malignancy. Colorectal cancer is the second leading cause of death from malignancies in the United States.

Animal studies have also confirmed the beneficial role of folate and other types of lipotropes (choline, methionine) in preventing the increased incidence of tumors and in the inhibition of tumor growth (24,25). An increased incidence of tumors of the liver, colon, esophagus and breast result from methyl group-deficient diets (25,26).

Cardiovascular Risk.—Cardiovascular diseases are a major cause of mortality and morbidity in the Western world. McCully (27) made the initial observation linking homocysteine concentrations and arteriosclerotic vascular disease more than 25 years ago. The association between plasma homocysteine concentration and atherosclerosis has more recently become the subject of a number of clinical studies that linked elevated blood homocysteine studies with coronary heart disease, cerebral vascular diseases, peripheral vascular disease and venous thromboembolism (20). Selhub et al. (28) noted the risk of extracranial carotid-artery stenosis in relation to both plasma homocysteine concentrations and nutritional determinants of hyperhomocysteinemia in elderly people.

Homocysteine is a highly reactive amino acid; it is toxic to vascular endothelium, can potentiate the auto-oxidation of low-density lipoprotein cholesterol and promotes thrombosis (29-31).

A nutritional link has been reported by several investigators (32-34) noting an inverse relationship between red-cell folate levels and serum vitamin B_{12} concentrations and hyperhomocysteinemia. In an extensive study with elderly patients, Selhub et al. (28) noted that the majority of persons with elevated plasma homocysteine concentrations showed insufficient concentrations of folate, vitamin B_{12}, or vitamin B_6.

Elevated homocysteine levels are amenable to nutritional intervention. Several investigators (35-38) have demonstrated that innocuous regimens of vitamin supplementation (including folate, vitamin B_{12} and vitamin B_6) effectively lowered moderately homocysteine concentrations to the normal range. Folic acid administered alone or with pyridoxine can reduce serum homocysteine concentrations (37).

Neural Tube Defects (NTD).—There is now strong scientific evidence supporting a link between folic acid intake and the prevention of neural tube defects in infants. The neural tube is embryonic tissue that forms the brain and spinal chord of a developing fetus. Because of the devastation of these defects, The Centers for Disease Control (39) have issued the following statement: "All women of childbearing age in the United States who are capable of becoming pregnant should consume 0.4 mg of folic acid per day for the purpose of reducing their risk of having a pregnancy affected with spina bifida or other neural tube defects. Because the effects of higher intakes are not well known but include complicating the diagnosis of vitamin B_{12} deficiency, care should be taken to keep total folate consumption at < 1 mg per day, except under the supervision of a physician. Women who have a prior neural tube defect-affected pregnancy are at high risk of having a subsequent affected pregnancy. When these women are planning to become pregnant, they should consult their physicians for advice. The Centers for Disease Control estimates that about 50% of all NTD can be prevented if women of childbearing age consume 0.4 mg of folic acid per day."

PROVITAMIN A PRECURSORS

Citrus and all other plant foods do not synthesize vitamin A, but form provitamin A compounds that can be converted to vitamin A. The most common forms of provitamin A compounds in citrus are the carotenoids. This large family of plant pigments is further subdivided into carotene (carotenoids containing only carbon and hydrogen) and xanthophylls (oxygenated carotenes). A structural condition of a carotenoid to possess provitamin A activity is an unsubstituted ß-ionone ring and an unchanged side chain. Sixteen carotenoids with provitamin A activity have been found in fruits (40). Of those 16 carotenoids, 11 have been identified in citrus, namely, α-carotene, ß-carotene, γ-carotene, mutatochrome, ß-semicarotenone, ß-cryptoxanthin, ß-cryptoxanthin-5, 6-epoxide, cryptoflavin, ß-apo-8'-carotenol, ß-apo-10'-carotenol and ß-apo-14'-carotenol. However, the provitamin A activity of citrus fruit is primarily derived from only four carotenoids, namely, α-carotene, ß-carotene, ß-cryptoxanthin and ß-apo-8^{1}-carotenol (concentrated in the peel).

Provitamin A carotenoids are cleaved in the intestinal mucosa by 15, 15^{1}-dioxygenase (41) to vitamin A aldehyde. Thereafter, aldehyde reductase reduces this aldehyde to the all trans vitamin A (retinol). The retinol molecule is then esterified with long-chain fatty acids, transported in the lymph and stored in the liver.

Fig. 11.2 depicts the conversion of ß-carotene to vitamin A. Although one molecule of ß-carotene may be converted into two molecules of vitamin A, the actual conversion is much less efficient because of several competing reactions that cleave ß-carotene nonsymmetrically (Fig. 11.2). ß-Carotene is degraded through oxidation at one or the other end of the polyene chain; the intermediates are the homologous carotenols. Bioassays confirm that only one-half of the ß-carotene molecule is active, thus 0.6 mg ß-carotene = 0.3 µg vitamin A = 1 IU vitamin A (40).

Determination and Content

Carotenoid compositional data is often difficult to compare due to the various methods used to quantify the carotenoids. Values from older studies employing spectroscopic methods to measure certain carotenoids were the most tenuous because they usually relied on converting the measured absorbance from a sample at a wavelength around 440 nm to a carotenoid composition using the molar absorptivity of the carotenoid of interest. However, since they often used liquid-liquid extraction to separate the carotenoids from the sample matrix, they generally had more than a single carotenoid in the measured solution and the results might have been high. Conversely, if care was not taken to protect the sample from light and oxygen during sample preparation, the reported values could be low due to carotenoid decomposition. Carotenoids in citrus occur mainly as esters. For ease of separation, they are saponified with a strong base to their alcohols. During this reaction, traces of acetone or other ketones will react with the aldo carotenoids to form artifacts (42).

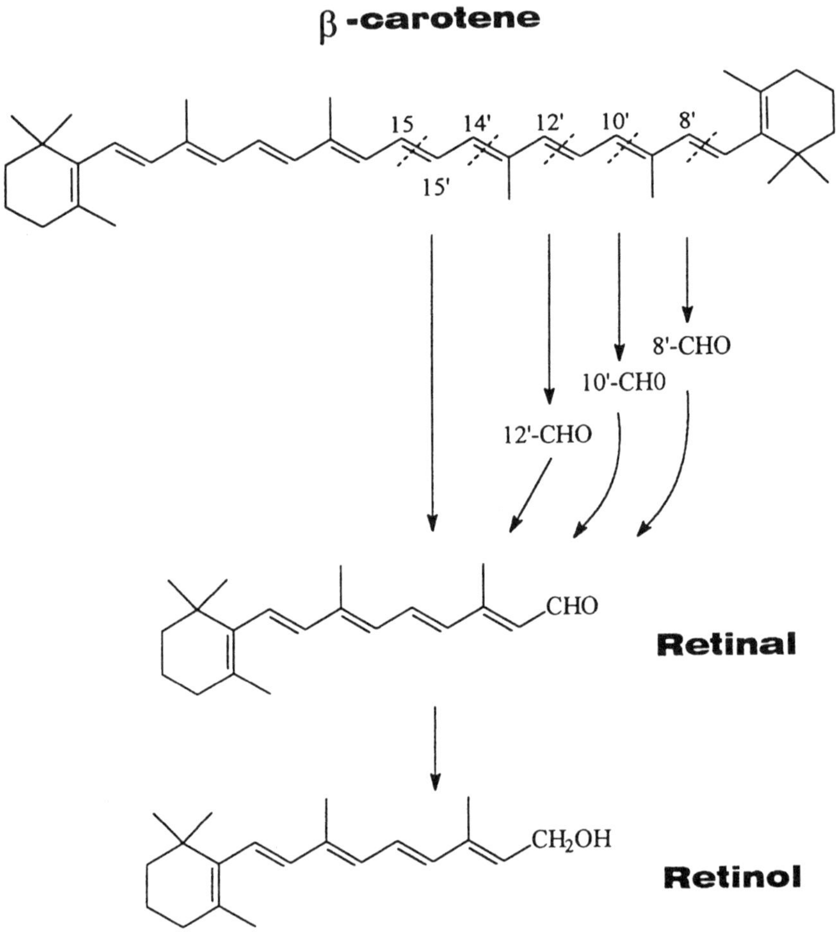

FIG. 11.2. CONVERSION OF ß-CAROTENE TO RETINOL (VITAMIN A).

With the advent of HPLC, it has been possible to separate individual citrus carotenoids in a relatively rapid manner. Used in combination with photodiode array detectors it has been possible to quantify each carotenoid from a single chromatographic separation using the absorbance at or near the absorbance maxima of each carotenoid of interest.

HPLC determinations of citrus provitamin A contents were effectively determined by Stewart (43). The provitamin A contents of citrus juices were primarily derived from α-carotene, ß-carotene and ß-cryptoxanthin. The following formula indicates that each of these carotenoids has a different provitamin A activity, namely:

$$\text{Total retinol equivalents} = \frac{\mu\text{g ß-carotene}}{6} + \frac{\mu\text{g } \alpha\text{-carotene} + \mu\text{g ß-carotene}}{12}$$

The values from Stewart's HPLC study of citrus juices are noted in Table 11.2. Orange juices were found to contain the least amount of provitamin A, whereas the tangerine (Dancy) and the tangerine hybrids (Robinson and Murcott) contained the most. Most of the vitamin A activity in tangerines derives from the high concentrations of ß-cryptoxanthin. All samples were taken from mature fruit, except Valencia. When mature, Valencia juice normally contains more provitamin A than Hamlin or Pineapple orange juices. Processing effects on individual carotenoids and vitamin A contents of citrus juices have not been ascertained.

There is a wide difference in provitamin A contents between white-fleshed grapefruit cultivars (Duncan, Marsh, Walters) and pigmented cultivars (Ruby Red, Flame, Ray Ruby, Star Ruby, Thompson) (44). White grapefruit contain only about 8 I.U. of vitamin A per 100 g juice (45). Ting and Deszyck (46) reported red and pink grapefruit juice to contain 1.0 to 1.4 mg of ß-carotene per 100 g of juice. These values when converted to a serving size of 8-fl. oz. would equal 3951 to 5508 I.U. of vitamin A. Rouseff et al. (47) showed the ß-carotene contents of the edible portion of pigmented grapefruit to contain:

Ruby Red (4.2 μg/g)	Ray Ruby (7.0 μg/g)
Flame (8.6 μg/g)	Star Ruby (9.6 μg/g)

These value would approximate 1680 to 3840 I.U. of vitamin A per 8-fl. oz. serving.

As noted by Fig. 11.3, oranges (Valencia and Washington Navel) are poor sources of ß-carotene. White grapefruit (Marsh) contains virtually no ß-carotene (40), whereas the red grapefruit (Ruby Red) is an excellent source for this nutrient. As a general rule, whitefleshed oranges, lemons, limes and white

TABLE 11.2. PROVITAMIN A CONTENT OF CITRUS JUICES

Juice	Vitamin A (I.U.)[1]	RDI percentage[2]
Hamlin	107	2.1
Pineapple	177	3.5
Valencia	111	2.2
Robinson	1523	30.5
Dancy	1287	25.7
Orlando	315	6.3
Murcott	4262	85.2

[1]Calculations based on ß-carotene equal to 1.66% International Units vitamin A/ug-equals 100%; α-carotene, 52.7%; ß-cryptoxanthin, 57%. Values based on 8-fl. oz. serving.
[2]Values based on 8-fl. oz. juice serving and calculated to a Reference Daily Intake value of 5000 I.U.

grapefruit contain minimal amounts of provitamin A carotenoids, whereas tangerines, tangerine hybrids, and red and pink grapefruit contain significant amounts.

DISEASE CONDITIONS

Possible Mechanistic Function

Retinoids possess powerful effects on cell differentiation and proliferation. They affect the differentiation of neoplastic and non-neoplastic cells and can act directly on non-neoplastic cells to suppress malignant transformation induced by chemical carcinogens, radiation, or transforming growth factors (1). Studies over the years have implicated a metabolite of retinol, retinoid acid, in the regulation of cellular differentiation. The mechanism of action of retinoids began with the discovery of nuclear receptor proteins that bind retinoic acid (48). Retinoic acid receptors are highly similar in structure to receptors that mediate steroid hormone effects. These binding receptors are thought to have important regulatory roles during embryogenesis and in maintaining the differentiated state of more mature cells (49). Very few of the genes regulated by retinoic acid recep-

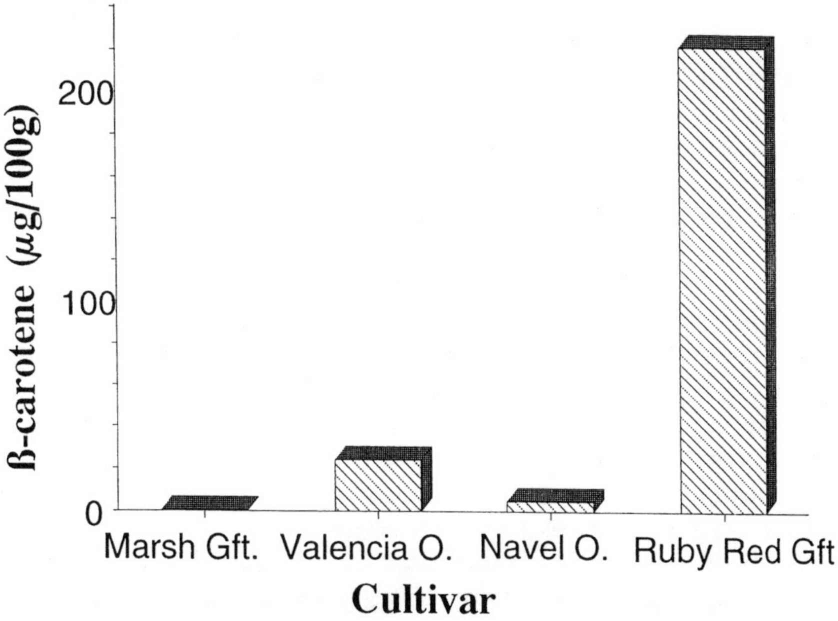

FIG. 11.3. COMPARISON OF THE ß-CAROTENE CONTENT AMONG MARSH GRAPEFRUIT, VALENCIA ORANGE, WASHINGTON NAVEL ORANGE AND RUBY RED GRAPEFRUIT.

tors (RAR) have been identified; however, the dysfunction of the RAR-gene leads to a dysfunction of retinoid acid in cell regulations and, thus, is implicated in the development of this type of leukemia. Of interest is the finding that treatments with vitamin A or other retinoids in pharmacologic quantities have had some success in producing remissions of leukemia (51).

Cancer Risk

In 1981, Peto and colleagues (52) reviewed the literature at that time and presented the question "Can dietary ß-carotene materially reduce cancer rates?" Since that time there has been a proliferation of experiments designed to discriminate between the potential capabilities of preformed vitamin A versus provitamin A carotenoids to modulate different human cancer states.

ß-Carotene is a strong antioxidant, and high dietary intakes may prevent cancers arising from oxygen-free radicals that damage DNA. Free radicals readily react with the many double bonds in lipids of the membranes surrounding cells as well as inside the cell. Cell membranes can be damaged or even destroyed in this process, producing cell breakdown and finally death. Free radicals can also damage the chromosomal material in the nucleus of the cell and the resulting damage to the genetic code could lead to the development of cancerous cells.

ß-Carotene has been shown to be effective in protecting lipid membranes from free radical damage (53), particularly under low oxygen partial pressure (54). The latter finding is of particular interest as enzyme or chainbreaking antioxidants are most effective at high oxygen pressures, whereas lower oxygen concentrations are typically found in capillary beds of tissues far removed from direct exposure to oxygen.

Both the Surgeon General's Report (55) and the NRC Report (1) concluded that the consumption of foods that are high in ß-carotene may protect against some epithelial cancers, and both reports concurred that the evidence is strongest in the case of lung cancer. The evidence presented in the Surgeon General's Report and the NRC Report did not support a significant, positive association between the amount of preformed vitamin A in the diet or the levels of retinol in blood and reduced cancer rates.

Evidence appears to favor foods rich in ß-carotene or provitamin A carotenoids over preformed vitamin A in cancer chemoprevention (1,52). There is an emerging concept implying that retinol (vitamin A) and ß-carotene should be treated as distinct entities. The metabolic activity of ß-carotene and its putative function in cancer chemoprevention may be quite different from retinol (56). ß-Carotene has been shown in chemical studies to have antioxidant properties that are not shared by retinol (57). Additionally, ß-carotene may modulate membrane properties important to cell-cell signaling or possibly serve as an intracellular precursor to retinoic acid (58). Napoli and Race (59) demonstrated that rodent tissues are capable of converting ß-carotene to retinoic acid that by-passes formation of retinol. Wang (60) has suggested that ß-carotene may prevent cancer because of the way humans convert it into the potent agent, retinoic acid. Whereas ß-carotene is a strong antioxidant and can prevent cancers arising from oxygen-free radicals, retinoic acid is a weak antioxidant. However, retinoic acid is very effective at treating tumors caused by agents that do not form oxygen radicals, such as cancers of the blood and bladder (60).

Both ß-carotene and retinoids have an inhibitory effect on cancers of the mouth, lung, bladder and breast (61). The consensus of opinion, based on many epidemiological studies, is that diets rich in provitamin A carotenoids are protective against a variety of epithelial cancers.

Heart Disease

In the ten-year Physicians' Health Study, 22,000 male doctors were given ß-carotene, aspirin, a placebo, or a combination of the three. Preliminary results (62) adjusted for aspirin and age found that those subjects given ß-carotene experienced only about half the number of major cardiovascular events as those subjects given a placebo. The men in this study were given 50 mg ß-carotene every other day.

It has been strongly recommended that the amount of dietary ß-carotene be increased in human diets. Lachance (63) has reported that the average American typically consumes only about 1.5 mg a day of ß-carotene.

CONCLUSION

Folate, primarily because of its critical role as a versatile carrier of activated one-carbon units, has ben implicated in a number of devastating disease disorders. Low levels of dietary folate (methyl-deficient diets) translate to low serum levels. Deficiencies of folate result in chromosomal damage, hypomethylation of DNA and neural tube defects in infants. More recent research findings have implicated low levels of serum folate with elevated levels of homocysteine. The link between elevated blood homocysteine levels and various cardiovascular disorders have been noted. Frequent consumption of fruits (especially citrus) and vegetables reduces cancer risk (1,64). Whether this benefit results from the presence of ß-carotene, other carotenoids, antioxidant vitamins and/or other factors in fruits and vegetables remains to be established. What has been ascertained for ß-carotene are the following (65):

A. Dietary carotenoid intake is positively associated with serum carotene concentrations.

B. Cigarette smoking, alcohol consumption and diets low in fruits and vegetables containing carotenoids continues to be strongly associated with lower circulating carotenoid concentrations.

C. Several studies have consistently reported an inverse association of dietary ß-carotene intake and the risk of lung cancer.

D. Several studies have strongly inferred that serum carotenoid levels especially ß-carotene, are negatively associated with oral, pharyngeal, esophageal and squamous cell lung cancers.

The data of Napoli and Race (58) are intriguing and may indicate that different biochemical mechanisms are operative. These Napoli-Race data suggest that ß-carotene metabolism is not simply a process for producing retinaldehyde, that is subsequently metabolized to either retinol or retinoic acid, but rather, a complex metabolism that can generate retinoic acid without cleavage of ß-carotene to retinaldehyde.

BIBLIOGRAPHY

1. National Research Council. "Cancer." *In* Diet and Health: Implications for Reducing Chronic Risk. National Academy Press: Washington, D.C., 1989.
2. GREGORY, J. F.; SARTAIN, D. B.; DAY, B. P. F. "Fluorometric determination of folacin in biological materials using high performance liquid chromatography." *J. Nutr.* 1984, 114, 341-353.
3. WHITE, D. R.; LEE, H. S.; KRUGER, R. E. "Reversed-phase HPLC/EC determination of folate in citrus juice by direct injection with column switching." *J. Agric. Food Chem.* 1991, 39, 714-717.

4. AOAC. *Official Methods of Analysis, 15th Ed.* Association of Official Analytical Chemists: Washington, D.C., 1990, Vol. 2, 1080-1084.
5. HERBERT, V. "Aseptic addition method for *Lactobacillus casei* assay of folate activity in human serum." *J. Clin. Pathol.* 1966, 19, 12-16.
6. STREIFF, R. R. "Folate levels in citrus and other juices." *Am. J. Clin. Nutr.* 1971, 24, 1390-1392.
7. TAMURA, T.; SHIN, Y. S.; WILLIAMS, M. A.; STOKSTAD, E. L. R. "*Lactobacillus casei* response to pteroylpolyglutamates." *Anal. Biochem.* 1972, 49, 517-520.
8. ENGELHARDT, R.; GREGORY, J. F. "Adequacy of enzymatic deconjugation in quantification of folate in foods." *J. Agric. Food Chem.* 1990, 38, 154-158.
9. ROUSEFF, R. "The use of dual detectors for HPLC multivitamin analysis of citrus juices." *In* Liquid Chromatographic Analysis of Foods and Beverages, Vol. 1. Charalambous, G., Ed. Academic Press: New York, 1979.
10. BAILEY, L. Unpublished results. University of Florida, Gainesville, 1994.
11. FELLERS, P. J.; NIKDEL, S.; LEE, H. S. "Five-year data base for the content of eleven essential vitamins and minerals for nutrition labeling in the major processed Florida citrus juice products." *Proc. Fla. State Hortic. Soc.* 1991, 104, 89-94.
12. SOUCI, S. W.; FACHMANN, W.; KRAUT, H. *Food Composition and Nutrition Table 1989/90.* Wissenschaftliche Verlagsgesellschaft mbH: Stuttgart, Germany, 1989.
13. CLAY, C. Unpublished results. Florida Department of Citrus, Lake Alfred, 1994.
14. RHODE, B. M.; COOPER, B. A.; FARMER, F. A. "Effect of orange juice, folic acid and oral contraceptives on serum folate in women taking a folate-restricted diet." *J. Am. Coll. Nutr.* 1983, 2, 221-230.
15. ABAD, A. R.; GREGORY, J. F. "Determination of folate bioavailability with a rat bioassay." *J. Nutr.* 1987, 117, 866-873.
16. BAILEY, L. B. "The role of folate in human nutrition." *Nutr. Today.* 1990, Sept./Oct., 12-19.
17. COLEMAN, N.; GREEN, R.; METZ, J. "Prevention of folate deficiency by food fortification. II. Absorption of folic acid from fortified staple foods." *Am. J. Clin. Nutr.* 1975, 28, 459-464.
18. GREGORY, J. F. Unpublished results. University of Florida, Gainesville, 1995.
19. GREGORY, J. F. "Chemical and nutritional aspects of folate synthesis, stability and bioavailability of dietary folats." *In* Advances in Food Research. Kinsella, J., Ed. Academic Press: New York, 1989.
20. TILLOTSTON, J. E.; GERSHOFF, S. M.; HUMBER, A. M.; CRIM, M. C. "Review of the medical and nutritional literature pertaining to the health and nutritional benefits of citrus fruits and juices." Food Policy Institute: Tufts University: Medford, Mass, 1993.
21. BUTTERWORTH, C. E.; HATCH, K. D.; GORE, H.; MUELLER, H.; KRUMDIECK, C. L. "Improvement in cervical dysplasia associated

with folic acid therapy in users of oral contraceptives." *Am. J. Clin. Nutr.* 1982, 35, 73-82.
22. POTISCHMAN, N. "Nutritional epidemiology of cervical neoplasia." *J. Nutr.* 1983, 123, 424-429.
23. GIOVANNUCCI, E.; STAMPFER, J. J.; COLDITZ, G. A.; RIMM, E. B.; TRICHOPOULOS, D.; RSNER, B. A.; SPEIZER, F. E.; WILLETT, W. C. "Folate, methionine and alcohol intake and risk of colorectal adenoma.": *J. Natl. Cancer Inst.* 1993, 85, 875-884.
24. LEUCHTENBERGER, R.; LEUCHTENBERGER, C.; LASZLO, D.; LEWISOHN, R. "The influence of folic acid on spontaneous breast cancers in mice." *Science.* 1945, 101, 46.
25. HOOVER, K. L.; LYNCH, P. H.; POIRIER, L. A. "Profound postinitiation enhancement by short-term severe methionine, choline, vitamin B_{12}, and folate deficiency of hepatocarcinogensis in F 344 rats given a single low-dose diethylnitrosamine injection." *J. Natl. Cancer, Inst.* 1984, 73, 1327-1336.
26. MIKOL, Y. B.; HOOVER, K. L.; CREASIA, D.; POIRIER, L. A. "Hepatocarcinogenesis in rats fed methyl-deficient, amino acid-defined diets." *Carcinogensis.* 1993, 4, 1619-1629.
27. MCCULLY, K. S. "Vascular pathology of homocysteinemia: implications for the pathogensis of arteriosclerosis." *Am. J. Pathol.* 1969, 56, 111-128.
28. SELHUB, J. et al. "Association between plasma homocysteine concentrations and extacranial carotid-artery stenosis." *N. Engl. J. Med.* 1995, 332, 286-291.
29. HARKER, L. A.; ROSS, R.; SLICHTER, S. J.; SCOTT, C. R. "Homocystine-induced arteriosclerosis: the role of endothelial cell injury and platelet response in its genesis." *J. Clin. Invest.* 1976, 58, 731-741.
30. PARTHASARATHY, S. "Oxidation of low density lipoprotein by thiol compounds leads to its recognition by the acetyl LDL receptor." *Biochim. Biophys. Acta.* 1987, 917, 337-340.
31. GRAEBER, J. E.; SLOTT, J. H.; ULANE, R. E.; SCHULMAN, J. D.; STUART, M. J. "Effect of homocysteine and homocystine on platelet and vascular arachidonic acid metabolism." *Pediatr. Res.* 1982, 16, 490-493.
32. COREY, M. C.; FENNELLY, J. J.; FITZGERALD, O. "Homocystinuria. II. Subnormal serum folate levels, increased folate clearance and effects of folic acid therapy." *Am. J. Med.* 1968, 45, 26-31.
33. WILCKEN, D. E. L.; WILCKEN, B. "The pathogenesis of coronary artery disease: A possible role for methionine metabolism. *J. Clin. Invest.* 1976, 57, 1079-1082.
34. KANG, S. S.; WONG P. W.; NORUSIS, M. "Homocysteinemia due to folate deficiency." *Metabolism.* 1987, 36, 458-462.
35. BRATTSTROM, L. E.; ISRAELSSON, B.; JEPPSSON, J. O.; HULTBERG, B. L. "Folic acid - an innocuous means of reducing plasma homocysteine." *Scand. J. Clin. Lab. Invest.* 1988, 48, 215-221.

36. BRATTSTROM, L.; ISRAELSSON, B.; NOPRRVING, B. "Impaired homocysteine metabolism in early-onset cerebral and peripheral occlusive arterial disease: effects of pyridoxine and folic acid treatment." *Atherosclerosis.* 1990, 81, 51-60.
37. MALINOW, M. R. "Hyperhomocysteinemia: A common and easily reversible risk factor for occlusive atherosclerosis." *Circulation.* 1990, 6, 2004-2006.
38. UBBINK, J. B.; VERMAAK, W. J.; VAN DER MERWE, A.; BECKER, P. J. "Vitamin B_{12}, vitamin B_6 and folate nutritional status in men with hyperhomocysteinemia." *Am. J. Clin. Nutr.* 1993, 57, 47-53.
39. Centers for Disease Control. "Recommendations for the use of folic acid to reduce the number of cases of spina bifida and other neural tube defects." MMWR. 1992, 41, 1-7.
40. GROSS, J. *Pigments in Fruits.* Academic Press: New York, 1987.
41. LAKSHMANAN, M. E.; CHANSANG, N.; OLSON, J. A. "Purification and properties of carotene 15, 15'-dioxygenase of rabbit intestine." *J. Lipid Res.* 1972, 13, 477-482.
42. STEWART, I.; WHEATON, T. A. "Conversion of -citraurin to reticulalaxanthin and -apo-8'-carotenal to citranaxanthin during the isolation of carotenoids from citrus." *Phytochemistry.* 1973, 12, 2947-2951.
43. STEWART, I. "Provitamin A and carotenoid content of citrus juices." *J. Agric. Food Chem.* 1977, 25, 1132-1137.
44. SHAW, P. E.; NAGY, S. "Grapefruit juices." *In* Fruit Juice Processing Technology. Nagy, S.; Chen, C. S.; Shaw, P. E., Eds. AgScience, Inc: Auburndale, Florida, 1993.
45. ADAMS, C. F. Agriculture Handbook No. 456; Agricultural Research Service, USDA: Washington, D. C., 1975.
46. TING, S. V.; DESZYCK, E. J. "The internal color and carotenoid pigments of Florida red and pink grapefruit." *Proc. Am. Soc. Hortic. Sci.* 1958, 712, 271-277.
47. ROUSEFF, R. L.; SADLER, G. D.; PUTMAN, T. J.; DAVIS, J. E. "Determination of ß-carotene and other hydrocarbon carotenoids in red grapefruit cultivars." *J. Agric. Food Chem.* 1992, 40, 47-51.
48. PETKOVICH, M.; BRAND, N. J.; DRUST, A.; CHAMBON, P. "A human retinoic acid receptor which belongs to the family of nuclear receptors." *Nature.* 1987, 330, 444-450.
49. ROSS, A. C. "Vitamin A: Current understanding of the mechanisms of action." *Nutr. Today.* 1991, 26, 6-12.
50. CHANG, K. S.; TRUJILLO, J. M.; OGURA, T.; CASTIGLIONE, C. M.; KIDD, K. K.; ZHAO, S.; FREIREICH, E. J.; STASS, S. A. "Rearrangement of the retinoic acid receptor gene in acute promyelocytic leukemia." *Leukemia.* 1991, 5, 200-204.
51. CASTAIGNE, S.; CHOMIENNE, C.; DANIEL, M. T.; BALLERINI, P.; BERGER, R.; FENAUX, P.; DEGOS, L. "All trans retinoic acid as a differentiation therapy for acute promyelocytic leukemia." *Blood.* 1990, 76, 1704-1709.

52. PETO, R.; DOLL, R.; BUCKLEY, J. D.; SPORN, M. B. "Can dietary beta-carotene materially reduce human cancer rates." *Nature.* 1981, 290, 201-208.
53. KRINSKY, N. I.; DENEKE, S. M. "Interaction of oxygen and oxyradicals with carotenoids." *J. Natl. Cancer Inst.* 1982, 69, 205-210.
54. BURTON, G. W.; INGOLD, G. W. "Beta-carotene: an unusual type of lipid antioxidant." *Science.* 1984, 224, 569-573.
55. U.S. Department of Health and Human Services. The Surgeon General's Report on Nutrition and Health. U.S. Govt. Printing Office: Washington, D. C., 1988.
56. ZIEGLER, R. G. "Vegetables, fruits, and carotenoids and the risk of cancer." *Am. J. Clin. Nutr.* 1991, 53, 251S-259S.
57. BENDICH, A.; OLSON, J. A. "Biological actions of carotenoids." *FASEB J.* 1989, 3, 1927-1932.
58. NAPOLI, J. L; RACE, K. R. "Biogenesis of retinoic acid from ß-carotene: differences between the metabolism of -carotene and retinal." *J. Biol. Chem.* 1988, 263, 17372-17377.
59. NAPOLI, J. L.; RACE, K. R. "The biosynthesis of retinoic acid from retinol by rat tissues *in vitro. Arch. Biochem. Biophys.* 1987, 255, 95-101.
60. WANG, X. D. "Anti-cancer effects of beta-carotene linked to metabolism." *Food Chem. News.* 1992, October 19, 48.
61. HONG, W. K.; LOTAN, R. Retinoids in Oncology. Marcel Dekker, Inc: New York, 1993.
62. GAZIANO, J. M.; MANSON, J. E.; RIDKER, P. M.; BURING, J. E.; HENNEKENS, C. H. "Beta-carotene therapy for chronic stable angina." *Circulation.* 1990, 92 (4) (Suppl. III), 201.
63. LACHANCE, P. "Dietary intake of carotenes and the carotene gap." *Clin. Nutr.* 1988, 7(3) 118-122.
64. BLOCK, G.; PATTERSON, B.; SUBAR, A. "Fruit, vegetables and cancer prevention: a review of the epidemiological evidence." *Nutr. Cancer.* 1992, 18, 1-29.
65. ROSS, A. C. "Vitamin A and cancer." *In* Nutrition and Disease Update: Cancer. Carroll, K. K.; Kritchevsky, D., (Eds.). AOCS Press: Champaign, IL, 1993.

12

The Importance of the B-Ring of the Limonoid Nucleus to the Cancer Chemopreventive Activity of Citrus Limonoids

Edward G. Miller
Jo Lynn Porter-Wright
William H. Binnie
Ingrid Y. Guo
Shin Hasegawa

Three citrus limonoids—limonol, deoxylimonic acid, and limonin carboxymethoxime—were tested for cancer chemopreventive activity. Each of these chemicals can be formed from limonin, a potential by-product of the citrus industry. In each case, the B-ring of the limonoid nucleus is modified. The solutions of the limonoids, like the solution of the carcinogen were applied topically to the tissues. For each experiment, there was a total of 71 applications, 35 with the carcinogen and 36 with the solution of the limonoid. The treatments with limonin carboxymethoxime significantly reduced both tumor number and tumor burden.

The treatments with deoxylimonic acid and limonol were ineffective. These results suggest that an intact B-ring and the double bond at C-7 are critical to antineoplastic activity.

Limonoids, such as limonin and nomilin, have long been a problem for the citrus industry. Both of these chemicals are extremely bitter (1, 2) and their presence in citrus juices and other processed products can easily affect consumer acceptance. For this reason, early research on the citrus limonoids centered on the metabolism of these chemicals (3-5), on techniques to reduce the concentration of limonin and nomilin in the final product (6), and on variations in the concentration of these two chemicals throughout the growing season and in different cultivars (7, 8). Recently, it has been found that the citrus limonoids may have commercial importance. Studies conducted primarily at the University of Maine have shown that limonin and several related compounds are effective insect control agents (9, 10). The data showed that these chemicals have antifeedant activity against the spruce budworm, the Colorado potato beetle, the fall armyworm, and the corn earworm. Several laboratories have also shown that some of these chemicals can inhibit the development of cancer in a variety of different animal models (11-18). Antineoplastic activity has been observed in carcinogen-induced tumor models for the forestomach, lung, skin, and oral mucosa. The carcinogens used in these experiments were benzo[a]pyrene and 7,12-dimethylbenz[a]anthracene (DMBA). How these citrus chemicals might be affecting the action of the carcinogen is still not clear. Some studies (11, 16, 17, 19) suggest that the active limonoids are type A blocking agents, inducers of increased glutathione S-transferase activity (20). Other studies (14) question whether changes in glutathione S-transferase activity can account for the inhibitory effect of limonoids in some tumor models.

Using the hamster cheek pouch model, we have tested five citrus limonoids for cancer chemopreventive activity (12-15). The results showed that two of these chemicals, limonin and limonin 17-ß-D-glucopyranoside, could inhibit by 55 to 60% the development of the DMBA-induced tumors. The other chemicals, nomilin, nomilin 17-ß-D-glucopyranoside and nomilinic acid 17-ß-D-glucopyranoside were inactive. As a continuation of this research, limonin carboxymethoxime, deoxylimonic acid and limonol have now been tested for cancer chemopreventive activity. A brief preliminary report of the results with limonin carboxymethoxime and deoxylimonic acid was included in an earlier publication (15). Each of the test chemicals can be prepared from limonin. A simple chemical reaction is used to form limonin carboxymethoxime. The substrates for this reaction are limonin and carboxymethoxylamine hemihydrochloride. Certain strains of bacteria can convert limonin into either deoxylimonic acid or limonol (6). Since large amounts of limonin can be extracted from a waste product of the citrus industry, seeds (21), each of these limonoids could be produced in quantity.

The structures of limonin, limonin carboxymethoxime, deoxylimonic acid, and limonol are noted in Fig. 12.1. In each of the new limonoids, the major modification and in two cases (limonin carboxymethoxime and limonol) the only modification is to the B-ring of the limonoid nucleus. In limonin, the limonoid nucleus is a collection of five rings. As illustrated, these rings are the A, A', B, C, and D rings.

HAMSTER CHEEK POUCH MODEL

One of the advantages of this tumor model for oral carcinogenesis is that the suspected cancer chemopreventive agent can be added to the diet or applied topically to the pouch. Topical treatments are especially important when only a small amount of the chemical is available. Topical applications were used in the experiments with limonin carboxymethoxime, deoxylimonic acid and limonol.

The same basic procedure was used for the two experiments. Sixty female Syrian golden hamsters (Lak:LVG) were used in the first experiment with limonin carboxymethoxime and deoxylimonic acid. Forty hamsters were used in the second experiment with limonol. All of the animals were purchased from the Charles River Breeding Laboratories (Wilmington, MA). The

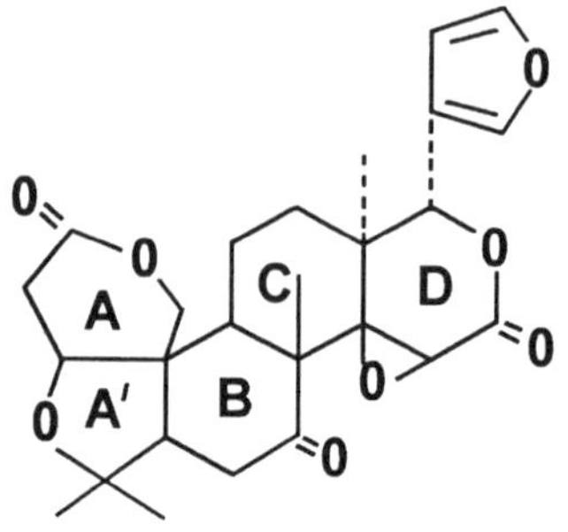

LIMONIN

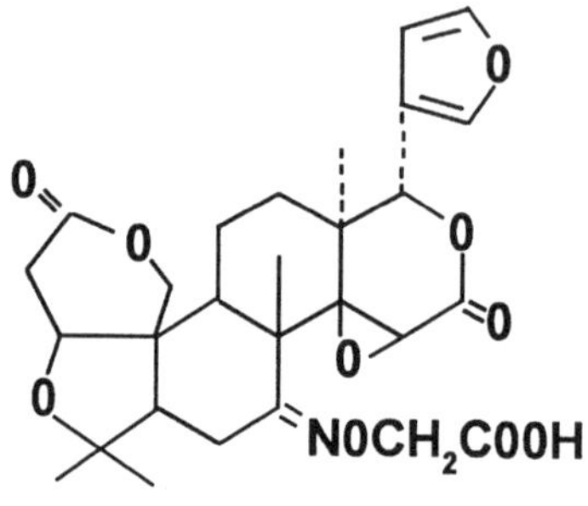

LIMONIN CARBOXYMETHOXIME

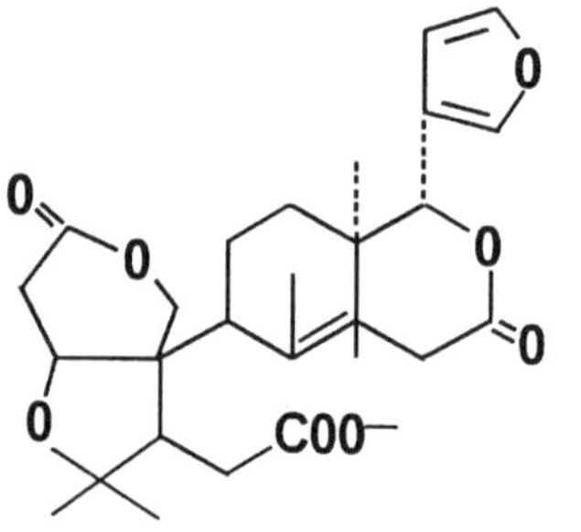

DEOXYLIMONIC ACID

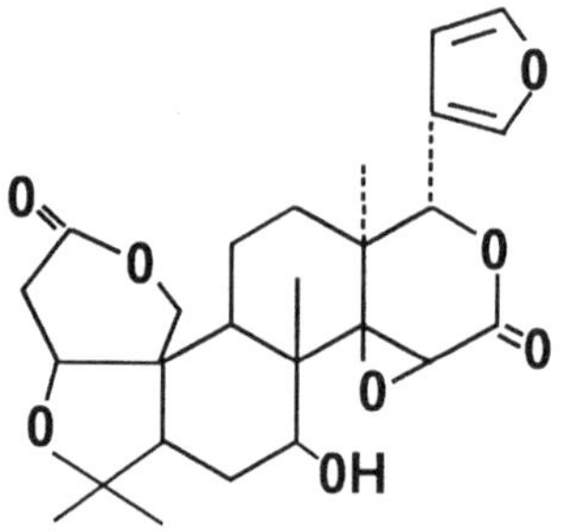

LIMONOL

FIG. 12.1. CHEMICAL STRUCTURE OF LIMONIN, LIMONIN CARBOXYMETHOXIME, DEOXYLIMONIC ACID, AND LIMONOL.

animals were housed in stainless steel cages in a room maintained at 22°C with a 12 hour light-dark cycle. After arriving, the hamsters were given 8 days to adjust to their new surroundings. During this time and throughout the rest of the experiment, water and food were provided *ad libitum*.In the first experiment, the hamsters were separated into three equal groups. The left buccal pouches of the animals in these three groups were pretreated with two separate daily applications of either water (group 1), a solution of limonin carboxymethoxime (group 2), or a solution of deoxylimonic acid (group 3). To evaluate stoichiometric changes, the concentration of the solution of limonin carboxymethoxime was adjusted to 3% (w/v) and the solution of deoxylimonic acid was set at 2.5% (w/v). The two limonoids were dissolved in water. Following the two initial treatments, 17 hamsters were selected from each group. The left buccal pouches of these experimental animals were painted 5 times per week. On an alternating week-to-week basis, the left buccal pouches of all of the animals were treated with two or three applications of a 0.5% solution of the carcinogen, DMBA, dissolved in heavy mineral oil. On alternate days, the pouches were either treated with water (group 1), a 3% solution of limonin carboxymethoxime (group 2), or a 2.5% solution of deoxylimonic acid (group 3). The other animals, three per group, served as controls. The left buccal pouches of these hamsters were also painted 5 times per week. Two or three times per week all of the pouches were treated with heavy mineral oil. On alternate days, the pouches of the control animals were either treated with water (group 1), a 3% solution of limonin carboxymethoxime (group 2), or a 2.5% solution of deoxylimonic acid (group 3).

In the second experiment, the hamsters were divided into two equal groups (20 animals/group).The left buccal pouches were pretreated with two separate daily applications of a 50:50 mixture of DMSO and propylene glycol (group 1) or a 2.5% solution of limonol (group 2), dissolved in a 50:50 mixture of DMSO and propylene glycol. Each group was then separated into 17 experimental animals and 3 controls. The left buccal pouches of all of the hamsters were again treated 5 times per week. For the experimental animals, the pouches were painted every other day with the 0.5% solution of DMBA. On alternate days, the pouches were either treated with the 50:50 mixture of DMSO and propylene glycol (group 1) or a 2.5% solution of limonol (group 2). The treatment pattern for the control animals was slightly different. Every other day the left buccal pouches were painted with heavy mineral oil, the solvent used to dissolve the carcinogen. On alternate days, the left buccal pouches were either treated with the 50:50 mixture of DMSO and propylene glycol (group 1) or the 2.5% solution of limonol (group 2). In each experiment, the solutions of the citrus limonoids were prepared on the day of use. All of the solutions were painted on the pouches with a camel hair brush. Each application places approximately 50 ml of the solution on the surface of the pouch (23).

Four experimental animals died during the two experiments. The deaths occurred early before the hamsters had a chance to develop tumors. All of these animals were excluded from the study. In each experiment, there was a total of 71 treatments, 35 with either the 0.5% solution of DMBA (experimental animals) or heavy mineral oil (control animals) and 36 with either the solvent used to dissolve the limonoids or one of the solutions of the citrus limonoids. Two or three days after the last treatment, all of the hamsters were sacrificed. The left buccal pouches were excised and the tumors, when present, were counted and measured (length, width, and height). The sum of the three measurements divided by six was used to calculate an average radius for each tumor. Using the formula for the volume of a sphere, an approximation of the volume of each tumor was determined. The sum of the volumes of all the tumors in one pouch was defined to be the animal's total tumor burden (12, 22, 23). Once the gross tumor data had been collected, the pouches were fixed in 10% formalin. The tissues were embedded in paraffin and processed by routine histological techniques. The data from the macroscopic and microscopic observations were used to assess differences in tumor incidence, number, burden, and type. Chi-square analysis and the Student's t-test were used to compare the data from the experimental groups. The procedures used in these two experiments were identical to the procedures used in our earlier work with limonin, nomilin, and the three limonoid glucosides (12-15).

Limonin Carboxymethoxime and Deoxylimonic Acid

At the end of the first experiment, the number of hamsters in the three experimental groups was 17 (group 1), 16 (group 2), and 17 (group 3). All of the pouches from the animals in group 2 had visible tumors. Two of the pouches, one from an animal in group 1 and another from a hamster in group 3, were free of tumors. Most of the pouches, 15 of 17 in group 1, 13 of 16 in group 2, and 15 of 17 in group 3, contained multiple tumors. Since the tumors were exophytic, well defined, and tended to be spherical in shape (23, 24), the three measurements (length, width, and height) were used to calculate an average radius for each tumor. These values ranged from 0.7 to 4.8 mm. The values for tumor volume ranged from 1.3 to 472 mm^3.

The gross tumor data for the first experiment is given in Table 12.1. As illustrated, the number of tumors ranged from a low of 49 (group 2) to a high of 79 (group 1). Comparing the data for group 2 to the data for group 1, it can be seen that the treatments with limonin carboxymethoxime led to a 35% decrease in average tumor number and a similar decrease in average tumor burden. The difference in average tumor number (group 1 vs. group 2) was significant, $p<0.025$. A similar comparison, group 3 vs. group 1, showed that the treatments with deoxylimonic acid led to a 25% reduction in average tumor number. This effect on tumor number was offset by the fact that the tumors in this group were slightly larger. Overall this led to an increase in average tumor burden for group 3 (10%). These difference in average tumor number and burden were not significant.

Further analysis of the data suggested that one of the animals in group 2 was a potential outlier. An extremely large tumor was found in the pouch from this animal. The tumor radius was 4.8 mm and the tumor volume was 472 mm^3. This one tumor accounted for 34% of the total tumor burden for

TABLE 12.1. EFFECT OF LIMONIN CARBOXYMETHOXIME AND DEOXYLIMONIC ACID ON ORAL CARCINOGENESIS

Group[a]	No. of animals	Total no. of tumors	Avg. no. of tumors[b]	Avg. tumor burden (mm^3)[b]
1	17	79	4.6±0.7	131±25
2	16	49	3.1±0.3*	86±31
3	17	59	3.5±0.5	144±25

[a]The control group, group 1, was treated with the solvent, water. Groups 2 and 3 were treated with the 3% solution of limonin carboxymethoxime and the 2.5% solution of deoxylimonic acid, respectively.
[b]Values are means ± S.E.
*$p<0.025$ when group 2 is compared to group 1.

group 2. To test for outliers, a number of statistical programs (box and whisker plots, analysis of variance, and Tukey's multiple comparison tests) were run. The results showed that there were actually three outliers, two in group 2 and one in group 3.

Table 12.2 gives the modified and unmodified tumor burden data for the first experiment. For comparison, the original average tumor burden data is given in the first column of figures. Removing just two outliers, one from group 2 and the other from group 3, produced the second column of figures. A more conservative way to handle extreme results is to winsorize the data (23). This technique forces the investigator to do the same thing to all of the experimental groups. In addition, both the high and the low values for each group have to be modified. Winsorizing the data one time, the high and low values for each group were replaced, respectively, by the next to the highest and next to the lowest values, yielded the data in the last column of Table 12.2. Comparing the modified and unmodified tumor burden data (Table 12.2), it can be seen that the treatments with deoxylimonic acid (group 3) were ineffective. A similar comparison (group 2 vs. group 1) shows that once the data is modified the treatments with limonin carboxymethoxime produced a 45 to 55% reduction in average tumor burden. In both cases, this decrease in average tumor burden proved to be significant ($p<0.01$ and $p<0.025$).

TABLE 12.2. UNMODIFIED AND MODIFIED TUMOR BURDEN DATA (EXPERIMENT ONE)

Group[a]	Original data	Outliers removed	Winsorized data
1	131±25	131±25	130±24
2	86±31	58±13*	69±16**
3	144±25	125±18	135±17

Values are means ± S.E.

[a]Group 1 was treated with the solvent, water. Group 2 was treated with the 3% solution of limonin carboxymethoxime and group 3 with the 2.5% solution of deoxylimonic acid.

*$p<0.01$ when group 2 is compared to group 1.

**$p<0.025$ when group 2 is compared to group 1.

Chi-square analysis can also be used to compare tumor burden data. In the past, we have found that the tumor burden data for the control group, in this case group 1, can be divided fairly evenly into two subgroups. The number of animals with large tumor burden values (greater than 100 mm^3) is one subgroup, while the number of animals with small tumor burden values (less than 100 mm^3) is the second subgroup. In this experiment, using the unmodified tumor burden data, the number of hamsters with large tumor burden values was 8 (group 1), 2 (group 2), and 10 (group 3). The number of hamsters with small tumor burden values was 9 (group 1), 14 (group 2), and 7 (group 3). The chi-square analysis showed that the differences between the three groups were significant ($p<0.05$). Like the data in Table 12.2, these results suggest that the treatments with limonin carboxymethoxime were effective in reducing tumor burden.

Limonol

At the end of the experiment with limonol, the number of animals in the two experimental groups was 15 (group 1) and 16 (group 2). Visible tumors were found in all of the pouches from the hamsters in group 1 and 14 of the 16 pouches from the hamsters in group 2. Multiple tumors were found in 11 of the 15 pouches from group 1 and 13 of the 16 pouches from group 2. The values for tumor radii ranged from 0.6 to 5.5 mm. The values for tumor volume went from a low of 0.8 to a high of 697 mm^3.

The tumor data for the second experiment is given in Table 12.3. Comparing the data for the two groups, it can be seen that the treatments with limonol (group 2) led to a moderate decrease in average tumor number (15%). Since the tumors in group 2 were slightly larger, there was no affect on average tumor burden. Histologically, it was found that all of the sections taken from the control pouches for the animals in the two experiments were normal. Throughout the course of the two experiments the gross appearance of the hamsters in the different groups remained normal. During each experiment, the weight gain profiles for the hamsters in the experimental groups were similar.

TABLE 12.3. EFFECT OF LIMONOL ON ORAL CARCINOGENESIS

Group[a]	No. of animals	Total no. of tumors	Avg. no. of tumors[b]	Avg. tumor burden (mm^3)[b]
1	15	67	4.5±0.7	144±56
2	16	60	3.8±0.6	144±60

[a]Group 1 was treated with a 50:50 mixture of DMSO and propylene glycol; group 2 with the 2.5% solution of limonol.
[b]Values are means ± S.E.

The B-Ring of the Limonoid Nucleus

Until information is available on how the citrus limonoids are metabolized by the cells in the oral mucosa, it will be impossible to make accurate predictions on the possible relationship between structure and cancer chemopreventive activity. Still it is obvious that some of these chemicals are active in this tumor model and others are inactive. This suggests that certain modifications to the limonoid nucleus may be important to antineoplastic activity. Considering our earlier work (12-15) with limonin, nomilin, limonin 17-ß-D-glucopyranoside, nomilin 17-ß-D-glucopyranoside, and nomilinic acid 17-ß-D-glucopyranoside, it would appear that changes in either the A and/or the A' ring of the limonoid nucleus can lead to a loss of cancer chemopreventive activity. Similarly, the results with limonin and limonin 17-ß-D-glucopyranoside suggest that an intact D-ring is not required for antineoplastic activity.

The results with limonin carboxymethoxime, deoxylimonic acid, and limonol give us some clues as to the potential relevance of the B-ring of the limonoid nucleus to cancer chemopreventive activity. Comparing the structures of limonin carboxymethoxime and limonol to limonin (see Fig. 12.1), it can be seen that in each molecule there is a structural change at carbon number seven in the B-ring. With limonol, a minor modification leads to a complete loss of cancer chemopreventive activity. With limonin carboxymethoxime, a major modification does not affect antineoplastic activity. These results indicate that the double bond at carbon number seven is critical to activity. Some evidence suggests that if this double bond is changed into a single bond, the relationship of the B-ring to the rest of the rings in the limonoid nucleus is altered (Hasegawa, S., U.S. Department of Agriculture, personal communication, 1994). Such a change in spatial configuration might account for the loss of antineoplastic activity.

With deoxylimonic acid, the situation is complicated by the fact that there is not one but three structural changes. Compared to limonin (see Fig. 12.1), there is a major modification to the B-ring and additional changes to the C- and D-rings. However, when one compares the data with deoxylimonic acid to the data with limonin carboxymethoxime, limonol, limonin, and limonin 17-ß-D-glucopyranoside (12-15), one is left with the distinct possibility that the critical modification is to the B-ring. Further experimental evidence is required, but an intact B-ring would appear to be a prerequisite for antineoplastic activity.

POTENTIAL RELEVANCE FOR HUMANS

Several factors suggest that citrus limonoids may prove to be of benefit to humans. As indicated (11-18), research using several different animal models has shown, in each case, that citrus limonoids can inhibit the development of carcinogen-induced tumors. In addition, evidence from a large number of epidemiological studies (25) has shown that the consumption of fruit, especially citrus fruit, is protective against a wide range of non-hormone-dependent cancers in humans. Significant reductions in risk have been found for cancers of the esophagus, larynx, oral cavity, rectum, lung, pancreas, colon, and stomach. One interesting aspect of these two sets of data is that three of the four animal models were for cancers of the stomach, lung, and oral cavity. It has been assumed that most, if not all, of the protective effect in humans is due to vitamin C and its antioxidant activity. However, in two of the epidemiological studies (26, 27) the investigators provided evidence on the relative importance of citrus fruit consumption to vitamin C intake. In both cases, citrus fruit consumption was more closely linked to risk reduction. These findings suggest that citrus fruits probably contain not one but several chemicals with cancer chemopreventive activity.

Until recently, it was unlikely that the limonoids might be contributing to the anticancer activity of citrus. Research with the aglycones had shown that these limonoids were concentrated in the seeds (7, 8, 18, 21). Their concentration in citrus fruits and products was extremely low, usually less than 1 to 2 ppm. The situation changed with the discovery of the limonoid glucosides (28, 29). Research with these chemicals has shown that the limonoid glucosides are present in high concentrations in the seed, peel, citrus molasses, and the fruit (8, 18, 21, 30). Some of the limonoid glucosides are lost during processing; however, even in commercial products the concentration of these chemicals remains high. For example, commercial samples of orange juice contain on average over 300 ppm (31, 32). The concentration of vitamin C in orange juice is only slightly higher. These same studies (31, 32) have also shown that the predominant limonoid glucoside both in oranges and in orange juice is limonin 17-ß-D-glucopyranoside, one of the three limonoids with cancer chemopreventive activity in the hamster cheek pouch model (13-15).

Taken together, all of this data supports the idea that citrus limonoids may be of benefit to humans. The data even suggests that these chemicals may already be contributing to the protective effect associated with the consumption of citrus.

Acknowledgments

The authors wish to thank Marjorie E. Steakley and Josephine E. Taylor for their technical assistance. J. L. Porter-Wright was supported by the National Institutes of Health (Bethesda, MD) Traineeship DE07188-05. The research was funded by a grant from the Florida Citrus Commission.

BIBLIOGRAPHY

1. ROUSEFF, R. L. "Nomilin, a New Bitter Component in Grapefruit Juice". *J. Agric. Food Chem.* 1982, 30, 504-507.

2. ROUSEFF, R. L.; MATTHEWS, R. F. "Nomilin, Taste Threshold and Relative Bitterness". *J. Food Sci.* 1984, 49, 777-779.
3. HASEGAWA, S.; HERMAN, Z. "Biosynthesis of Obacunone from Nomilin in Citrus Limon". *Phytochemistry* 1985, 24, 1973-1974.
4. HASEGAWA, S.; HERMAN, Z.; ORME, E.; OU, P. "Biosynthesis of Limonoids in Citrus: Sites and Translocation". *Phytochemistry* 1986, 25, 2783-2785.
5. OU, P.; HASEGAWA, S.; HERMAN, Z.; FONG, C. H. "Limonoid Biosynthesis in the Stem of Citrus Limon". *Phytochemistry* 1988, 27, 115-118.
6. HASEGAWA, S. "Limonoid Debittering of Citrus Juices Using Immobilized Bacterial Cell Systems". *Food Biotech.* 1987, 1, 249-261.
7. MCINTOSH, C. A.; MANSELL, R. L.; ROUSEFF, R. L. "Distribution of Limonin in the Fruit Tissues of Nine Grapefruit Cultivars". *J. Agric. Food Chem.* 1982, 30, 689-692.
8. HASEGAWA, S.; OU, P.; FONG, C. H.; HERMAN, Z.; COGGINS, C. W., JR.; ATKIN, D. R. "Changes in the Limonate A-Ring Lactone and Limonin 17-D-Glucopyranoside Content of Navel Oranges during Fruit Growth and Maturation". *J. Agric. Food Chem.* 1991, 39, 262-265.
9. KLOCKE, J. A.; KUBO, I. "Citrus Limonoid By-Products as Insect Control Agents". *Entomol. Exp. Appl.* 1982, 32, 299-301.
10. ALFORD, A. R.; BENTLEY, M. D. "Citrus Limonoids as Potential Antifeedants for the Spruce Budworm (Lepidoptera: Tortricidae)". *J. Econ. Entomol.* 1986, 79, 35-38.
11. LAM, L. K. T.; HASEGAWA, S. "Inhibition of Benzo[a]pyrene-Induced Forestomach Neoplasia in Mice by Citrus Limonoids". *Nutr. Cancer* 1989, 12, 43-47.
12. MILLER, E. G.; FANOUS, R.; RIVERA-HIDALGO, F.; BINNIE, W. H.; HASEGAWA, S. "The Effect of Citrus Limonoids on Hamster Buccal Pouch Carcinogenesis". *Carcinogenesis* 1989, 10, 1535-1537.
13. MILLER, E. G.; GONZALES-SANDERS, A. P.; COUVILLON, A. M.; WRIGHT, J. M.; HASEGAWA, S.; LAM, L. K. T. "Inhibition of Hamster Buccal Pouch Carcinogenesis by Limonin 17-D-Glucopyranoside". *Nutr. Cancer* 1992, 17, 1-7.
14. MILLER, E. G.; GONZALES-SANDERS, A. P.; COUVILLON, A. M.; BINNIE, W. H.; HASEGAWA, S.; LAM, L. K. T. "Citrus Limonoids as Inhibitors of Oral Carcinogenesis". *Food Technol.* 1994a, 48, 110-114.
15. MILLER, E. G.; GONZALES-SANDERS, A. P.; COUVILLON, A. M.; WRIGHT, J. M.; HASEGAWA, S.; LAM, L. K. T.; SUNAHARA, G. I. "Inhibition of Oral Carcinogenesis by Green Coffee Beans and Limonoid Glucosides". In Food Phytochemicals for Cancer Prevention I. Fruits and Vegetables, Huang, M. T., Osawa, T., Ho, C. T., Rosen, R. T., Eds.; American Chemical Society: Washington, DC, 1994b; pp. 220-229.
16. LAM, L. K. T.; ZHANG, J.; HASEGAWA, S. "Citrus Limonoid Reduction of Chemically Induced Tumorigenesis". *Food Technol.* 1994a, 48, 104-108.
17. LAM, L. K. T.; ZHANG, J.; HASEGAWA, S.; SCHUT, H. A. J. "Inhibition of Chemically Induced Carcinogenesis by Citrus Limonoids". In Food Phy-

tochemicals for Cancer Prevention I. Fruits and Vegetables, Huang, M. T., Osawa, T., Ho, C. T., Rosen, R. T., Eds.; American Chemical Society: Washington, DC, 1994b; pp. 209-219.

18. HASEGAWA, S.; MIYAKE, M.; OZAKI, Y. "Biochemistry of Citrus Limonoids and Their Anticarcinogenic Activity". In Food Phytochemicals for Cancer Prevention I. Fruits and Vegetables, Huang, M. T., Osawa, T., Ho, C. T., Rosen, R. T., Eds.; American Chemical Society: Washington, DC, 1994; pp. 198-208.
19. LAM, L. K. T.; LI, Y.; HASEGAWA, S. "Effects of Citrus Limonoids on Glutathione S-Transferase Activity in Mice". *J. Agric. Food Chem.* 1989, 37, 878-880.
20. WATTENBERG, L. W. "Inhibition of Neoplasia by Minor Dietary Constituents". *Cancer Res.* 1983, 43, 2448s-2453s.
21. OZAKI, Y.; FONG, C. H.; HERMAN, Z.; MAEDA, H.; MIYAKE, M.; IFUKU, Y.; HASEGAWA, S. "Limonoid Glucosides in Citrus Seeds". *Agric. Biol. Chem.* 1991, 55, 137-141.
22. NIUKIAN, K.; SCHWARTZ, J.; SHKLAR, G. "Effect of Onion Extract on the Development of Hamster Buccal Pouch Carcinomas as Expressed in Tumor Burden". *Nutr. Cancer* 1987, 9, 171-176.
23. MILLER, E. G.; MCWHORTER, K.; RIVERA-HIDALGO, F.; WRIGHT, J. M.; HIRSBRUNNER, P.; SUNAHARA, G. I. "Kahweol and Cafestol: Inhibitors of Hamster Buccal Pouch Carcinogenesis". *Nutr. Cancer* 1991, 15, 41-46.
24. MILLER, E. G.; FORMBY, W. A.; RIVERA-HIDALGO, F.; WRIGHT, J. M. "Inhibition of Hamster Buccal Pouch Carcinogenesis by Green Coffee Beans". *Oral Surg.* 1988, 65, 745-749.
25. BLOCK, G. "Vitamin C and Cancer Prevention: The Epidemiologic Evidence". *Am. J. Clin. Nutr.* 1991, 53, 270s-282s.
26. METTLIN, C.; GRAHAM, S.; PRIORE, R.; MARSHALL, J.; SWANSON, M. "Diet and Cancer of the Esophagus". *Nutr. Cancer* 1981, 2, 143-147.
27. RISCH, H. A.; JAIN, M.; CHOI, N. W.; FODOR, J. G.; PFEIFFER, C. J.; HOWE, G. R.; HARRISON, L. W.; CRAIB, K. J. P.; MILLER, A. B. "Dietary Factors and the Incidence of Cancer of the Stomach". *Am. J. Epidemiol.* 1985, 122, 947-957.
28. BENNETT, R. D.; HASEGAWA, S.; HERMAN, Z. "Glucosides of Acidic Limonoids in Citrus". *Phytochemistry* 1989, 28, 2777-2781.
29. HASEGAWA, S.; BENNETT, R. D.; HERMAN, Z.; FONG, C. H.; OU, P. "Limonoid Glucosides in Citrus". *Phytochemistry* 1989, 28, 1717-1720.
30. MAEDA, H.; OZAKI, Y.; MIYAKE, M.; IFUKU, Y.; HASEGAWA, S. "Limonoid Glucosides in Hassaku". *Nippon Nogeikagaku Kaishi* 1990, 64, 1231-1234.
31. FONG, C. H.; HASEGAWA, S.; HERMAN, Z.; OU, P. "Limonoid Glucosides in Commercial Citrus Juices". *J. Food Sci.* 1990, 54, 1505-1506.
32. HERMAN, Z.; FONG, C. H.; OU, P.; Hasegawa, S. "Limonoid Glucosides in Orange Juices by HPLC". *J. Agric. Food Chem.* 1990, 38, 1860-1861.

13

The Citrus Flavonoid Tangeretin Inhibits Invasion of Human Breast Cancer Cells

Marc E. Bracke
Stefan J. Vermeulen
Erik A. Bruyneel
Krist'l Vennekens
Marc M. Mareel

MCF-7/6 are human breast carcinoma cells which are invasive after confrontation *in vitro* with embryonic chick heart fragments or with Matrigel, a gelified mixture of basement membrane molecule, and give rise to invasive tumors in immunodeficient laboratory mice. This invasiveness is due to the defective function of the cell-cell adhesion molecule E-cadherin. The citrus flavonoid tangeretin corrects the function of E-cadherin within minutes and does not require *de novo* protein synthesis. In its action mechanism tangeretin differs from another activator of the E-cadherin function (insulin-like growth factor-I). In experiments with immunodeficient mice inoculated with MCF-7/6 cells, oral tangeretin treatment results in a group of long-term survivors, some of which have reached the age of three years.

THE ROLE OF THE E-CADHERIN/CATENIN COMPLEX IN HUMAN BREAST CANCER INVASION AND METASTASIS

Breast cancer is a major challenge in medicine for several reasons. The disease is more prevalent among the female population than any other type of cancer. Many therapeutic approaches have proven to be effective in increasing the life expectancy of breast cancer patients. While therapy was initially restricted to radical removal of the affected breast and its surrounding tissues, modern treatment regimens include the application of radiotherapy, chemotherapy and adjuvant therapy. These modalities have both reduced surgical aggressiveness and improved therapeutic efficiency. Furthermore, a lively debate is actually pointing to the possibility of preventing the development of breast cancer by oral administration of the antiestrogen tamoxifen.

As for many other diseases, therapeutic progress in breast cancer greatly depends on our understanding of its mechanisms. The cellular phenomena implicated in the dissemination of cancer have been described for more than one decade. In the primary breast tumor, cells escape from control mechanisms for growth and invasion. Uncontrolled cell growth leads to the formation of a local tumor mass, while invasion of this cell population results in occupation and destruction of the surrounding normal tissues. One consequence of this invasion is that the tumor cells gain access to the circulation, and are transported to sites distant from the primary tumor. Eventually, from these cells secondary tumors (metastases) arise, which are usually responsible for the poor prognosis for the disease (1-3).

During recent years some of the molecular mechanisms of invasion and metastasis have been elucidated. In this context proteases (4,5) and motility factors (6) have been shown to be implicated. From a therapeutical point of view, the discovery of natural invasion-suppressor molecules has gained widespread interest. One example was found in protease inhibitors, that counteract the enzymatic destruction of the surrounding normal tissues (7-9). A potent invasion-suppressor was also found among a family of cell surface molecules which are responsible for the adhesion between normal epithelial cells. Indeed, E-cadherin was found to be present as a cell-cell adhesion molecule at the surface of normal epithelial cells (10). In carcinomas, however, cell-cell adhesion is disturbed either because the expression of E-cadherin at the cell surface is downregulated (11), or because its function is impaired (12).

E-cadherin is a calcium-dependent cell-cell adhesion molecule, which possesses an extracellular domain that is involved in the homophilic recognition of another E-cadherin, present on the surface of a neighboring epithelial cell. This extracellular domain is connected to an intracellular part of the molecule which in turn, is connected to the actin cytoskeleton via the catenins (13-15). We have shown the presence of an apparently complete, though functionally inactive E-cadherin/catenin complex in invasive human breast cancer cells (16). One of the goals of our current research is to find agents that can activate this complex. Such agents would increase the adhesion between breast cancer cells and inhibit their invasion. This approach is aimed to reveal the regulatory mechanisms of cancer invasion, and will hopefully be useful in cancer therapy.

SELECTION OF AGENTS THAT ACTIVATE THE E-CADHERIN/CATENIN COMPLEX

We have been using an assay *in vitro* to select agents that can inhibit invasion of tumor cells. Such agents are further investigated to reveal the mechanism of their anti-invasive effect.

The assay for invasion consists of confronting tumor cells with a fragment of normal tissue in organ culture (17). For the present studies human MCF-7/6 breast cancer cells were used to confront with normal embryonic chick heart fragments. MCF-7/6 cells reproducibly invade into the heart fragments within an incubation period of eight days. This is inferred from histological analysis, showing progressive occupation and destruction of the heart by the tumor cells (18). A number of compounds added to the culture medium was found to inhibit invasion *in vitro*. Up to now, these compounds are: insulin-like growth factor I (IGF-I) (16)], the vitamin A derivative all-*trans*-retinoic acid (RA) (18), the anti-estrogen tamoxifen (19) and the citrus flavonoid tangeretin (20). Two comments can be made here. First, at anti-invasive concentrations (e.g. 10^{-4} to 10^{-5} M tangeretin) these compounds were cytotoxic for neither the MCF-7/6 cells nor the chick heart fragments. Second, other citrus flavonoids (nobiletin, hesperedin and naringin) did not show an anti-invasive effect in this assay.

IGF-I, RA, tamoxifen and tangeretin all activate the E-cadherin complex in MCF-7/6 cells (19, 21), although the signal transducing pathways appear to be different. Spontaneous adhesion between MCF-7/6 cells is poor, as demonstrated by their inefficient formation of aggregates from a cell suspension. Addition of any of the above mentioned compounds leads to a dramatic increase of aggregation. The evidence that activation of E-cadherin is implicated in this phenomenon stems from the neutralizing effect of antibodies against E-cadherin. Two monoclonal antibodies (HECD-1 and MB2), directed against extracellular functional domains of E-cadherin, were indeed able to block the effect of IGF-I, RA, tamoxifen and tangeretin on cell aggregation (Fig. 13.1).

Another piece of evidence to relate the effect of these compounds on cell aggregation to activation of E-cadherin is the strict dependence on the presence of calcium in the medium. In the absence of calcium, which is an ion essential for functional integrity of E-cadherin, none of the compounds, including tangeretin, was able to stimulate MCF-7/6 cell aggregation *in vitro* (21).

SIGNAL TRANSDUCTION FROM THE TRIGGERING BY TANGERETIN TO THE E-CADHERIN/CATENIN COMPLEX

Only in the case of IGF-I has the initial steps of the signal transduction pathway been elucidated. IGF-I triggers its spe-

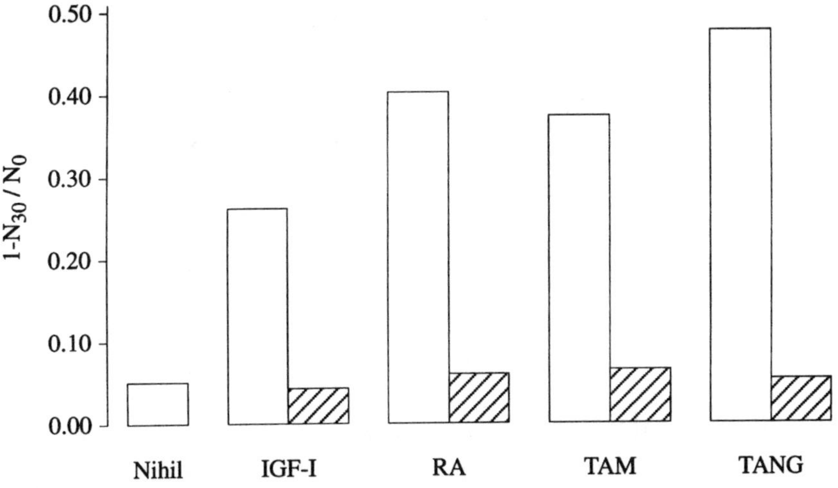

FIG. 13.1. EFFECT OF INSULIN-LIKE GROWTH FACTOR I (IGF-I), ALL-*TRANS*-RETINOIC ACID (RA), TAMOXIFEN (TAM) AND TANGERETIN (TANG) ON HUMAN MCF-7/6 BREAST CANCER CELL AGGREGATION *IN VITRO*. Aggregation was measured by first bringing the cells in suspension with a method that does not abrogate the function of the E-cadherin/catenin complex. Then the number of particles is counted initially (N_0) and after 30 min (N_{30}). Cell aggregation is expressed as $1\text{-}N_{30}/N_0$. The cells were not pretreated (0.5 g/ml IGF-I or 10^{-6} M TAM), or pretreated for 24 h (10^{-6} M RA or 10^{-5} M TANG), and the agents remained present in the medium during the assay (30 min). The hatched bars indicate that for each agent the effect could be neutralized by a monoclonal antibody (HECD-1) against the extracellular part of E-cadherin.

cific receptor at the surface of MCF-7 cells (22). The potency of IGF-I for this triggering is modulated outside the cell by at least three binding proteins secreted by MCF-7/6 (21, 23). Part of the ambiant IGF-I is neutralized by these proteins, and will lose its triggering activity before reaching the receptor. The remaining fraction of IGF-I, however, binds to the extracellular domains of the IGF-I receptor, and this results in an immediate upregulation of the tyrosine kinase activity of its intracellular domains (24, 25). Tyrosine kinase leads to phosphorylation of the receptor itself and of a series of intracellular substrates. Whether this signal eventually results in alterations in the phosphorylation of the E-cadherin/catenin complex is the matter of our ongoing experiments.

Experimental data suggest that tangeretin uses a different signal transducing pathway than IGF-I. First, the kinetics of the activation of the E-cadherin/catenin complex differ substantially: while the effect of IGF-I is very rapid (within 30 min), tangeretin needs 24 h to exert its maximal effect, with a half-maximal effect reached after 4 h of treatment. Second, the extracellular domain of the IGF-I receptor does not appear to be involved in the effect of tangeretin on cell-cell adhesion. A monoclonal antibody (aIR3) that binds to this receptor and blocks triggering by IGF-I, does not inhibit the tangeretin effect (12). Furthermore, treatment of MCF-7/6 cells with tangeretin does not result in increased phosphorylation of the intracellular domains of the receptor (Fig. 13.2). One common characteristic of the effects of IGF-I, RA, tamoxifen and tangeretin is that they are not sensitive to cycloheximide, which indicates that they do not require *de novo* protein synthesis.

Combined treatment of MCF-7/6 cells with tangeretin and tamoxifen showed their effects on cell-cell adhesion to be slightly additive (Fig. 13.3). This finding is not without practical importance, since the potency of both compounds is limited by their individual solubility in aqueous media.

EFFECT OF TANGERETIN ON ARTIFICIAL MCF-7/6 LIVER METASTASIS IN LABORATORY MICE

Understanding the molecular mechanisms of tumor invasion is a major topic of our research, and tangeretin has been found to be an interesting tool in this regard. Our ultimate goal, however, is to find compounds that can be applied as therapeutic agents in oncology. So, we wondered whether tangeretin would be useful to treat tumor-bearing laboratory animals. We preferred to stick to the same type of tumor cells as we had been using in our experiments *in vitro*, namely the invasive MCF-7/6 variant. Because these cells are of human origin, they would be rejected by any acceptor animal, except by a peculiar type of

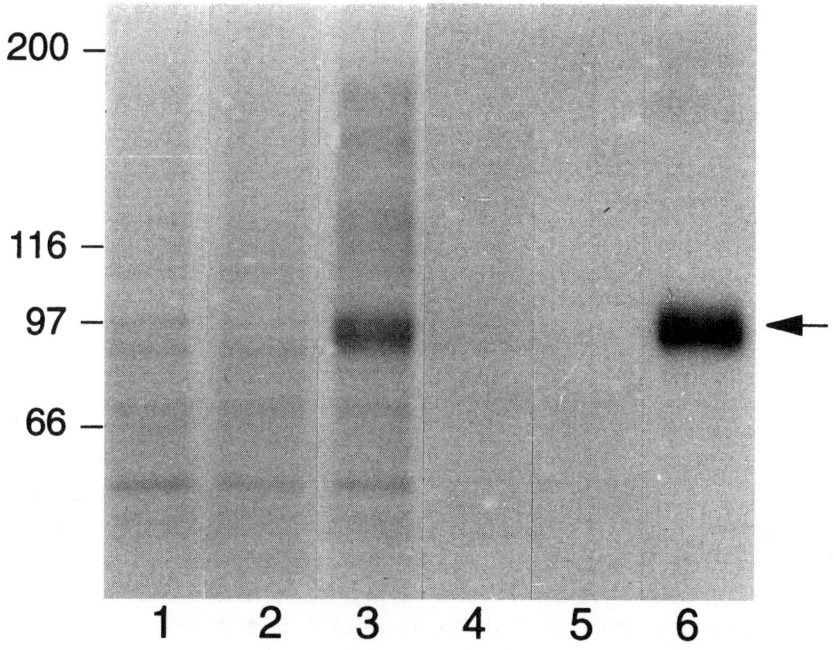

FIG. 13.2. EFFECT OF TANGERETIN ON TYROSINE PHOSPHORYLATION OF THE IGF-I RECEPTOR. MCF-7/6 cells were left untreated (lanes 1 and 4), or treated with 10^{-5} M tangeretin for 4 h (lanes 2 and 5) or with 0.5 g/ml IGF-I for 12 min (lanes 3 and 6). Tyrosine phosphorylation was revealed by first labeling the cells metabolically with ^{32}P, then precipitating with a monoclonal antibody against phosphotyrosine (PY20) and finally separating the precipitate by SDS gel electrophoresis followed by autoradiographic detection of the labeled molecules (lanes 1, 2 and 3). In lanes 4, 5, and 6, a second precipitation step (on phosphotyrosine immunoprecipitated proteins) was included with a monoclonal antibody (IR3) against the IGF-I receptor. Arrow indicates the phosphorylated-subunit of the IGF-I receptor after treatment with IGF-I. Molecular weights (left) are in kilodalton. Tangeretin does not trigger autophosphorylation of the IGF-I receptor.

mouse: the hairless nude mouse. These animals are genetically immunodeficient, and for this reason they do not reject transplanted human cells.

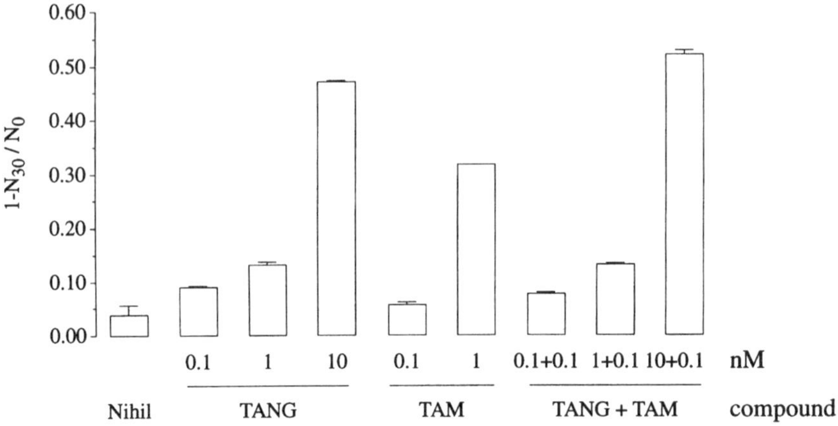

FIG. 13.3. EFFECT OF COMBINED TREATMENT WITH TAMOXIFEN (TAM) AND TANGERETIN (TANG) ON MCF-7/6 CELL AGGREGATION. The assay principle was described in Fig. 13.1. Some of the cell cultures were pretreated with TANG for 24 h at different concentrations. During the assay (30 min) these concentrations of TANG were combined with different concentrations of TAM. The effects of TANG and TAM appear to be slightly additive.

In a pharmacodynamic study in laboratory mice different administration routes of tangeretin were tried out: the flavonoid was injected into the peritoneal cavity, or intravenously, or it was given orally with the drinking water. The distribution of tangeretin in different organs was examined via extraction and reverse-phase high performance liquid chromatography. We found that after oral administration of tangeretin significant levels of the flavonoid could be detected in the liver (26). In this study intact tangeretin and at least 5 metabolites were found in the liver extracts of orally treated mice. Inspired by this result, we decided to study the effect of oral tangeretin treatment on the formation of MCF-7/6 metastases in the liver.

The model to study liver metastasis consisted of injecting invasive MCF-7/6 cells into the spleen of nude mice (27). The cells are then transported in the splenic veins and colonize the liver. MCF-7/6 cells appeared to give rise to tumoral enlargement of the spleen as compared to the spleen of normal nude mice. Mice inoculated with MCF-7/6 cells in the spleen also developed liver metastases, which was obvious from the enlargement of the organ. Histologically multiple liver metastases were observed. They could be detected on sections stained with a routine hematoxylin-eosin technique, and even better after specific staining with a monolonal antibody against MCF-7/6 cells.

Nude mice were thus injected with MCF-7/6 cells into the spleen, randomly distributed into two groups, and treated orally either with tangeretin or with the solvent dimethyl sulfoxide only. The survival time of these animals was noted, and every mouse was examined *post mortem* to evaluate the extent of liver metastasis at the moment of death. Up to now, no differences between the treated and the control group were found, as far as the number and the size of the liver metastases are concerned. However, in every experiment a small number of long-term survivors was observed, and this number was always higher in the tangeretin-treated group than in the control group (12). We have to be very careful about the interpretation of these preliminary results, because they are extracted from ongoing experiments. Yet, some of the treated animals have already survived more than three years. We are now trying to find out whether this phenomenon is due to a direct effect of tangeretin on the tumor cells, or to an increase of the resistance of the mice against tumor formation. In view of the latter possibility we have tried to explain the effect of tangeretin on survival of nude mice by studying a number of parameters in the blood of these animals. Two groups of female nude mice were allowed to drink sterilized tap water containing 0.1 mM tangeretin or the solvent only. After 4 months a blood sample was taken.

The following analyses were done:

A. Parameters evaluating host resistance and health status in a general way: hemoglobin, hematocrit, enumeration of red and white blood cells, differentiation of the leukocytes, platelet count, folate, vitamin B12, cholesterol, triglycerides, blood urea nitrogen, creatinin, creatin kinase, uric acid, phosphorus and total protein.

B. Parameters evaluating liver and pancreas condition: gamma-glutamyl transpeptidase, transaminases, lactate dehydrogenase and amylase.
C. Parameters evaluating the hormonal status: free triiodothyronin, cortisol, dehydroepiandrosteron sulfate, testosteron, progesteron and estradiol. It should be emphasized that tumorigenicity of MCF-7/6 cells is estrogen-dependent, and that some flavonoids can act as weak estrogens, and possibly disturb the normal hormonal status (28).

The mean values of tangeretin-treated and solvent-treated mice were not significantly different for all analyses, except for amylase. The mean value of amylase in the tangeretin group was 146 units/l, and was 84 units/l in the solvent group. This difference is significant at the $0.025 < p < 0.050$ level (Student's t-test). Amylase is a serum compound, which finds its origin in either the salivary glands or the pancreas. Further analyses are now in progress to confirm the effect of tangeretin on either organ.

CONCLUSION

The citrus flavonoid tangeretin is able to activate the E-cadherin/catenin complex in human MCF-7/6 breast carcinoma cells *in vitro*. Tangeretin shares this property with insulin-like growth factor I, all-*trans*-retinoic acid and tamoxifen. The action mechanism of tangeretin appears to differ from the one of insulin-like growth factor, and the effects of tangeretin and tamoxifen are slightly additive. Activation of the E-cadherin/catenin complex results in increased cell-cell adhesion and in inhibition of invasion of MCF-7/6 cells *in vitro*. Studies in laboratory mice indicate that substantial concentrations of tangeretin can be obtained in the liver after oral administration with the drinking water. After inoculation of MCF-7/6 into the spleen of nude mice, artificial liver metastases develop both in tangeretin-drinking and solvent-drinking animals. The number of long-term survivors, however, was higher in the groups treated with tangeretin.

ACKNOWLEDGEMENTS

This work was supported by the Citrus Department of the State of Florida. We thank George De Bruyne for his help in preparing the manuscript, and Jean Roels-Van Kerckvoorde for preparing the illustrations.

BIBLIOGRAPHY

1. NICOLSON, G. L.; BIRDWELL, C. R.; BRUNSON, K. W.; ROBBINS, J. C.; BEATTIE, G.; FIDLER, I. J. "Cell interactions in the metastatic process: some cell surface properties associated with successful blood-borne tumor spread". In *Cell and Tissue Interactions*; Lash, J. W., Burger, M. M., Eds.; Raven Press: New York, 1977; pp. 225-241.
2. FIDLER, I.; HART, I. "Biological diversity in metastatic neoplasms: origins and implications". *Science* 1982, 217, 998-1003.
3. MAREEL, M.M.; VAN ROY, F.M.; BRACKE, M.E. "How and when do tumor cells metastasize?". *Crit. Rev. Oncogenesis* 1993, 4, 559-594.
4. DANØ, K.; ANDREASEN, P. A.; GRONDAHL-HANSEN, G.; KRISTENSEN, P.; NIELSEN, L. S.; SKRIVER, L. "Plasminogen activators, tissue degradation and cancer". *Adv. Cancer Res.* 1985, 44, 139-266.
5. MURPHY, G.; REYNOLDS, J. J.; HEMBRY, R. M. "Metalloproteinases and cancer invasion and metastasis". *Int. J. Cancer* 1989, 44, 757-760.
6. STOKER, M.; GHERARDI, E. "Regulation of cell movement: the motogenic cytokines". *Biochem. Biophys. Acta* 1991, 1072, 81-102.
7. MOTTONEN, J.; STRAND, A.; SYMERSKY, J.; SWEET, R. M.; DANLEY, D. E.; GEOGHEGAN, K. F.; GERARD, R. D.; GOLDSMITH, E. J. "Structural basis of latency in plasminogen activator inhibitor-1". *Nature* 1992, 355, 270-273.
8. KHOKHA, R.; WATERHOUSE, P.; YAGEL, S.; LALA, P. K.; OVERALL, C. M.; NORTON, G.; DENHARDT, D. T. "Antisense RNA induced reduction in murine TIMP levels confers oncogenicity on Swiss 3T3 cells". *Science* 1989, 243, 947-950.
9. ZOU, Z.; ANISOWICZ, A.; HENDRIX, M. J.; THOR, A.; NEVEU, M.; SHENG, S.; RAFIDI, K.; SEFTOR, E.; SAGER, R. "Maspin, a serpin with tumor-suppressing activity in human mammary epithelial cells". *Science* 1994, 263, 526-529.
10. KEMLER, R. "Classical cadherins". *Semin. Cell Biol.* 1992, 3, 149-155.
11. TAKEICHI, M. "Cadherins in cancer: implications for invasion and metastasis". *Current Opin. Cell Biol.* 1993, 5, 806-811.
12. BRACKE, M. E.; BRUYNEEL, E. A.; VERMEULEN, S. J.; VENNEKENS, K.; VAN MARCK, V.; MAREEL, M. "Citrus flavonoid effect on tumor invasion and metastasis: The citrus flavonoid tangeretin may inhibit the processes that shorten the life expectancy of tumor-bearing patients". *Food Technol.* 1994a, 48, 121-124.

13. CUNNINGHAM, B. A.; LEUTZINGER, Y.; GALLIN, W. J.; SORKIN, B. C.; EDELMAN, G. M. "Linear organization of the liver cell adhesion molecule L-CAM". *Proc. Natl. Acad. Sci. USA* 1984, 81, 5787-5791.
14. HINCK, L.; NÄTHKE, I. S.; PAPKOFF, J.; NELSON, W. J. "Dynamics of cadherin/catenin complex formation: novel protein interactions and pathways of complex assembly". *J. Cell Biol.* 1994, 125, 1327-1340.
15. NÄTHKE, I. S.; HINCK, L.; SWEDLOW, J. R.; PAPKOFF, J.; NELSON, W. J. "Defining interactions and distributions of cadherin and catenin complexes in polarized epithelial cells". *J. Cell Biol.* 1994, 125, 1341-1352.
16. BRACKE, M. E.; VYNCKE, B. M.; BRUYNEEL, E. A.; VERMEULEN, S. J.; DE BRUYNE, G. K.; VAN LAREBEKE, N. A.; VLEMINCKX, K.; VAN ROY, F. M.; MAREEL, M. M. "Insulin-like growth factor I activates the invasion suppressor function of E-cadherin in MCF-7 human mammary carcinoma cells in vitro". *Br. J. Cancer* 1993, 68, 282-289.
17. MAREEL, M.; KINT, J.; MEYVISCH, C. "Methods of study of the invasion of malignant C3H mouse fibroblasts into embryonic chick heart in vitro". *Virchows Arch. B Cell Pathol.* 1979, 30, 95-111.
18. BRACKE, M. E.; VAN LAREBEKE, N. A.; VYNCKE, B. M.; MAREEL, M. M. "Retinoic acid modulates both invasion and plasma membrane ruffling of MCF-7 human mammary carcinoma cells in vitro". *Br. J. Cancer* 1991, 63, 867-872.
19. BRACKE, M. E.; CHARLIER, C.; BRUYNEEL, E. A.; LABIT, C.; MAREEL, M. M.; CASTRONOVO, V. "Tamoxifen restores the E-cadherin function in human breast cancer MCF-7/6 cells and suppresses their invasive phenotype". *Cancer Res.* 1994b, 54, 4607-4609.
20. BRACKE, M. E.; VYNCKE, B. M.; VAN LAREBEKE, N. A.; BRUYNEEL, E. A.; DE BRUYNE, G. K.; DE PESTEL, G. H.; DE COSTER, W. J.; ESPEEL, M. F.; MAREEL, M. M. "The flavonoid tangeretin inhibits invasion of MO4 mouse cells into embryonic chick heart in vitro". *Clin. Exp. Metastasis* 1989, 7, 283-300.
21. BRACKE, M. E.; VERMEULEN, S. J.; BRUYNEEL, E. A.; VENNEKENS, K. M.; DE BRUYNE, G. K.; VAN ROY, F. M.; MAREEL, M. M. "The invasion suppressor function of E-cadherin in mammary epitheloid cells. In *Prospects in Diagnosis and Treatment of Breast Cancer*, Schmitt, M., Graeff H., and Kindermann, G. Eds.; Exerpta Medica International Congress Series N 1050, Elsevier Science B.V.: Amsterdam, 1994c; pp. 107-115.
22. DE LEON, D. D.; BAKKER, B.; WILSON, D. M.; HINTZ, R. L.; ROSENFELD, R. G. "Demonstration of insulin-like growth factor (IGF-I and -II) receptors and binding protein in human breast cancer cell lines". *Biochem. Biophys. Res. Commun.* 1988, 152, 390-405.
23. FIGUEROA, J. A.; YEE, D. "The insulin-like growth factor binding proteins (IGFBPs) in human breast cancer". *Breast Cancer Res. Treat.* 1992, 22, 81-90.
24. JACOBS, J.; KULL, F. C. JR.; EARP, H. S.; SVOBODA, M. E.; VAN WYCK, J. J.; CUATRECASAS, P. "Somatomedine-C stimulates the

phosphorylation of the ß subunit of its own receptor". *J. Biol. Chem.* 1983, 258, 9581-9584.
25. KADOWAKI, T.; KOYASU, S.; NISHIDA, E.; TOBE, K.; IZUMI, T.; TAKAKU, F.; SAKAI, H.; YAHARA, I.; KASUGA, M. "Tyrosine phosphorylation of common and specific sets of cellular proteins rapidly induced by insulin, insulin-like growth factor I, and epidermal growth factor in an intact cell". *J. Biol. Chem.* 1987, 262, 7342-7350.
26. BRACKE, M. E.; VYNCKE, B.; DE PESTEL, G.; VAKAET, L. JR; BOURGOIS, L.; VAN LAREBEKE, N.; BORTIER, H.; MAREEL, M. M. "Effect of flavonoids on cancer cell invasiveness. In *Plant Flavonoids in Biology and Medicine. III. Current Issues in Flavonoid Research*; Das, N. P., Ed.; National University of Singapore Press: Singapore, 1990; pp. 279-292.
27. KOPPER, L.; VAN HAHN, T.; LAPIS, K. "Experimental model for liver metastasis formatting using Lewis lung tumor". *J. Cancer Res. Clin. Oncol.* 1982, 103, 31-38.
28. MARTIN, P. M.; HORWITZ, K. B.; RYAN, D. S.; MCGUIRE, W. L. "Phytoestrogen interaction with estrogen receptors in human breast cancer cells". *Endocrinol.* 1978, 103, 1860-1867.

14

The Phenolic Phytochemicals in Wine, Fruit and Tea: Dietary Levels, Absorption and Potential Nutritional Effects

Andrew L. Waterhouse
J. Bruce German
Edwin N. Franke
Rosemary L. Walzem
Pierre Louis Teissedre
John Folts

Recent epidemiological studies demonstrate correlations between consumption of either wine, foods high in flavonols, or vitamin E, rich dietary sources of phenolic compounds—with reduced coronary heart disease (CHD) mortality. In addition, *in vitro* studies have revealed several plausible mechanisms by which phenolic phytochemicals could inhibit atherosclerosis or thrombosis. A comparison of the published levels of phenolic substances in foods shows that wine, tea and fresh fruits are a rich source of these substances, but fruit juices are not. Absorption data on phenolics from food are sparse, but a recent study at University of California, Davis demonstrates that humans absorb catechin readily from red wine. The epidemiological, mechanistic and absorption data make a compelling case that some phenolic compounds could provide nutritional benefits that may reduce CHD mortality rates.

There appears to be a clear link between diet and health (1). Diets high in fruits and vegetables appear to offer many benefits in reducing heart disease and cancer and there is considerable interest in the dietary constituents which may cause these effects. The nutritional benefits of beta-carotene (2), vitamin C (3), and fiber (4) have been extensively studied with respect to cancer. New studies have focused on the effects of dietary phenolics on both cancer and coronary heart disease. The reader is referred to a recent review that deals with phenolics and cancer (5)-this review will focus on CHD. Historically the nutritional value of these substances was discounted (6), and much of the research carried out on phenolic compounds has investigated the *anti-nutritive* effects of these substances, one example being a paper by Butler and Rogler (7).

DIETS HIGH IN PHENOLIC SUBSTANCES APPEAR TO CORRELATE WITH REDUCED CORONARY HEART DISEASE

Interest in the potential health benefits of phenolic compounds has been stimulated by a number of studies that have shown correlations between the consumption of foods high in phenolic content and reduced CHD mortality. The 1992 “French paradox” study of Renaud and de Lorgeril (8) demonstrates a better correlation between CHD mortality and dairy fat consumption when wine consumption was included as a factor that reduced disease. Another report showed an association between high doses of the phenolic compound a-tocopherol (vitamin E) and reduced CHD mortality (9). Vitamin E is known to be an essential antioxidant in blood (10).

A direct correlation was observed between reduced CHD mortality in elderly men and dietary flavonols, one of the major classes of phenolics. The investigators divided the subjects into three groups based on their consumption of flavonols. Consumption of flavonols was based on their reported diets and the flavonol content of those foods (11). The best correlation between reduced CHD mortality and specific dietary components was found with tea, onions and apples. The best correlation between CHD mortality and chemical constituents of the diet was found with quercetin (11). This was an interesting outcome because previous studies demonstrated negligible absorption and rapid clearance of pure quercetin in humans (12).

Recently, a study compared the mortality of subjects who consumed different levels of specific alcoholic beverages (13). Increasing wine consumption was related to decreasing mortality, while increasing consumption of other alcoholic beverages was related to either a neutral effect or increased mortality. The authors concluded that the "J-curve" associated with alcohol consumption was a combination of decreasing mortality at moderate consumption levels due to wine consumption and increasing mortality due to spirits consumption at high consumption levels.

EFFECTS OF PHENOLICS ON ATHEROSCLEROSIS MECHANISMS

Atherosclerosis and CHD are associated with elevated levels of cholesterol in circulating low density lipoproteins (LDL). Brown and Goldstein (14) and Steinberg et al. (15) proposed that during circulation a transformation of a small proportion of these lipoproteins are converted from native particles into modified and atherogenic LDL. Modification of LDL occurs primarily through oxidation of the polyunsaturated lipids and thence modification of the apoprotein (15). In addition, the net yield of oxidized LDL particles *in vitro* can be decreased by the presence of antioxidants either in blood or in the lipoproteins themselves (16).

Frankel *et al.* (17) showed that a wine fraction containing phenolic compounds was a potent antioxidant for LDL oxidation *in vitro*, and, based on this finding, formulated the hypothesis that protection from CHD by wine consumption was due in part to the phenolic substances. Frankel *et al.* (18) subsequently reported that three specific phenolic compounds found in wine, resveratrol, epicatechin and quercetin were antioxidants for LDL. Thus, the phenolic constituents in wine are most likely providing the majority of wine's antioxidant activity. Kinsella *et al.* (19) elaborated mechanisms by which phenolic antioxidants compounds could provide significant protection from CHD.

EFFECTS OF PHENOLICS ON PLATELETS

When an atherosclerotic lesion in a coronary artery causes a significant blockage, there is a risk of developing a partial or totally occlusive platelet mediated coronary thrombus that can lead to fatal or nonfatal myocardial infarction (20). Therefore, reduced platelet activity should reduce CHD mortality, and any dietary habit that reduces platelet activity is likely to be beneficial.

An *in vivo* animal model for studying the interaction of platelets with damaged and stenosed coronary arteries has been developed. In this model, periodic acute platelet-mediated thrombosis occurs in a mechanically stenosed artery, followed by embolization distally. This produces cyclic flow reductions (CFRs) and cyclic periods of myocardial ischemia. This animal model is a good model for studying the thrombotic events that occur in patients with unstable angina because a similar pattern of events has been observed in such patients (21).

The model demonstrated that an average of 1.0 mL/kg body wt. of pure ethanol given intravenously, dissolved in saline (producing an average blood alcohol content (BAC) of 0.24 g/dL) inhibits *in vivo* platelet activity and prevents coronary thrombosis (22) in the canine model. Red wine, dissolved in saline, given intravenously or by stomach tube, significantly inhibited *in vivo* platelet activity and prevented experimental coronary thrombosis (23). However, when wine was administered in place of pure alcohol, CFR inhibition required a BAC level of only 0.04 g/dL. This was provided by 4 mL/kg of red wine, the equivalent of approximately two glasses of wine (10 fluid ounces or 280 mL) in an average adult person. Thus, red wine was a more effective platelet inhibitor than pure alcohol since the wine was effective with a BAC of 0.04 g/dL while pure alcohol required a BAC of 0.24 g/dL (23), and the effect was observed at a level comparable to typical mealtime consumption.

An explanation for this effect may be that the naturally occurring flavonoids found in wine have been shown to decrease platelet aggregation in vitro (24), and the flavonoids found in beer and wine inhibit platelet activity, in part by elevating cyclic AMP levels in the platelet (25, 26). In addition, Seigneur showed that the consumption of red wine for a 15-day period significantly decreased ADP-induced platelet aggregation (27). Thus, during circulation in blood, the phenolic components from wine may decrease platelet activity and consequently decrease thrombotic CHD.

EFFECTS OF PHENOLICS ON VASCULATURE

The first report of the nutritional properties of flavonoids (vitamin P), describes the effects of a flavonoid preparation on the resistance and permeability of the capillary wall (28). A new report links the effects of grapes and wine to vasorelaxing activity (29), and this activity may reduce hypertension, another factor in CHD mortality by interfering with NO-dependent receptors.

TOXICITY

Not all phenolic substances are beneficial and some are toxic. Singleton (30) attributed 123 U.S. poisonings during one year to phenolic plant toxicants. The authors point out that while most common flavonoids are nontoxic, they can be toxic if administered at high levels for a long time. One striking example is that catechin, perhaps the most common flavonoid in food, found in wine, tea, and many fruits, was used at high doses as a drug to treat hepatic diseases, but after acute hemolytic anemia was associated with the use of the drug, its use was discontinued (31).

PHENOLIC COMPOUNDS DEFINED

Phenolic compounds are a class of phytochemicals widely distributed in plants, and ubiquitous in the diet (32). Because these compounds are secondary metabolites in plants, their levels are subject to wide variation. For instance, a recent study showed that increased sun exposure on grapes dramatically increased the levels of a particular flavonoid, quercetin (33). Thus, the very large sample sizes are required to determine the content of phenolic compounds in a particular food. Reports which rely on small sample sizes clearly show poor precision (34).

There are several chemical classes of phenolic compounds found in food, broadly separated into two classes, the flavonoids and the nonflavonoids. The phenolic compounds are dietary constituents of only plants, except for vitamin E, which also occurs in animal tissues.

In grapes, the most significant sub-classes of the flavonoids are the catechins (also called flavan-3-ols), including oligomers (the procyanidins) and polymers (the tannins) of this sub-class, the flavonols, and the anthocyanins (Fig. 14.1). There are numerous other classes of flavonoids, however, the quantities of these other classes in food are generally low; these latter classes generally occur as biosynthetic intermediates in the production of the major classes.

The classes of flavonoids are distinguished by differences in the central oxygen-containing "C" ring (Fig. 14.1). The "A" ring rarely has a different substitution pattern, typically having hydroxyl groups at positions 5 and 7. In most cases, class members are distinguished by differences in substitution on the "B" ring. Here, one, two or three hydroxy or methoxy substituents at the 3, 4, and 5 positions are most common.

Nearly 8000 individual flavonoids have been characterized (35). However, differences in the flavonoid nucleus account for only a few of these. In most cases, the nucleus is often glycosylated or otherwise substituted, and very large number of different sugars have been found to substitute flavonoids, in particular the flavonol class (32). The presence of specific flavonoids, based largely on the presence of specific glycosides can be used to verify the identity of the fruit species or occasionally the variety used to make a processed product such as juice or wine (36, 37).

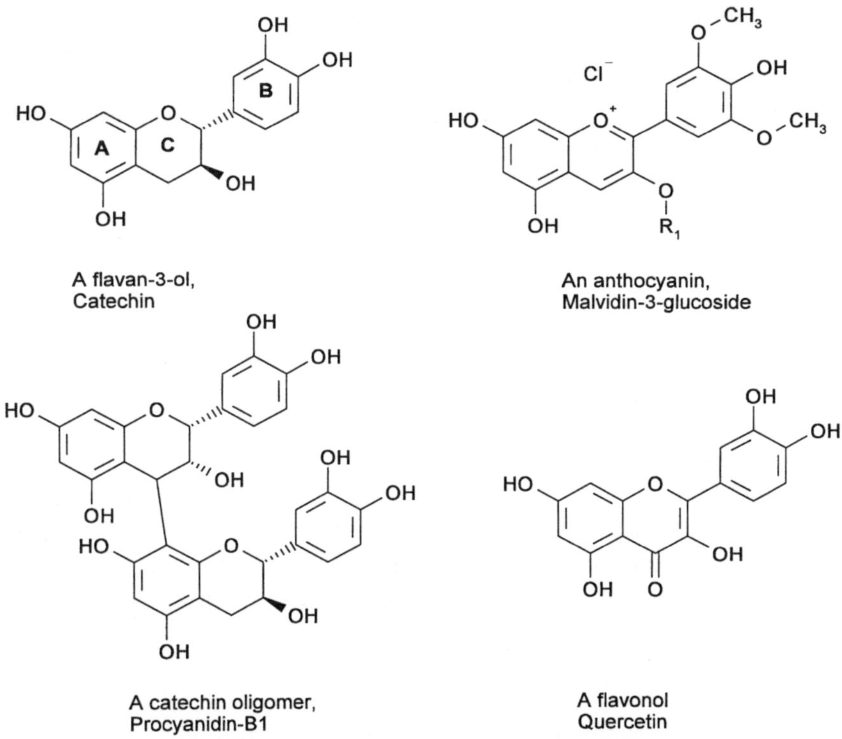

FIG. 14.1. A SELECTION OF THE FLAVONOIDS FOUND IN WINE, FRUIT, TEA AND OTHER MANY FOOD SOURCES. THE FLAVONOID LETTER DESIGNATION ARE SHOWN ON CATECHIN.

There are also several classes of nonflavonoids, dominated by a few groups including the benzoic acids and the hydroxycinnamates. There are other classes, such as the stilbene derivatives, but again the levels of these other components is low (Fig. 14.2).

PRINCIPAL DIETARY SOURCES OF PHENOLIC COMPOUNDS

To compare the amounts of phenolic compounds from a selection of common food sources, the levels of classes of phenolic compounds in various fruits or beverages have been normalized to the amount that would be found in either 200 grams fresh weight of fruit or 200 mL of beverage, a nominal serving. These amounts have been derived from the literature concentrations of individual phenolic compounds or totals of particular classes (32, 34, 37-42). In many cases, the amounts of the compounds reported for a particular fruit or beverage came from multiple publications. Since these levels are derived from chromatographic analysis of individual compounds, they must be seen as a lower limit for each fruit, since some compounds may have been missed. In addition, specific data on the concentrations of the polymeric substances are difficult to find, largely because these materials are difficult to quantitate chromatographically.

Dividing the phenolics into a limited number of classes or groups of materials allows for a simple and informative comparison (Fig. 14.3 to 14.8) of the relative constitution of the selected food products. However, a comparison of nutritional value, if such a value can be attached to these substances, will require definitive information on the chemistry of each specific compound-to date, and even the nature of this critical information

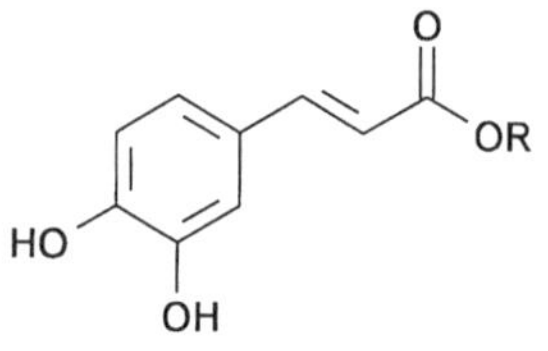

A Hydroxy-Cinnamate,
Substituted Caffeic Acid, R=various

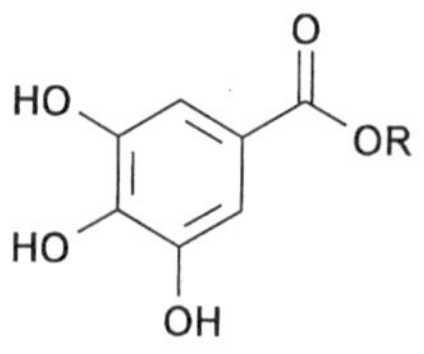

A Benzoid Acid,
Substituted Gallic Acid, R=various

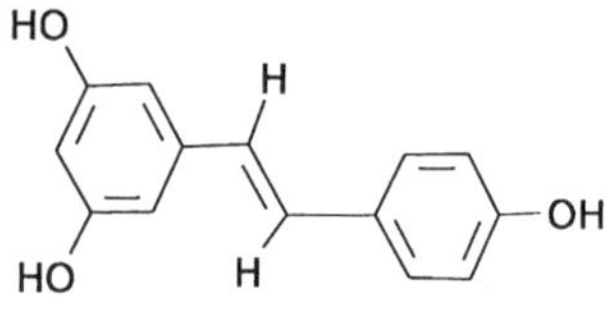

A Stilbene,
trans-resveratrol

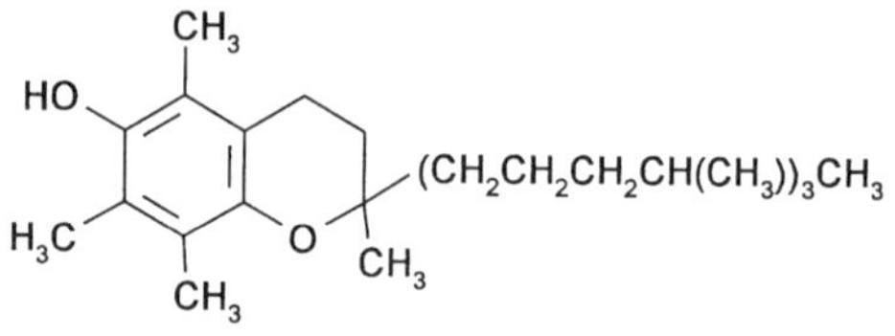

A Vitamin E,
a-tocopherol

FIG. 14.2. A SELECTION OF THE NONFLAVONOID PHENOLICS FOUND IN WINE, FRUIT AND TEA.

is poorly defined. The groups have been selected based on chemical classes, but to limit the number of groups, some are more expansive than a strict chemical system would allow. The groups are 1) the catechins, which include all monomeric flavan-3-ols and gallates thereof; 2) the oligomers, the oligomeric catechin forms (proanthocyanidins), and polymeric catechins (condensed tannins), as well as the hydrolyzable tannins; 3) the flavonols and the flavanones, including all glycosides; 4) the anthocyanins; 5) the cinnamates; and 6) the benzoic acid derivatives.

The specific fruit tissues analyzed are often not clearly identified. This creates a limitation in a comparison of the levels of phenolic compounds in a selection of food sources because it is known that these compounds are often localized into specific tissues. For instance, in oranges the flavonols are found exclusively in the white pulp (44). Where the data is unambiguous, the phenolic materials in nonedible fruit tissues, such as grape seeds, have been excluded from the tabulated totals in Fig. 14.3 to 14.8. Controlled phenolic intake experiments using fresh fruit would have to take into account the specific fruit portions

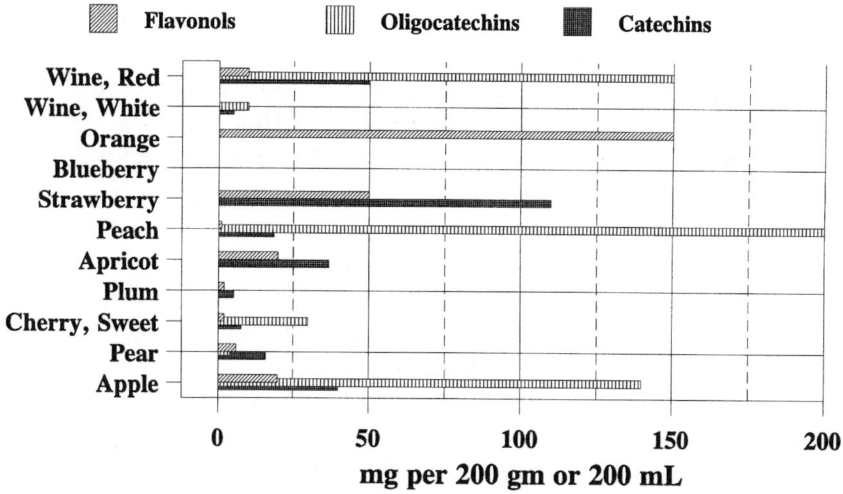

FIG. 14.3. LEVELS OF THE ANTHOCYANINS, BENZOIC ACIDS AND CINNAMATES IN WINES AND A SELECTION OF WHOLE FRUITS.

eaten and the phenolic composition of the eaten portions. Since the levels of these substances is so variable in fresh fruit, fresh fruit is a problematic source of these substance in experimentally defined diets. Homogeneous, processed food sources such as wine, avoid this experimental difficulty.

In the first grouping shown in Fig. 14.3, the catechins, oligomers and flavonols of wine and whole fruits, it is clear that red wine has relatively high levels of both catechins and oligomers/polymers and moderate amounts of flavonols. White wine has lower levels of all these classes. Among the whole fruits, oranges are notable in having solely flavonols/flavanones and blueberries are notable in having very low levels of all three compounds. Among the stone fruits, peaches are the richest and plums the poorest sources. Apples have higher levels than pears.

In acid solutions such as wine, the catechins slowly polymerize to higher molecular weight tannins, so that as wine ages, it gradually changes from a solution high in monomers and oligomers of the flavan-3-ols to one that has mostly polymers. Since very high molecular weight tannins are insoluble in aqueous solutions, bottles of old wine will form a precipitate of high molecular weight tannins. However, even fresh fruit products contain the oligomeric and polymeric forms and apples and peaches are notable for high levels of these materials (Fig. 14.3).

The anthocyanins are the red and blue pigments in most fruits, and their levels are related to color density and pH. Thus, as seen in Fig. 14.4, red wine has anthocyanins and white wine has none. Fruit sources high in anthocyanins include blueberries, strawberries and cherries. Blueberries are also a very rich source of hydroxycinnamates and plums and cherries both have high levels. Wines and most other fruits also contain the hydroxycinnamates. In general, fruits have low levels of the benzoic acids while wine has moderate amounts because these acids generally occur as esters in fresh fruit, but the aqueous acid environment of wine (pH 3.5) causes a slow hydrolysis of these phenolic fruit esters.

Fig. 14.5 compares the levels of the catechins, oligomers and flavonols in beverages. The levels in fruit juices are strikingly low compared to either wine or tea, and are lower than the lev-

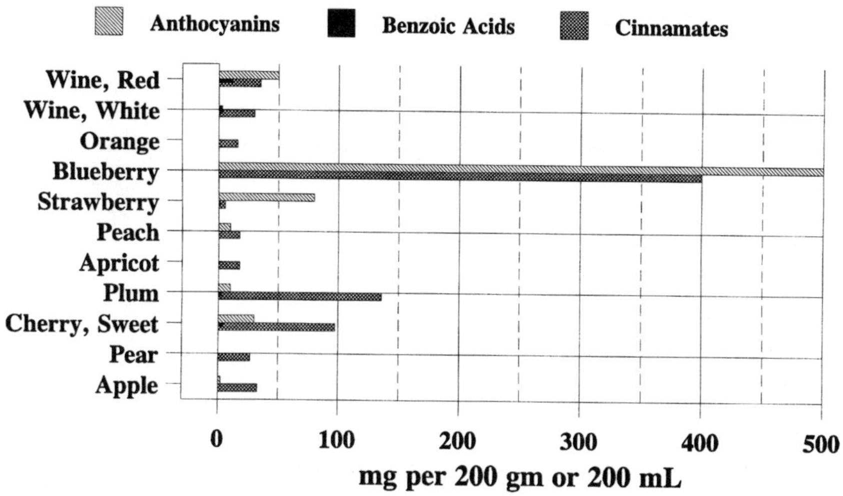

FIG. 14.4. LEVELS OF THE CATECHINS, OLIGOMERS/POLYMERS AND FLAVONOLS IN WINES AND A SELECTION OF WHOLE FRUITS.

els in similar whole fruits. Red wines have high levels of catechins and other phenolics because they are made by fermenting the whole fruit, including the seeds, and the flavonoids are extracted from these tissues by the alcohol produced during the fermentation. Even white wines contain relatively high concentrations of these substances compared to juices, because wines are protected from the oxygen that would oxidize the phenolic compounds.

The two teas are very rich sources of the catechins although the specific composition of each is quite different. Green tea, which is tea leaves that have simply been picked and dried, contains largely the monomeric catechins, while black tea, which has been fermented, has largely the oligomeric theaflavins and thearubigens, along with tannins. The catechins in tea are also somewhat different from fruit catechins, being largely of the gallotannin series. The gallo-derivatives have three hydroxyl groups on the "B" ring at the 3', 4', and 5' positions.

Fig. 14.6 compares the concentrations of anthocyanins and phenolic acids in beverages and shows that red wine contains

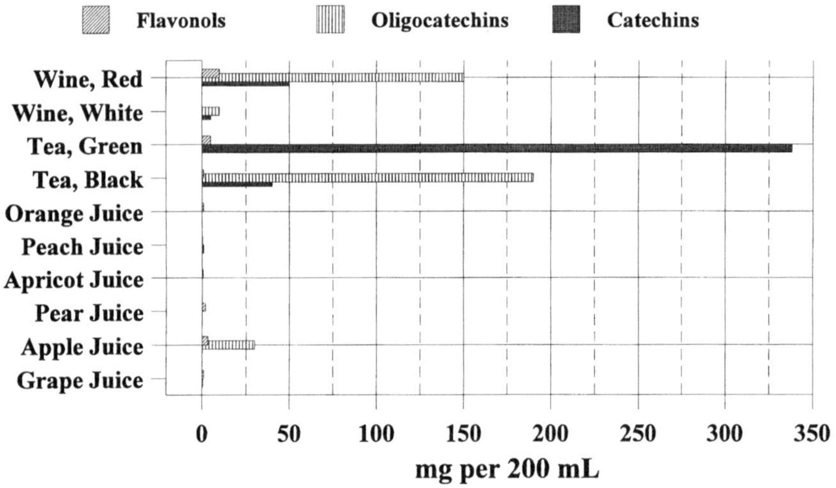

FIG. 14.5. LEVELS OF THE CATECHINS, OLIGOMERS/POLYMERS AND FLAVONOLS IN WINES, TEAS AND SELECTED FRUIT JUICES.

more anthocyanins than any other beverage. Both red and white wine and some juices contain the cinnamates, wine being a richer source than any juice. The cinnamates of grapes are somewhat unique among fruits, existing as the tartrate ester, while in many other fruits, the ester is with quinic acid (45). The free hydroxycinnamate acids are rare in fruit, but are found in wines due to acid hydrolysis.

In 1976 Kuhnau (32) estimated the average intake of flavonoids in the U.S. to be 1 g/day based on data obtained from 1955-71. Hertog et al. (11) disputed this amount, but they considered only the class of flavonols. From the totals shown in Fig. 14.7 and 14.8 it is clear that wine, fresh fruits and tea are rich sources of phenolic compounds, and the flavonoids comprise most of the total. A glass (5 ounces or 140 mL) of red wine or tea contains approximately 0.3 g of phenolic materials, largely flavonoids. Since wine and tea are preserved products and thus are available throughout the year, they can provide a constant source of these substances in the diet, while any particular fresh fruit will be seasonal.

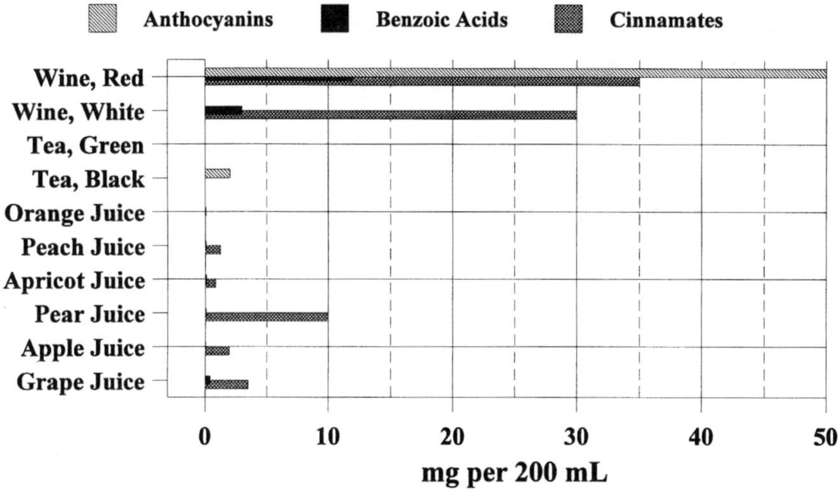

FIG. 14.6. LEVELS OF THE ANTHOCYANINS, BENZOIC ACIDS AND CINNAMATES IN WINES, TEAS AND SELECTED FRUIT JUICES.

DIETARY ABSORPTION AND METABOLISM STUDIES

The metabolism of flavonoids by mammals has been studied but is not completely understood (46, 47). Metabolism studies have been carried out on pure compounds as opposed to the compounds in a food matrix, and the available studies address a few flavonoids.

The most recent study of catechin metabolism in man was designed to utilize 2-g doses of ^{14}C-labeled catechin (47). This investigation showed that 55% of the dose was excreted in urine and that 90% of the administered radioactivity was excreted within 24 hr of oral administration of the catechin. The major urinary metabolites were the glucuronides of catechin and 3-methylcatechin, as well as the sulfate of the latter. Unchanged catechin in the urine was only 0.1 to 1.4% of the dose. Unchanged catechin was detected in plasma between 30 min and 12 hr after administration, and peak plasma levels of 1 to 2 μg/mL unchanged catechin were observed at 3 hr.

The pharmacokinetics of ^{14}C-labeled quercetin were studied by Gugler *et al.* (12) in 6 volunteers after single 100 mg intravenous doses and after single 4 g oral doses. After intravenous

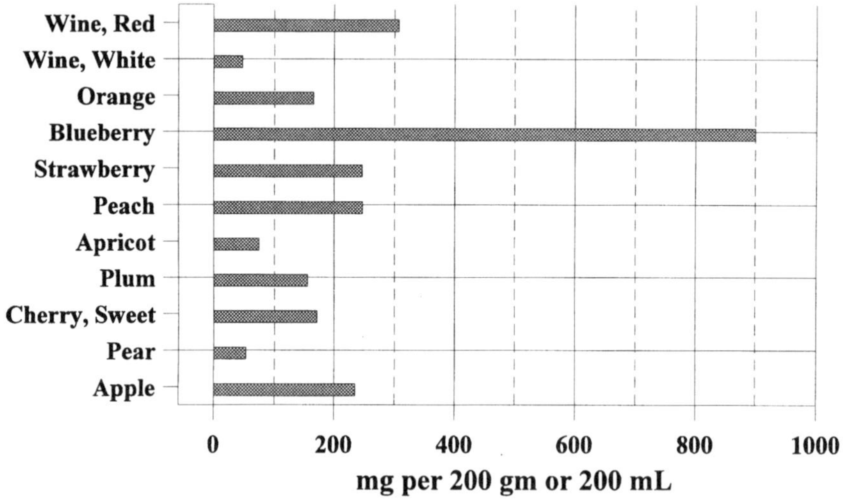

FIG. 14.7. TOTALS OF THE COMPILED AMOUNTS OF ALL PHENOLIC COMPOUNDS IN WINES AND A SELECTION OF WHOLE FRUITS.

administration, a two-phase plasma clearance was observed with half-lives of 8 min and 2.4 hr. After oral administration no quercetin was detected in plasma or urine, either unchanged or in a metabolized form. These results exclude absorption of more than 1% of quercetin; recovery in feces after the oral doses was 55%, which suggests extensive degradation by gut microorganisms to CO_2. The authors conclude that oral administration of quercetin for pharmacologic purposes may be of questionable value. However, in a canine model, gastric administration of quercetin in an animal thrombosis model reduced clo-forming activity (reduced cyclic flow reduction) (49), suggesting that absorption had occurred.

We have recently observed that when wine is consumed, a large proportion of the catechin is absorbed into the bloodstream (50). After 48 hr on a catechin-depleted diet, four subjects consumed wine that contained 80 mg total catechin. Three hours later, the average concentration of unchanged catechin in their plasma was 10 μM, approximately 20% of the catechin from the wine (Fig. 14.9). After 24 hr, over half of the catechin

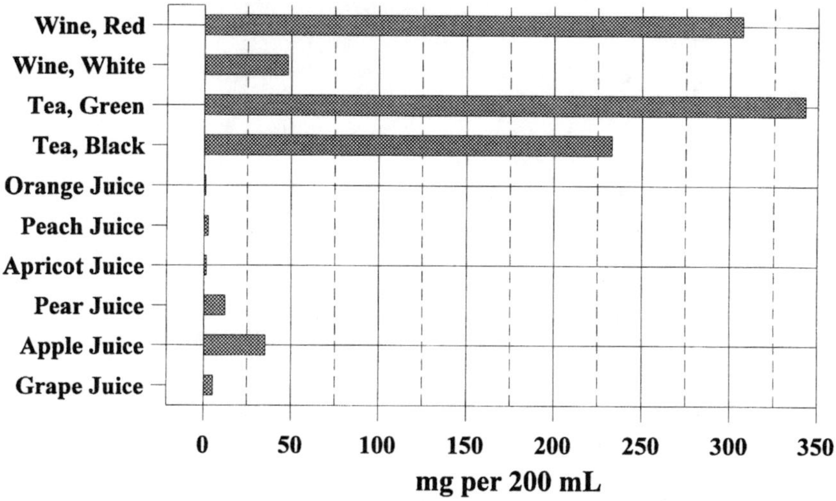

FIG. 14.8. TOTALS OF THE COMPILED AMOUNTS OF ALL PHENOLIC COMPOUNDS IN WINES, TEAS AND SELECTED FRUIT JUICES.

was eliminated from the plasma. The concentration found in the plasma were higher than the amount needed to inhibit the oxidation of LDL in vitro (51).

CONCLUSIONS

Epidemiological studies suggest a reduction in CHD mortality for those who consume wine or diets otherwise rich in flavonoids. Some of these compounds have been demonstrated as antioxidants for LDL, and some have been shown to inhibit platelet activity and reduce thrombotic events. Consequently, the hypothesis has been advanced that the phenolic compounds may explain the "French paradox" (18, 23) wherein CHD mortality rates are much lower than expected based on the daily fat consumption and serum lipid levels.

Summaries of the amounts of these compounds found in particular foods are of limited value for several reasons. The fundamental data on the levels of these substance in the numerous dietary sources is very limited. Much of the data presented

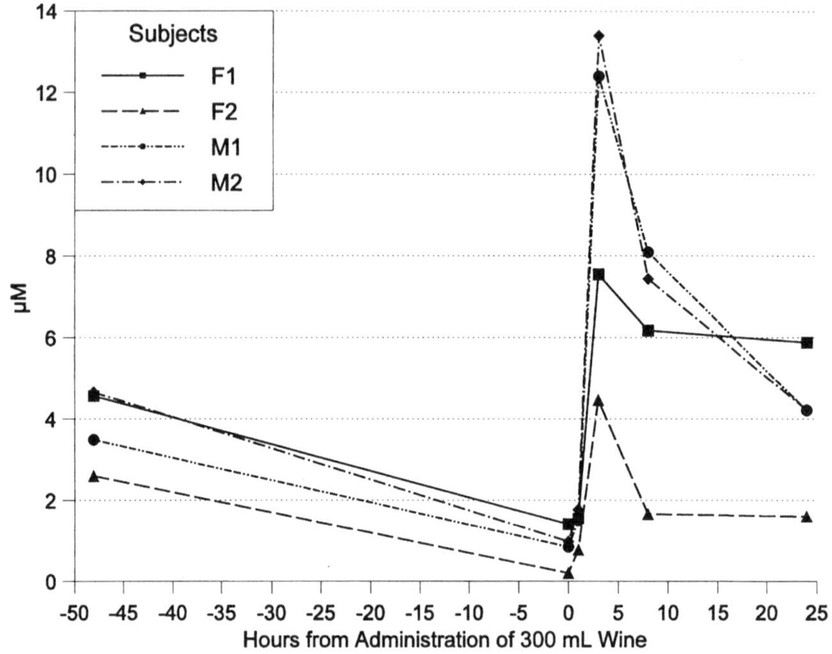

FIG. 14.9. CATECHIN LEVELS IN PLASMA IN FOUR HUMAN SUBJECTS BEFORE AND AFTER CONSUMPTION OF 300 ML CARMINE WINE. LDL OXIDATION WAS INHIBITED BY 80% AT 2 µM CATECHIN.

above was based on notably few samples, and given the large variability of phenolic compounds in plants, much better sampling is necessary and may be necessary in each market due to different sources. The terms *"phenolic compounds"* or *"phenolics"* encompasses thousands of individual chemicals, and while groupings of these substances based on chemical nomenclature are useful organizational tools, these groupings may be poor predictors of physiological activity. In order to understand the basis of any health benefits of these substances, it is critical to identify the specific actions of individual compounds and then study how these activities are altered by interactions (*i.e.* synergism) with other substances, in particular other antioxidants including other phenolics. It is just as important to identify which compounds may have detrimental effects and at what level these effects occur. In addition, the literature on absorption and metabolism of these compounds is remarkably thin and not well corroborated.

Because both epidemiology and mechanistic studies strongly suggest that some of the phenolic substances may partially explain the reduced CHD mortality correlated with increased fruit, vegetable, and wine consumption, a significant research effort is warranted to demonstrate or disprove any value for these substances as "beneficial nutrients." Bioavailability and well developed molecular mechanisms of action must be clearly defined before large scale human intervention studies can be properly designed to ascertain the physiological effects of dietary phenolic substances on humans.

BIBLIOGRAPHY

1. WILLETT, W. C. "Diet and health-what should we eat". *Science* 1994, 264, 532-537.
2. FONTHAM, E. T. "Protective dietary factors and lung cancer". *Int. J. Epidemiol.* 1990, 19 (suppl.), S32-42.
3. BLOCK, G. "Vitamin C status and cancer. Epidemiologic evidence of reduced risk". *Ann. N.Y. Acad. Sci.* 1992, 669, 280-290.
4. BAGHURST, P. A.; ROHAN, T. E. "High-fiber diets and reduced risk of breast cancer". *Int. J. Cancer* 1994, 56, 173-176.
5. HUANG, M. T.; HO, C. T.; LEE, C. Y., Eds. Phenolic Compounds in Food and Their Effect on Health; American Chemical Society: Washington, DC, 1992; Vol. 1 and 2.
6. ENSMINGER, A. H.; ENSMINTER, M. E.; KONLANDE, J. E.; ROBSON, J. R. K. Food and Nutrition Encyclopedia, 2nd ed.; CRC Press: Boca Raton, 1994; Vol. 1; pp. 206-210.
7. BUTLER, L. G.; ROGLER, J. C. "Biochemical mechanisms of the antinutritional effects of tannins". In Phenolic Compounds in Food and Their Effects on Health; Ho, C.-T.; Lee, C. Y.; Huang, M.-T., Eds.; American Chemical Society: Washington, DC, 1992; Vol. 1, pp. 298-304.
8. RENAUD, S.; DE LORGERIL, M. "Wine, alcohol, platelets, and the French paradox for coronary heart disease". *Lancet* 1992, 339, 1523-1526.
9. RIMM, E. B.; STAMPFER, M. J.; ASCHERIO, A.; GIOVANNUCCI, E.; COLDITZ, G. A.; WILLETT, W. C. "Vitamin E consumption and the risk of coronary heart disease in men". *N. Engl. J. Med.* 1993, 328, 1450-1456.
10. TRABER, M. G.; BURTON, G. W.; HUGHES, L.; INGOLD, K. U.; HIDAKA, H.; MALLOY, M.; KANE, J.; HYAMS, J.; KAYDEN, H. J.

"Discrimination between forms of vitamin E by humans with and without genetic abnormalities of lipoprotein metabolism". *J. Lipid Res.* 1992, 33, 1171-1182.

11. HERTOG, M. G. L.; FESKENS, E. J. M.; HOLLMAN, P. C. H.; KATAN, J. B.; KROMHOUT, D. "Dietary antioxidant flavonoids and risk of coronary heart disease: the Zutphen elderly study". *Lancet* 1993a, 342, 1007-1011.
12. GUGLER, R.; LESCHIK, M.; DENGLER, H. J. "Disposition of quercetin in man after single oral and intravenous doses". *Eur. J. Clin. Pharmacol.* 1975, 9, 229-234.
13. GRONBAEK, M.; DEIS, A.; SORENSEN, T. I. A.; BECKER, U.; SCHNOHR, P.; JENSEN, G. "Morality associated with moderate intakes of wine, beer and spirits". *Br. Med. J.* 1995, 310, 1165-1169.
14. BROWN, M. S.; GOLDSTEIN, J. L. "Receptor-mediated control of cholesterol metabolism". *Science* 1976, 191, 150-154.
15. STEINBERG, D.; PARTHASARATHY, S.; CAREW, T. E.; KHOO, J. C.; WITZTUM, J. L. "Beyond cholesterol. Modification of low-density lipoproteins that increase its atherogenicity". *N. Engl. J. Med.* 1989, 320, 915-924.
16. ESTERBAUER, M.; PUHL, H.; DIEBER-ROTHENEDER, M.; WAEG, G.; RAHL, H. "Effects of antioxidants on oxidative modification of LDL". *Ann. Med.* 1991, 23, 573-581.
17. FRANKEL, E. N.; KANNER, J.; GERMAN, J. B.; PARKS, E.; KINSELLA, J. E. "Inhibition of oxidation of human low-density lipoprotein by phenolic substances in red wine". *Lancet* 1993a, 341, 454-457.
18. FRANKEL, E. N.; WATERHOUSE, A. L.; KINSELLA, J. E. "Inhibition of human LDL oxidation by resveratrol". *Lancet* 1993b, 341, 1103-1104.
19. KINSELLA, J. E.; FRANKEL, E. N.; GERMAN, J. B.; KANNER, J. "Possible mechanisms for the protective role of antioxidants in wine and plant foods". *Food Technol.* 1993, 47 (4), 85-89.
20. WOOLF, N.; DAVIES, M. J. "Interrelationship between atherosclerosis and thrombosis". In Thrombosis in Cardiovascular Disorders; Fuster, V.; Verstraete, M., Eds.; 1992; pp. 50-55; N.
21. FOLTS, J. D. "An in vivo model of experimental arterial stenosis, intimal damage and periodic thrombosis". *Circulation* 1991, 83 [suppl IV], IV-3-IV-4.
22. KELLER, J.; FOLTS, J. D. "Relative effects of cigarette smoke and ethanol on acute platelet thrombosis formation in stenosed canine coronary arteries". *Cardiovasc. Res.* 1988, 22, 73-78.
23. DEMROW, H. S.; FOLTS, J. D. Gastric or IV administration of French red wine but not white wine inhibits in vivo platelet activity and thrombosis in stenosed canine coronary arteries, *J. Am. Coll. Card.* 1994, February, 49A.
24. MOWER, R.; LANDOLFI, R.; STEINER, M. "Inhibition in vitro of platelet aggregation and arachidonic acid metabolism by flavone". *Biochem. Pharmacol.* 1984, 36, 317-322.

25. FERRELL, J. E.; PETER, D. G.; SING, C.; LOEW, G.; KING, R.; MANSOUR, J. M.; MANSOUR, T. E. "Structure-activity studies of flavonoids as inhibitors of cAMP phophodiesterase and relationship to quantum chemical indices". *Mol. Pharmacol.* 1979, 16, 556-568.
26. HERTOG, M. G. L.; HOLLMAN, P. C. H.; KATAN, M. B.; KROMHOUT, D. "Intake of potentially anticarcinogentic flavonoids and their determinants in adults in the Netherlands". *Nutr. Cancer* 1993b, 20, 21-29.
27. SEIGNEUR, M.; BONNET, J.; DORIAN, B.; BENCHIMOL, D.; DROUILLET, F.; GOUVERNEUR, G.; LARRUE, J.; CROCKETT, R.; BOISSEAU, M.; RIBEREAU-GAYON, P.; BRICAUD, H. "Effect of the consumption of alcohol, white wine, and red wine on platelet function and serum lipids". *J. Appl. Card.* 1990, 5, 215-222.
28. BENSÁTH, A.; RUSZNYÁK, ST.; SZENT-GYÖRGYI, A. "Vitamin nature of flavones". *Nature* 1936, 138, 798.
29. FITZPATRICK, D. F.; HIRSCHFIELD, S. L.; COFFEY, R. G. "Endothelium-dependent vasorelaxing activity of wine and other grape products". *Am. J. Physiol.* 1993, 265, H774-H778.
30. SINGLETON, V. L.; KRATZER. "Plant phenolics". In Toxicants Occurring Naturally in Foods, 2nd ed.; Anon., Ed.; National Academy of Sciences: Washington DC, 1971; pp. 309-345.
31. ROTOLI, B.; BIBLIO, F.; BILE, M.; FORMISANO, S. "Immune-mediated acute intravascular haemolysis caused by cianidanol". *Haematologica* 1985, 70, 495-499.
32. KÜHNAU, J. "The flavonoids, a class of semi-essential food components: their role in human nutrition". *Wld Rev. Nutr. Diet* 1976, 24, 117-191.
33. PRICE, S. F.; BREEN, P. J.; VALLADAO, M.; WATSON, B. T. "Cluster sun exposure and quercetin in Pinot noir grapes and wine". *Am. J. Enol. Vitic.* 1995, 46, 187-194.
34. HERRMANN, K. "Occurrence and content of hydroxycinnamic and hydrocybenzoic acid compounds in foods". *Crit. Rev. Food Sci. Nutr.* 1989, 28, 315-347.
35. HARBORNE, J. B., Ed. The Flavonoids: Advances in Research Since 1986; Chapman and Hall: London, 1993.
36. ALBACH, R. F.; KEPNER, R. E.; WEBB, A. D. "Comparison of anthocyanin pigments of red vinifera grapes, II". *Am. J. Enol. Vitic.* 1959, 10, 164-172.
37. FERNÁNDEZ DE SIMON, B.; PÉREZ-ILZARBE, J.; HERNÁNDEZ, T.; GÓMEZ-CORDOVÉS, C.; ESTRELLA, I. "Importance of phenolic composition for the characterization of fruit juices". *J. Agric. Food Chem.* 1992, 40, 1531-1535.
38. SINGLETON, V. L. "Grape and Wine Phenolics; Background and Prospects". Proc. Symposium Univ. Calif. Davis, Grape & Wine Centennial, 1980 1982, 215-227.
39. PILANDO, L. S.; WROLSTAD, R. E.; HEATHERBELL, D. A. "Influence of Fruit composition, maturity, and mold contamination of the color and appearance of strawberry wine". *J. Food Sci.* 1985, 50, 1121-1125.

40. BILYK, A.; SAPERS, G. M. "Varietal differences in the quercetin, kaempherol and myricetin contents of highbush blueberry, cranberry and thornless blackberry fruits". *J. Agric. Food Chem.* 1986, 34, 585.
41. SPANOS, G. A.; WROLSTAD, R. E. "Influence of Variety, maturity processing, and storage on the phenolic composition of pear juice". *J. Agric. Food Chem.* 1990, 38, 817-824.
42. PELEG, H.; NAIM, M.; ROUSEFF, R. L.; ZEHAVI, U. "Distribution of bound and free phenolic acids in oranges (*Citrus sinensis*) and grapefruits (*Citrus paradisi*)". *J. Sci. Food Agric.* 1991, 57, 417-426.
43. BALENTINE, B. A. Manufacturing and Chemistry of Tea, ACS Symp. Ser. 1992, 506, 102-117.
44. JORUDAN, P. S.; WEILER, E. W.; MANSELL, R. L. "Naringen levels in citrus tissues. I. Comparison of different antibodies and tracers for the radioimmunoassay of naringin". *Plant Physiol.* 1985, 77, 696.
45. MOLGAARD, P.; RAVN, H. "Evolutionary aspect of caffeoyl ester distribution in dicotyledons". *Phytochemistry* 1988, 27, 2411.
46. DE EDS, F. "Flavonoid metabolism". In Comprehensive Biochemistry; Florkin, M.; Stotz, E. H., Eds.; Elsevier: Amsterdam, 1968; Vol. 20, pp. 127-171.
47. HACKETT, A. M. "The metabolism of flavonoid compounds in mammals". In Plant Flavonoids in Biology and Medicine: Biochemical Pharmacologocal and Structure-Activity Relationships; Progress in clinical and biological research 213; Cody, V.; Middleton, E. J.; Harborne, J. B., Eds.; Liss: New York, 1986; pp. 177-194.
48. HACKETT, A. M.; GRIFFITHS, L. A.; BROILLET, A.; WERMEILLE, M. "The metabolism and excretion of (+)-[14C]cyanidanol-3 in man following oral administration". *Xenobiotica* 1983, 13, 279-283.
49. SLANE, P. R.; FOLTS, J. D. "Platelet inhibition in stenosed canine arteries by quercetin, an antioxidant flavonoid found in red wine". *Clin. Res.* 1994, 42, 394.
50. WALZEM, R. L.; TEISSEDRE, P. L.; GERMAN, J. B.; HANSEN, R. J.; FRANKEL, E. N.; WATERHOUSE, A. L. "Absorption of the polyphenolic catechin from red wine". *J. Agric. Food Chem.* 1996, (submitted).
51. FRANKEL, E. N.; GERMAN, J. B.; DAVIS, P. A. "Headspace gas chromatography to determine human low density lipoprotein oxidation". *Lipids* 1992, 27, 1047-1051.

15

Tea and Cancer Prevention

Zhi Y. Wang
Laishun Chen
Mao-Jung Lee
Chung S. Yang

Inhibition of tumorigenesis by tea preparations has been observed in many animal models. This information has been propagated in the news media and popular magazines, sometimes with over-interpretations and inappropriate extrapolations concerning the cancer prevention activities of tea in humans. In this chapter, we examine the available evidence from laboratory and epidemiological studies, and discuss the possible mechanisms by which tea components inhibit carcinogenesis. Future research that is required to elucidate the possible role of tea consumption in the prevention of human cancers is also discussed.

The possible cancer prevention activity of tea is receiving a great deal of recent attention. Since our previous review on the topic "Tea and Cancer" in 1993 (1), about one hundred new research articles have been published. In this chapter, we intend to examine the available evidence from laboratory and epidemiological studies, and to discuss the possible mechanisms by which tea components inhibit carcinogenesis.

INHIBITION OF CARCINOGENESIS BY TEA IN ANIMAL MODELS

Tea extracts and tea polyphenols have been demonstrated to inhibit tumorigenesis in a variety of animal models covering different organ sites. Some recent studies from our and other laboratories are discussed herein.

Protection Against *N*-nitrosodiethylamine (NDEA)-induced Lung and Forestomach Tumorigenesis in Mice

Administration of 0.63% or 1.25% of green tea infusion (0.63 g or 1.25 g of tea leaves brewed in 100 ml of boiling water) as the sole source of drinking fluid to A/J mice during the NDEA-treatment period (10 mg/kg, i.g., once weekly for 8 weeks), the post NDEA-treatment period, or the entire experimental period significantly decreased the forestomach tumor multiplicity (by 31% to 63%) and lung tumor multiplicity (by 36% to 60%). The 1.25% green tea also decreased lung tumor incidence in all three protocols (by 36% to 44%) and significantly decreased forestomach tumor incidence when given during the initiation period or the entire experimental period. Inhibitory effects on lung and forestomach tumorigenesis by green tea were also observed in a similar experiment using a higher dosage of NDEA (20 mg/kg). Histopathological examination showed that almost all lung tumors were pulmonary adenomas. Most of the forestomach lesions were hyperplasia, papillomas, carcinomas *in situ*, and squamous cell carcinomas. In all the tea treatment groups, the incidence of papilloma was lower and the tumor size was smaller than those in the positive control group (2).

Protection Against 4-(methylnitrosamino)-1-(3-pyridyl)-1-butanone (NNK)-induced Lung Tumorigenesis in Mice

When 0.6% decaffeinated green tea (DGT) or decaffeinated black tea (DBT) extracts (0.6 g of dehydrated tea extract reconstituted in 100 ml of distilled water) were given to female A/J mice starting 2 weeks before the treatment with NNK (103 mg/kg, i.p., one dose) and ending 1 week later, the tumor multiplicity was reduced by 67% or 65%, respectively. When the tea preparation was given after the NNK-treatment period until the end of the experiment, 0.3% and 0.6% DGT reduced the tumor multiplicity by 74% and 85% and the tumor incidence by 14% and 30%, respectively. Under the same conditions, DBT decreased tumor multiplicity by about 63%, but did not significantly reduce the tumor incidence (2). In order to gain mechanistic information, mice were administrated DGT in different time periods before or after the NNK treatment (3). Treatment with DGT starting 2 weeks before and until 1 week after the NNK injection was more effective in the reduction of tumor multiplicity than treatment for 2 days before NNK injection. When tea was given after NNK treatment for a period of 1 week, tumor multiplicity was also reduced (by 20%). Tumor multiplicity was also inhibited (by 54%) even when DGT administration started at 5 weeks after NNK treatment.

Protection Against *N*-nitrosomethylbenzylamine (NMBzA)-induced Esophageal Tumorigenesis in Rats

When 0.6% DGT or DBT extracts were given to male Sprague-Dawley rats as the drinking fluid during the NMBzA treatment period (2.5 mg/kg, s.c., twice weekly for 5 weeks), esophageal tumor incidence and multiplicity were reduced by approximately 70%. When the tea preparations were given after the NMBzA treatment period, the esophageal papilloma incidence and multiplicity were reduced by approximately 50%. The volume per tumor was also reduced in rats which received DBT after the carcinogen treatment period. In a second experiment, the rats received 0.9% regular green tea or DGT (0.9 g of dehydrated tea extract in 100 ml of water) after the NMBzA treatment period (3.5 mg/kg, s.c., twice weekly for 5 weeks), and the tumor multiplicity was decreased by more than 55% at 16 weeks after the first dose of NMBzA. The volume per tumor was reduced by approximately 60% in the rats receiving 0.9% regular green tea. Histological analysis indicated that both the incidence and multiplicity of esophageal carcinoma were decreased by treatment with either regular green tea or DGT (4).

Protection Against Chemically- and Ultraviolet-induced Carcinogenesis in Murine Skin

In a two-stage skin tumorigenesis model in CD-1 mice, using either 7,12-dimethylbenz(a)anthracene (DMBA) or benzo(a)pyrene as an initiator and 12-O-tetradecanoylphorbol-13-acetate (TPA) as a promotor, topical application of green tea polyphenol fraction (GTPF) 5 min prior to each application of the carcinogen inhibited skin papilloma multiplicity by 35 to 67% (5). With CD-1 mice, after initiation with DMBA, topical application of GTPF before the application of TPA inhibited skin papilloma incidence and multiplicity by 71% and 94%, respectively (5). In other studies with SKH-1 mice initiated by DMBA and promoted by TPA, administration of 1.25% green tea as the sole source of drinking fluid during the promotion period significantly reduced the multiplicity and incidence of skin tumors (6). These results clearly indicated that green tea inhibited skin tumor initiation and promotion.

Skin tumorigenesis initiated by ultraviolet B light (UVB) and promoted by TPA was inhibited by the administration of 1.25% green tea as the drinking fluid prior to and during the 10 days of UVB treatment period and 1 week afterward. In other experiments using DMBA as an initiator and UVB as the promotor, administration of 1.25% green tea as the drinking fluid, prior to and during the period of 30 weeks of UVB treatment, decreased the number and size of the skin tumors (6). Using a similar protocol, oral administration of 0.63% or 1.25% green tea, black tea, DGT and DBT also had a marked inhibitory effect on UVB-induced skin carcinogenesis in DMBA-initiated SKH-1 mice (7).

Inhibition of Tumor Growth in Mice and Rats

In 10 separate experiments, mice bearing chemically induced or UVB light-induced skin papillomas were administered green

TABLE 15.1. SUMMARY OF ANTI-CARCINOGENESIS EFFECT OF TEA IN EXPERIMENTAL ANIMALS

			Tea administration			
Target organs	Animals	Tumor-induction	Tea	Application	During the period	References
Skin	Balb/C mice	3-MC, topical	GTPF	topical	whole	(9)
	SKH-1 mice	UVB	GTPF	topical	whole	(10)
	SKH-1 mice	UVB	GTPF	drinking	whole	(10)
	Sencar mice	BPDE/TPA, topical	GTPF	topical	initiation	(11)
	Sencar mice	DMBA/TPA, topical	GTPF	topical	initiation	(9)
	Sencar mice	DMBA/TPA, topical	EGCG	topical	initiation	(12, 13)
	CD-1 mice	BP/TPA, topical	GTPF	topical	initiation	(5)
	CD-1 mice	DMBA/TPA, topical	GTPF	topical	initiation	(5)
	SKH-1 mice	UVB-TPA, topical	GT	drinking	initiation	(6)
	CD-1 mice	DMBA/teleocidin, topical	EGCG (85%)	topical	promotion	(14)

*GTPF, green tea polyphenol fraction; GT, green tea leaf water extract; BT, Black tea leaf water extract; 3-MC, 3-methylcholanthrene; BPDE, bezo(a)pyrene diolepoxide; BPO, benzoylperoxide; NQO, 4-nitroquinoline-*N*-oxide; MNNG, *N*-methyl -*N*'-nitro-*N*-nitroguanidine; ENNG, *N*-ethyl-*N*'-nitro-*N*-nitroguanidine; DMH, 1,2-dimethylhydrazine; and BOP, *N*-nitroso-bis-(2-oxoprpyl)-amine.

TABLE 15.1. (Con't) SUMMARY OF ANTI-CARCINOGENESIS EFFECT OF TEA IN EXPERIMENTAL ANIMALS

			Tea administration			
Target organs	Animals	Tumor-induction	Tea	Application	During the period	References
	CD-1 mice	DMBA/okadaic acid, topical	EGCG (85%)	topical	promotion	(15)
	Sencar mice	DMBA/TPA, topical	GTPF	topical	promotion	(16)
	CD-1 mice	DMBA/mezerein, topical	GTPF	topical	promotion	(17)
	CD-1 mice	DMBA/TPA, topical	GTPF	topical	promotion	(5)
	SKH-1 mice	DMBA/TPA, topical	GT	drinking	promotion	(6)
	SKH-1 mice	DMBA/UVB, topical	GT	drinking	promotion	(10)
	Sencar mice	DMBA/TPA/BPO, topical	GTPF	topical	progression	(18)
	Sencar mice	DMBA/TPA/4-NQO, topical	GTPF	topical	progression	(18)
Esophagus	Wistar rats	NMBzA, i.g.	GT, BT, oolong	drinking	whole	(19)

*GTPF, green tea polyphenol fraction; GT, green tea leaf water extract; BT, Black tea leaf water extract; 3-MC, 3-methylcholanthrene; BPDE, bezo(a)pyrene diolepoxide; BPO, benzoylperoxide; NQO, 4-nitroquinoline-*N*-oxide; MNNG, *N*-methyl-*N'*-nitro-*N*-nitroguanidine; ENNG, *N*-ethyl-*N'*-nitro-*N*-nitroguanidine; DMH, 1,2-dimethylhydrazine; and BOP, *N*-nitroso-bis-(2-oxoprpyl)-amine.

TABLE 15.1. (Con't) SUMMARY OF ANTI-CARCINOGENESIS EFFECT OF TEA IN EXPERIMENTAL ANIMALS

			Tea administration			
Target organs	Animals	Tumor-induction	Tea	Application	During the period	References
	Wistar rats	precursors of NBMzA, i.g.	GT, BT, oolong	drinking	whole	(20)
	Kuinming mice	precursors of NSACS, i.g.	GT	i.g.	whole	(21)
	S-D rats	NMBzA, i.g.	DGT, DBT	drinking	initiation	(4)
	S-D rats	NMBzA, i.g.	GT, DGT, DBT	drinking	post-initiation	(4)
Forestomach	Kunming mice	precursors of NMBzA, i.g.	GT	p.o.	whole	(22)
	Kunming mice	precursors of NSACS, i.g.	GT	p.o.	whole	(21)
	A/J mice	NDEA, or BP, i.g.	GT	drinking	whole	(23)
	A/J mice	NDEA, i.g.	GT	drinking	initiation	(2)
	A/J mice	NDEA, i.g.	GT	drinking	post-initiation	(2)
	A/J mice	NDEA or BP, i.g.	GTPF	p.o.	initiation	(24)
Stomach	S-D rats	MNNG, drinking	DGT	drinking	whole	(25)

*GTPF, green tea polyphenol fraction; GT, green tea leaf water extract; BT, Black tea leaf water extract; 3-MC, 3-methylcholanthrene; BPDE, bezo(a)pyrene diolepoxide; BPO, benzoylperoxide; NQO, 4-nitroquinoline-*N*-oxide; MNNG, *N*-methyl-*N'*-nitro-*N*-nitroguanidine; ENNG, *N*-ethyl-*N'*-nitro-*N*-nitroguanidine; DMH, 1,2-dimethylhydrazine; and BOP, *N*-nitroso-bis-(2-oxoprpyl)-amine.

TABLE 15.1. (Con't) SUMMARY OF ANTI-CARCINOGENESIS EFFECT OF TEA IN EXPERIMENTAL ANIMALS

Target organs	Animals	Tumor-induction	Tea administration: Tea	Application	During the period	References
Duodenum and small intestine	C57BL/6 mice	ENNC, i.g.	EGCG (85%)	drinking	post-initiation	(26)
	F344 rats	multiple carcinogens	GTPF	in diet	initiation	(27)
	F344 rats	multiple carcinogens	GTPF	in diet	post-initiation	(27)
Colon	Fisher rats	Azoxymethane, s.c.	GTPF	drinking	post-initiation	(28)
	Kunming mice	DMH, s.c.	GTPF or EGCG	i.g.	whole	(29)
Lung	A/J mice	NDEA or BP, i.g.	GT	drinking	whole	(23)
	A/J mice	NDEA, i.g.	GT	drinking	initiation	(2)
	A/J mice	NDEA, i.g.	GT	drinking	post-initiation	(2)
	A/J mice	NDEA or BP, i.g.	GTPF	p.o.	initiation	(24)
	A/J mice	NNK, i.p.	IDGT or IDBT	drinking	initiation	(2, 3)
	A/J mice	NNK, i.p.	IDGT or IDBT	drinking	post-initiation	(2,3)

*GTPF, green tea polyphenol fraction; GT, green tea leaf water extract; BT, Black tea leaf water extract; 3-MC, 3-methylcholanthrene; BPDE, bezo(a)pyrene diolepoxide; BPO, benzoylperoxide; NQO, 4-nitroquinoline-*N*-oxide; MNNG, *N*-methyl -*N'*-nitro-*N*-nitroguanidine; ENNG, *N*-ethyl-*N'*-nitro-*N*-nitroguanidine; DMH, 1,2-dimethylhydrazine; and BOP, *N*-nitroso-bis-(2-oxoprpyl)-amine.

TABLE 15.1. (Con't) SUMMARY OF ANTI-CARCINOGENESIS EFFECT OF TEA IN EXPERIMENTAL ANIMALS

			Tea administration			
Target organs	Animals	Tumor-induction	Tea	Application	During the period	References
	A/J mice	NNK, i.g.	GT, EGCG or caffeine	drinking	initiation	(30)
	LACA mice	MNNG, i.v.	GT	in diet	initiation	(31)
Liver	Wistar rats	NDEA, i.p.	GT	in diet	initiation	(32)
Pancreas	Syrian hamster	BOP, s.c.	GTPF	in diet	promotion	(33)
Mammary gland	S-D rats	DMBA, i.p.	GTPF	in diet	post-initiation	(27)
	C3H/HeN mice	spontaneous	GTPF-$Al(OH)_3$	in diet	post-initiation	(34)

*GTPF, green tea polyphenol fraction; GT, green tea leaf water extract; BT, Black tea leaf water extract; 3-MC, 3-methylcholanthrene; BPDE, bezo(a)pyrene diolepoxide; BPO, benzoylperoxide; NQO, 4-nitroquinoline-*N*-oxide; MNNG, *N*-methyl -*N'*-nitro-*N*-nitroguanidine; ENNG, *N*-ethyl-*N'*-nitro-*N*-nitroguanidine; DMH, 1,2-dimethylhydrazine; and BOP, *N*-nitroso-bis-(2-oxoprpyl)-amine.

tea in the drinking water, or GTPF or (-)-epigallocatechin gallate (EGCG) by i.p. injections three times weekly, for 4 to 10 weeks. Tumor regression or inhibition of tumor growth, as measured by changes in tumor volume per mouse, was observed (8).

Other Laboratory Studies

More than 20 laboratories in different countries have reported the inhibitory effect of tea against tumorigenesis in animal models on different organ sites, such as skin, esophagus, forestomach, stomach, duodenum and small intestine, colon, lung, liver, pancreas, mammary gland. A summary of these results is shown in Table 15.1.

EPIDEMIOLOGICAL STUDIES ON TEA AND CANCER

In a 1991 monograph of the International Agency for Research on Cancer (35), it was concluded that "There is inadequate evidence for the carcinogenicity in humans and experimental animals of tea drinking." In our review on "Tea and Cancer" in 1993, we concluded that no clear-cut conclusion could be drawn concerning the protective effects of tea against human cancers (1). The conclusion still held true after inclusion of the 16 new case-control studies (36-51) published after our review. A summary of case-control studies on the relationship between tea consumption and human cancers is shown in Table 15.2. Some recent results on esophageal and gastric cancer are discussed in more detail in this section.

Esophageal Cancer

In several earlier studies it was suggested that excessive consumption of tea may be a causative factor for esophageal cancer (52-54). Several case-control studies, however, showed that there was no association between drinking of tea at normal temperature and esophageal cancer; but ingestion of very hot tea was associated with a two- to three-fold increase in risk for esophageal cancer (55-59). It was suggested that the high tem-

TABLE 15.2. CASE-CONTROL STUDIES ON THE RELATIONSHIP BETWEEN TEA CONSUMPTION AND HUMAN CANCERS

	Number of reports		
Organs	Reduction	Causation	No relationship
Bladder and urinary tract	—	—	17
Breast	—	—	6
Colon and rectum	3	1	6
Esophagus	1	7*	6
Kidney	—	1	5
Liver	—	—	1
Lung	—	1	1
Nasopharynx	—	—	3
Oral and tongue	1	—	1
Pancreas	2	1	8
Prostate	—	—	1
Stomach	4	1	8

*6 cases were with hot tea.

perature of hot tea, rather than the chemicals in tea, is an important etiological factor in human esophageal cancer (35). Two recent small case-control studies conducted in Northern China, one with 112 cases and 112 controls (60) and the other with 196 cases and 392 controls (40), reported that high temperature of meals and drinks had a strong association with esophageal cancer risk, but after adjustment of the temperature, the strength of tea and the amount of tea consumption were still independent determinants of the risk. On the other hand, a recent report by Gao *et al.* (38) indicated that, in Shanghai, frequent consumption of green tea was associated with lower incidence of esophageal cancer. Of the 902 patients interviewed, 734 patients had their esophageal cancer pathologically confirmed and there were 1552 control subjects interviewed. After adjustment for age and other possible confounders, a protective effect of green tea drinking on esophageal cancer was observed among women: odds ratio (OR), 0.50; 95% confidence interval (CI), 0.30 to 0.83, and this risk decreased (p for trend 0.01) as the quantity of tea consumption increased. Among men, the protective effect was not statistically significant. Among nonsmokers and nonalcoholic drinkers, statistically significant decreases in risk among tea drinkers were observed for both men (69 cases and 192 controls) (OR, 0.43; 95% CI, 0.22 to 0.86; p for trend = 0.05) and women (194 cases and 564 controls) (OR, 0.40; 95% CI, 0.20 to 0.77; p for trend < 0.001).

Gastric Cancer

Early correlative studies suggested that tea consumption is a protective factor against stomach cancer (61, 62). Case-control studies also suggest that tea consumption reduced the risk of stomach cancer in Kyushu (Japan) (63), Shanghai (China) (64), northwestern Turkey (49) and central Sweden (44). In Kyushu (139 cases and 2574 controls), individuals consuming green tea more frequently or in larger quantities (10 or more cups a day) tended to have a lower risk for gastric cancer (63). In a population-based case-control study (669 cases and 880 controls) in central Sweden, tea (mostly black tea) consumption showed a protective effect for the development of gastric cancer (44).

On the other hand, case-control studies on stomach cancer and tea consumption conducted in Buffalo (65), Kansas City (66), Nagoya (Japan) (67), Piraeus (Greece) (68) Milan (Italy) (56), Spain (69), Canada (70) and Turkey (71) indicated that there was no significant association between tea consumption and cancer of the stomach. A small case-control study in Taiwan (10 cases and 14 controls) suggested that green tea consumption is a risk factor for gastric cancer (72). An earlier cohort study (172 cases in 14,453 men), also showed a trend of positive association between black tea consumption and stomach cancer in London (73).

MECHANISMS FOR THE INHIBITION OF TUMORIGENESIS BY TEA

The most noteworthy properties of tea polyphenols that may affect carcinogenesis are their antioxidative activities, inhibitory action against nitrosation, modulation of carcinogen-metabolizing enzymes, trapping of ultimate carcinogens, and inhibition of cell proliferation-related activities (1, 74-76). For example, topically applied GTPF inhibited TPA-induced hydrogen peroxide formation in mouse epidermis (5, 77). Xu *et al.* reported that oral administration of green tea inhibited NNK-induced formation of 8-hydroxydeoxyguanosine in mouse lung (30). The major green tea polyphenols are derivatives of flavan-3-ols (catechins) such as EGCG, (-)epigallocatechin, (-)epicatechin-3-gallate, and (-)epicatechin. In the flavonol structure, the 5- and 7- dihydroxy groups and 1-oxygen make the carbons at positions 6 and 8 strongly nucleophilic. This property enables tea polyphenols effectively to block nitrosoamine formation and interact with reactive oxygen species or ultimate carcinogens. It appears that many of the biological activities of tea are due to the combined effects of all these polyphenols rather than a specific active ingredient.

Tea polyphenols are also known to have high complexation affinity to metals, alkaloids, and biological macromolecules such as lipids, carbohydrates, proteins, and nucleic acids. It has been reported that catechins can interact with the bacterial membrane resulting in anti-bacterial actions (78), interfere with the binding of estrogen to its receptors in MCF7 cells (79), inhibit the invasive activity of MO4 cells (80), and the adsorption of influenza virus to MDCK cells (81). The relevance of these observations to the biological activities of catechins *in vivo* remains to be studied.

In black tea the levels of catechins are about 30% of that of green tea, but the inhibitory activity of black tea against tumorigenesis was comparable to green tea in several animal models (2, 4, 7). The effective components in black tea are not clearly understood. During the manufacturing of black tea, catechins are oxidized by phenol oxidase and condensed to form oligomeric proanthocyanidins (82) known as theaflavins and thearubigins. These compounds still contain multiple hydroxyl groups and possess antioxidant activity. Other non-polyphenolic constitutions may also play a role in the anti-tumorigenesis activities of tea. Our tumorigenesis study indicated that decaffeinated tea displayed similar inhibitory activity to regular green tea in some experiments, but was less effective in other experiments (4, 7), suggesting that caffeine also possesses inhibitory activities in some animal models. Xu *et al*. reported that oral feeding of caffeine to A/J mice also inhibited NNK-induced lung tumorigenesis (30). High molecular weight complexes of polyphenols-polysaccharide-protein have also been suggested to possess biological activities (83).

FUTURE DIRECTIONS OF RESEARCH

Although the inhibitory actions of tea preparations against tumorigenesis have been demonstrated repeatedly in different animal models, no clear-cut conclusion can be drawn on the effect of tea consumption in the prevention of human cancers. In order to elucidate the role of tea consumption in human cancers and other health parameters, the following studies are needed.

A. Additional studies on the chemical properties and biological activities of tea and tea components are needed to provide a sound background for examining the effects of tea on health. Although a large volume of data have been accumulated concerning the protective effects of tea on cancer in laboratory studies, a clear understanding of the mechanisms by which tea components affect the genesis, growth, and progression of specific cancers are essential. Of importance is the selection of relevant experimental models and the ability to correlate results obtained *in vitro* to the situations in whole animals and in humans. Possible harmful effects should also be noted. Black tea is the major form of tea consumed in the Western countries. The chemistry and biological activities of black tea components, however, are poorly understood. Research needs in this area are obvious.

B. The bioavailabilities of tea components and the dose-response relationship in the inhibition of tumorigenesis need to be studied systematically. We have begun to measure the plasma and urinary levels of green tea polyphenols in humans and animals after ingestion of different amounts of green tea. The bioavailabilities and interconversions of the different tea polyphenols are being studied. Similar studies on black tea components are also needed. Extension of these studies will enable us to establish the quantitative relationship among tea consumption, blood (tissue) levels, and inhibitory activities against tumorigenesis. This information is useful in evaluating the possible inhibitory effect of tea consumption against carcinogenesis in humans.

C. More epidemiological studies concerning the effect of tea consumption on human cancer risk are needed. Because the causative factors are various for different cancers or for the same cancer in different populations, tea consumption may affect carcinogenesis only in selected situations. Therefore, in future epidemiological studies, it is important to consider the etiological factors of the specific cancers and to collect more specific information on the qualitative and quantitative aspects of tea consumption. Definitive information on the protective effects of tea consumption on cancer will come from intervention studies. Based on the suggestive epidemiological data from Shizuoka, Kyushu, Shanghai, northwestern Turkey, and central Sweden, intervention studies on gastric cancer among higher risk populations should be very interesting. If we assume that *N*-nitroso compounds are important causative factors for gastric cancer, then the protective effect of tea may be partially due to its ability to inhibit the endogenous formation of these nitroso compounds via nitrosation reactions. In such future studies, exposure biomarkers such as the urinary excretion of tea polyphenols, endogenous nitrosation markers such as urinary *N*-nitrosoproline, and intermediate biomarkers such as sulfomucins and Lewis antigens (84) may be very useful.

BIBLIOGRAPHY

1. YANG, C. S.; WANG, Z. Y. "Tea and cancer". *J. Natl. Cancer Inst.* 1993, 85, 1038-49.

2. WANG, Z. Y.; HONG, J.-Y.; HUANG, M.-T.; REUHL, K. R.; CONNEY, A. H.; YANG, C. S. "Inhibition of *N*-nitrosodiethylamine- and 4-(methylnitrosamino)-1-(3-pyridyl)-1-butanone-induced tumorigenesis in A/J mice by green tea and black tea". *Cancer Res.* 1992, 52, 1943-1947.
3. SHI, S. T.; WANG, Z. Y.; SMITH, T.; HONG, J.-Y.; CHEN, W.-F.; HO, C.-T.; YANG, C. S. "Effects of green tea and black tea on 4-(methylnitrosamino)-1-(3-pyridyl)-1-butanone bioactivation, DNA methylation, and lung tumorigenesis in A/J mice". *Cancer Res.* 1994, 54, 4641-4647.
4. WANG, Z. Y.; WANG, L.-D.; LEE, M.-J.; HO, C.-T.; HUANG, M.-T.; CONNEY, A. H.; YANG, C. S. "Inhibition of *N*-nitrosomethylbenzylamine-induced esophageal tumorigenesis in rats by green and black tea". *Carcinogenesis* 1995, 16, 2143-2148.
5. HUANG, M.-T.; HO, C.-T.; WANG, Z. Y.; FERRARO, T.; FINNEGAN-OLIVE, T.; LOU, Y.-R.; MITCHELL, J. M.; LASKIN, J. F.; NEWMARK, H.; YANG, C. S.; CONNEY, A. H. "Inhibitory effect of topical application of a green tea polyphenol fraction on tumor initiation and promotion in mouse skin". *Carcinogenesis* 1992, 13, 947-954.
6. WANG, Z. Y.; HUANG, M. T.; FERRARO, T.; WONG, C. Q.; LOU, Y. R.; REUHL, K.; IATROPOULOS, M.; YANG, C. S.; CONNEY, A. H. "Inhibitory effect of green tea in the drinking water on tumorigenesis by ultraviolet light and 12-O-tetradecanoylphorbol-13-acetate in the skin of SKH-1 mice". *Cancer Res.* 1992, 52, 1162-1170.
7. WANG, Z. Y.; HUANG, M. T.; LOU, Y. R.; XIE, J. G.; REUHL, K. R.; NEWMARK, H. L.; HO, C. T.; YANG, C. S.; CONNEY, A. H. "Inhibitory effects of black tea, green tea, decaffeinated black tea, and decaffeinated green tea on ultraviolet B light-induced skin carcinogenesis in 7,12-dimethylbenz[a]anthracene-initiated SKH-1 mice". *Cancer Res.* 1994, 54, 3428-3435.
8. WANG, Z. Y.; HUANG, M. T.; HO, C. T.; CHANG, R.; MA, W.; FERRARO, T.; REUHL, K. R.; YANG, C. S.; CONNEY, A. H. "Inhibitory effect of green tea on the growth of established skin papillomas in mice". *Cancer Res.* 1992, 52, 6657-6665.
9. WANG, Z. Y.; KHAN, W. A.; BICKERS, D. R.; MUKHTAR, H. "Protection against polycyclic aromatic hydrocarbon-induced skin tumor initiation in mice by green tea polyphenols". *Carcinogenesis* 1989, 10, 411-415.
10. WANG, Z. Y.; AGARWAL, R.; BICKERS, D. R.; MUKHTAR, H. "Protection against ultraviolet B radiation-induced photocarcinogenesis in hairless mice by green tea polyphenols". *Carcinogenesis* 1991, 12, 1527-1530.
11. KHAN, W. A.; WANG, Z. Y.; ATHAR, M.; BICKERS, D. R.; MUKHTAR, H. "Inhibition of the skin tumorigenicity of (±)7B, 8a-epoxy-7, 8, 9, 10-tetrahydrobenzo(a)pyrene by tannic acid, green tea polyphenols and quercetin in Sencar mice". *Cancer Lett.* 1988, 42, 7-12.
12. WANG, Z. Y.; ZHOU, Z. C.; BICKERS, D. R.; MUKHTAR, H. "Inhibition of chemical and photocarcinogenesis in murine skin by green tea polyphenols". *Proc. Am. Assoc. Cancer Res.* 1990, 31, 159.

13. KATIYAR, S. K.; AGARWAL, R.; WANG, Z. Y.; BHATIA, A. K.; MUKHTAR, H. "(-)-Epigallocatechin-3-gallate in *Camellia sinensis* leaves from Himalayan region of Sikkim: inhibitory effects against biochemical events and tumor initiation in Sencar mouse skin". *Nutr. Cancer* 1992, 18, 73-83.
14. YOSHIZAWA, S.; HORIUCHI, T.; FUJIKI, H.; YOSHIDA, T.; OKUDA, T.; SUGIMURA, T. "Antitumor promoting activity of (-)-epigallocatechin gallate, the main constituent of "tannin" in green tea". *Phytother. Res.* 1987, 1, 44-47.
15. YOSHIZAWA, S.; HORIUCHI, T.; SUGIMURA, M.; NISHIWAKI, S.; YATSUNAMI, J.; OKABE, S.; OKUDA, T.; MUTO, Y.; FRENKEL, K.; TROLL, W.; FUJIKI, H. "Penta-o-galloyl—D-glucose and (-)-epigallocatechin gallate: cancer prevention agent". In *Phenolic Compounds in Foods and Health. II.*; Huang, M.-T.; Lee, C. Y.; Ho, C.-T., Eds.; American Chemical Society: Washington, 1992; pp. 316-325.
16. KATIYAR, S. K.; AGARWAL, R.; WOOD, G. S.; MUKHTAR, H. "Inhibition of 12-O-tetradecanoylphorbol-13-acetate-caused tumor promotion in 7,12-dimethylbenz[a]anthracene-initiated SENCAR mouse skin by a polyphenolic fraction isolated from green tea". *Cancer Res.* 1992, 52, 6890-6897.
17. KATIYAR, S. K.; AGARWAL, R.; MUKHTAR, H. "Inhibition of both stage I and stage II skin tumor promotion in SENCAR mice by a polyphenolic fraction isolated from green tea: inhibition depends on the duration of polyphenol treatment". *Carcinogenesis* 1993, 14, 2641-2643.
18. KATIYAR, S. K.; AGARWAL, R.; MUKHTAR, H. "Protection against malignant conversion of chemically induced benign skin papillomas to squamous cell carcinomas in SENCAR mice by a polyphenolic fraction isolated from green tea". *Cancer Res.* 1993, 53, 5409-5412.
19. HAN, C.; XU, Y. "The effect of Chinese tea on the occurrence of esophageal tumors induced by *N*-nitrosomethylbenzylamine in rats". *Biomed. Environ. Sci.* 1990, 3, 35-42.
20. XU, Y.; HAN, C. "The effect of Chinese tea on the occurrence of esophageal tumors induced by *N*-nitrosomethylbenzylamine formed *in vivo*". *Biomed. Environ. Sci.* 1990, 3, 406-412.
21. CHEN, S.-J.; DING, L.; ZHEN, Y.-S.; LIN, P.-Z.; ZHU, Y.-J.; CHEN, Y.-Q.; HU, X.-Z. "Progress in studies on the antimutagenicity and anticarcinogenicity of green tea epicatechins". *Chinese Med. Sci. J.* 1991, 6, 233-238.
22. GAO, G. D.; ZHOU, L. F.; QI, G.; WANG, H. S.; LI, T. S. "Initial study of antitumorigenesis of green tea (animal test and flow cytometry)". *Tumor (Chinese)* 1990, 10, 42-44.
23. WANG, Z. Y.; R., A.; KHAN, W. A.; MUKHTAR, H. "Protection against benzo(a)pyrene and N-nitrosodiethylamine-induced lung and forestomach tumorigenesis in A/J mice by water extracts of green tea and licorice". *Carcinogenesis* 1992, 13, 1491-1494.

24. KATIYAR, S. K.; AGARWAL, R.; ZAIM, M. T.; MUKHTAR, H. "Protection against *N*-nitrosodiethylamine and benzo[a]pyrene-induced forestomach and lung tumorigenesis in A/J mice by green tea". *Carcinogenesis* 1993, 14, 849-855.
25. YAN, Y. S. "The experiment of tumor-inhibiting effect of green tea extract in animal and human body". *Chung Hua Yu Fang I Hsueh Tsa Chih* 1993, 27, 129-131.
26. FUJITA, Y.; YAMANE, T.; TANAKA, M.; KUWATA, K.; OKUZUMI, J.; TAKAHASHI, T.; FUJIKI, H.; OKUDA, T. "Inhibitory effect of (-)-epigallocatechin gallate on carcinogenesis with *N*-ethyl-*N'*-nitro-*N*-nitrosoguanidine in mouse duodenum". *Jpn. J. Cancer Res.* 1989, 80, 503-5.
27. ITO, N.; HIROSE, M.; SHIRAL, T. "Carcinogenicity and modification of carcinogenic response by plant phenols". In *Phenolic Compounds in Foods and Health, II.*; Huang, M.-T.; Lee, C. Y.; Ho, C.-T., Eds.; American Chemical Society: Washington, D. C., 1992; pp. 269-281.
28. YAMANE, T.; HAGIWARA, N.; TATEISHI, M.; AKACHI, S.; KIM, M.; OKUZUMI, J.; KITAO, Y.; INAGAKE, M.; KUWATA, K.; TAKAHASHI, T. "Inhibition of azoxymethane-induced colon carcinogenesis in rat by green tea polyphenol fraction". *Jpn. J. Cancer Res.* 1991, 82, 1336-1339.
29. YIN, P.; ZHAO, J.; CHENG, S.; ZHU, Q.; LIU, Z.; ZHENGGUO, L. "Experimental studies of the inhibitory effects of green tea catechin on mice large intestinal cancers induced by 1,2-dimethylhydrazine". *Cancer Lett.* 1994, 79, 33-38.
30. XU, Y.; HO, C.-T.; AMIN, S. G.; HAN, C.; CHUNG, F.-L. "Inhibition of tobacco-specific nitrosamine-induced lung tumorigenesis in A/J mice by green tea and its major polyphenol as antioxidants". *Cancer Res.* 1992, 52, 3875-3879.
31. LUO, D.; LI, Y. "Preventive effect of green tea on MNNG-induced lung cancers and precancerous lesions in LACA mice". *Hua Hsi I Ko Ta Hsueh Hsueh Pao* 1992, 23, 433-437.
32. LI, Y. "Comparative study on the inhibitory effect of green tea, coffee and levamisole on the hepatocarcinogenic action of diethylnitrosamine". *Chung Hua Chung Liu Tsa Chih* 1991, 13, 193-195.
33. HARADA, N.; TAKABAYASHI, F.; OGUNI, I.; HARA, Y. "Anti-promotion effect of green tea extracts on pancreatic cancer in golden hamster induced by N-nitroso-bis(2-oxopropyl)amine". In *Proceedings of the Int. Sympo. on Tea Sci.*; Yamanishi, T., Eds.; Kurofune Printing Co., Ltd.: Shizuoka, Japan, 1991; pp. 200-204.
34. HARA, Y. "Prophylactic functions of tea polyphenols". In *Proceedings of the Int. Sympo. on Tea Sci.*; Yamanishi, T., Eds.; Shizuoka, Japan, 1991; pp. 200-204.
35. WHO INTERNATIONAL AGENCY FOR RESEARCH ON CANCER. "Coffee, tea, mate, methylxanthines, and methylgloxyal". *IARC Monogr. Carcinog. Risks. Hum.* 1991, 51, 207-271.

36. WAKAI, K.; OHNO, Y.; OBATA, K.; AOKI, K. "Prognostic significance of selected lifestyle factors in urinary bladder cancer". *Jpn. J. Cancer Res.* 1993, 84, 1223-1229.
37. SHIBATA, A.; MACK, T. M.; PAGANINI, H. A.; ROSS, R. K.; HENDERSON, B. E. "A prospective study of pancreatic cancer in the elderly". *Int. J. Cancer* 1994, 58, 46-49.
38. GAO, Y. T.; MCLAUGHLIN, J. K.; BLOT, W. J.; JI, B. T.; DAI, Q.; FRAUMENI, J. J. "Reduced risk of esophageal cancer associated with green tea consumption". *J. Natl. Cancer Inst.* 1994, 86, 855-8.
39. MELLEMGAARD, A.; ENGHOLM, G.; MCLAUGHLIN, J. K.; OLSEN, J. H. "Risk factors for renal cell carcinoma in Denmark. I. Role of socioeconomic status, tobacco use, beverages, and family history". *Cancer Causes Control* 1994, 5, 105-113.
40. HU, J.; NYREN, O.; WOLK, A.; BERGSTROM, R.; YUEN, J.; ADAMI, H. O.; GUO, L.; LI, H.; HUANG, G.; XU, X. "Risk factors for oesophageal cancer in northeast China". *Int. J. Cancer* 1994, 57, 38-46.
41. SLATTERY, M. L.; WEST, D. W. "Smoking, alcohol, coffee, tea, caffeine, and theobromine: risk of prostate cancer in Utah (United States)". *Cancer Causes Control* 1993, 4, 559-563.
42. EWERTZ, M. "Breast cancer in Denmark. Incidence, risk factors, and characteristics of survival". *Acta Oncol.* 1993, 32, 595-615.
43. DHAR, G. M.; SHAH, G. N.; NAHEED, B.; HAFIZA "Epidemiological trend in the distribution of cancer in Kashmir Valley". *J Epidemiol. Community Health* 1993, 47, 290-2.
44. HANSSON, L. E.; NYREN, O.; BERGSTROM, R.; WOLK, A.; LINDGREN, A.; BARON, J.; ADAMI, H. O. "Diet and risk of gastric cancer. A population-based case-control study in Sweden". *Int. J. Cancer* 1993, 55, 181-9.
45. OLSEN, J.; KRONBORG, O. "Coffee, tobacco and alcohol as risk factors for cancer and adenoma of the large intestine". *Int. J. Epidemiol.* 1993, 22, 398-402.
46. MASHBERG, A.; BOFFETTA, P.; WINKELMAN, R.; GARFINKEL, L. "Tobacco smoking, alcohol drinking, and cancer of the oral cavity and oropharynx among U.S. veterans". *Cancer* 1993, 72, 1369-1375.
47. ZATONSKI, W. A.; BOYLE, P.; PRZEWOZNIAK, K.; MAISONNEUVE, P.; DROSIK, K.; WALKER, A. M. "Cigarette smoking, alcohol, tea and coffee consumption and pancreas cancer risk: a case-control study from Opole, Poland". *Int. J. Cancer* 1993, 53, 601-607.
48. HUANG, C.; ZHANG, X.; QIAO, Z.; GUAN, L.; PENG, S.; LIU, J.; XIE, R.; ZHENG, L. "A case-control study of dietary factors in patients with lung cancer". *Biomed. Environ. Sci.* 1992, 5, 257-65.
49. MEMIK, F.; NAK, S. G.; GULTEN, M.; OZTURK, M. "Gastric carcinoma in northwestern Turkey: epidemiologic characteristics". *J Environ. Pathol. Toxicol. Oncol.* 1992, 11, 335-338.
50. MIZUNO, S.; WATANABE, S.; NAKAMURA, K.; OMATA, M.; OGUCHI, H.; OHASHI, K.; OHYANAGI, H.; FUJIKI, T.; MOTOJIMA, K. "A

multi-institute case-control study on the risk factors of developing pancreatic cancer". *Jpn. J. Clin. Oncol.* 1992, 22, 286-291.
51. FRANCESCHI, S.; SERRAINO, D. "Risk factors for adult soft tissue sarcoma in northern Italy". *Ann. Oncol.* 1992, 3, 85-88.
52. SEGI, M. "Tea-gruel as a possible factor for cancer of the esophageal cancer". *Gann.* 1975, 66, 199-202.
53. JOINT IRAN-INTERNATIONAL AGENCY FOR RESEARCH ON CANCER STUDY GROUP "Esophageal cancer studies in the Caspian Littoral of Iran: results of population studies-a prodrome". *J. Natl. Cancer Inst.* 1977, 59, 1127-1138.
54. KAPADIA, G. J.; RAO, S.; MORTON, J. F. "Herbal tea consumption and esophageal cancer". In *Carcinogens and Mutagens in the Environment*; Stich, H. F., Eds.; CRC Press. Inc.: Boca Raton, Florida., 1983; 3, pp. 3-12.
55. VICTORA, C. G.; MUNOZ, N.; DAYN.E.; BARCELOS, I. B.; PECCIN, D. A.; BRAGA, N. M. "Hot beverages and oesophageal cancer in southern Brazil: a case-control study". *Int. J. Cancer* 1987, 39, 710-716.
56. LA VECCHIA, C.; NEGRI, E.; FRANCESCHI, S.; D'AVANZO, B.; BOYLE, P. "Tea consumption and cancer risk". *Nutr. Cancer* 1992, 17, 27-31.
57. KAUFMAN, B. D.; LIBERMAN, I. S.; TYSHETSKY, V. I. "Some data concerning the incidence of oesophageal cancer in the Gurjev region of the Kazakh SSR (Russ.)". *Vopr. Onkol.* 1965, 11, 78-85.
58. BASHIROV, M. S.; NUGMANOV, S. N.; KOLYCHEVA, N. I. "Epidemiological study of oesophageal cancer in the Akhtubinsk region of the Kazakh Socialist Republic (Russ.)". *Vopr. Onkol.* 1968, 14, 3-7.
59. COOK-MOZAFFARI, P. J.; AZORDEGAN, F.; DAY, N. E.; RESSICAUD, A.; SABAI, C.; ARAMESH, B. "Oesophageal cancer studies in the Caspian littoral of Iran: results of a case-control study". *Br. J. Cancer* 1979, 39, 293-309.
60. REN, A.; HAN, X. "Dietary factors and esophageal cancer: a case-control study". *Chung Hua Liu Hsing Ping Hsueh Tsa Chih* 1991, 12, 200-204.
61. STOCKS, P. "Cancer mortality in relation to national consumption of cigarettes, solid fuel, tea and coffee". *Br. J. Cancer* 1970, 24, 215-225.
62. OGUNI, I.; CHEN, S. J.; LIN, P. Z.; HARA, Y. "Protection against cancer risk by Japanese green tea". *Prevent. Med.* 1992, 21, 332.
63. KONO, S. "Green tea and colon cancer [letter]". *Jpn. J. Cancer. Res.* 1992, 83, 669.
64. YU, G. P.; HSIE, C. C. "Risk factors for stomach cancer: a population-based case-control study in Shanghai. AD: Department of Epidemiology, School of Public Health, Shanghai Medical University, People's Republic of China". *Cancer Causes Control* 1991, 2, 169-174.
65. GRAHAM, S.; LILIENFELD, A. M.; TIDINGS, J. E. "Dietary and purgation: factors in the epidemiology of gastric cancer". 1967, 20, 2224-2234.
66. HIGGINSON, J. "Etiological factors in gastrointestinal cancer in man". *J. Natl. Cancer Inst.* 1966, 37, 527-545.

67. TAJIMA, K.; TOMINAGA, S. "Dietary habits and gastro-intestinal cancers: a comparative case-control study of stomach and large intestinal cancers in Nagoya, Japan". *Jpn. J. Cancer Res. (Gann)* 1985, 76, 705-716.
68. TRICHOPOULOS, D.; OURANOS, G.; DAY, N. E.; TZONOU, A.; MANOUSOS, O.; PAPADIMITRIOU, C.; TRICHOPOULOS, A. "Diet and cancer of the stomach: a case-control study in Greece". *Int. J. Cancer* 1985, 36, 291-297.
69. AGUDO, A.; GONZALEZ, C. A.; MARCOS, G.; SANZ, M.; SAIGI, E.; VERGE, J.; BOLEDA, M.; ORTEGO, J. "Consumption of alcohol, coffee, and tobacco, and gastric cancer in Spain". *Cancer Causes Control* 1992, 3, 137-43.
70. RISCH, H. A.; JAIN, M.; CHOI, N. W.; FODOR, J. G.; PFEIFFER, C. J.; HOWE, G. R.; HARRISON, L. A.; CRAIB, K. J. P.; MILLER, A. B. "Dietary factors and the incidence of cancer of the stomach". *A. J. Epidemiol.* 1985, 122, 947-959.
71. DEMIRER, T.; ICLI, F.; UZUNALIMOGLU, O.; KUCUK, O. "Diet and stomach cancer incidence. A case-control study in Turkey". *Cancer* 1990, 65, 2344-8.
72. LEE, H. H.; WU, H. Y.; CHUANG, Y. C.; CHANG, A. S.; CHAO, H. H.; CHEN, K. Y.; CHEN, H. K.; LAI, G. M.; HUANG, H. H.; CHEN, C. J. "Epidemiologic characteristics and multiple risk factors of stomach cancer in Taiwan". *Anticancer Res.* 1990, 10, 875-881.
73. KINLEN, L. J.; MCPHERSON, K. "Pancreas cancer and coffee and tea consumption: a case-control study". *Br. J. Cancer* 1984, 49, 93-96.
74. AGARWAL, R.; KATIYAR, S. K.; KHAN, S. G.; MUKHTAR, H. "Protection against ultraviolet B radiation-induced effects in the skin of SKH-1 hairless mice by a polyphenolic fraction isolated from green tea". *Photochem. Photobiol.* 1993, 58, 695-700.
75. KLAUNIG, J. E. "Chemopreventive effects of green tea components on hepatic carcinogenesis". *Prev. Med.* 1992, 21, 510-519.
76. YOKOZAWA, T.; OURA, H.; IWANO, M.; DOHI, K.; HATTORI, M. "Inhibitory effects of crude drug components on the proliferation of cultured human mesangial cells". *Nippon Jinzo Gakkai Shi.* 1993, 35, 321-327.
77. LASKIN, J. D.; HECK, D.; LASKIN, D. L.; MITCHELL, J. M.; HUANG, M.-T.; WANG, Z. Y.; YANG, C. S.; HO, C.-T.; CONNEY, A. H. "Inhibitory effects of a green tea polypheno fraction on 12-O-tetradecanoylphorbol-13-acetate-induced hydrogen peroxide formation in mouse epidermis". In *Phenolic Compounds in Foods and Health, II.*; Huang, M.-T.; Lee, C. Y.; Ho, C.-T., Eds.; American Chemical Society: Washington, D. C., 1992; pp. 308-314.
78. IKIGAI, H.; NAKAE, T.; HARA, Y.; SHIMAMURA, T. "Bactericidal catechins damage the lipid bilayer". *Biochimi. Biophys. Acta* 1993, 1147, 132-136.
79. KOMORI, A.; YATSUNAMI, J.; OKABE, S.; ABE, S.; HARA, K.; SUGANUMA, M.; KIM, S. J.; FUJIKI, H. "Anticarcinogenic activity of green tea polyphenols". *Jpn. J. Clin. Oncol.* 1993, 23, 186-190.

80. BRACKE, M. E.; VYNCKE, B.; OPDENAKKER, G.; FOIDART, J.-M.; PESTEL, G.; MAREEL, M. "Effect of catechins and citrus flavonoids on invasion in vitro". *Clin. Expl. Metastasis* 1991, 9, 13-25.
81. NAKAYAMA, M.; SUZUKI, K.; TODA, M.; OKUBO, S.; HARA, Y.; SHIMAMURA, T. "Inhibition of the infectivity of influenza virus by tea polyphenols". *Antiviral Res.* 1993, 21, 289-299.
82. HEMINGWAY, R. W. "Structural variations in proanthocyanidins and their derivatives". In *Chemistry and Significance of Condensed Tannins*; Hemingway, R. W.; Karchesy, J. J., Eds.; Plenum Press: New York, London, 1989; pp. 83-118.
83. NAKAMURA, Y.; HARADA, S.; KAWASE, I.; MASTUDA, M.; TOMITA, I. "Inhibitory effects of tea ingredients on the *in vivo* tumor promotion of mouse epidermal JB6 cells". In *Proceedings of the Int. Sympo. on Tea Sci.*; Yamanishi, T., Eds.; Kurofune Printing Co., Ltd.: Shizuoka, Japan, 1991; pp. 205-209.
84. CORREA, P. "Human gastric carcinogenesis: A multistep and multifactorial process-First American Cancer Society Award Lecture on Cancer Epidemiology and Prevention". *Cancer Res.* 1992, 52, 6735-6740.

16

The Chemistry and Health Benefits of Organosulfur and Organoselenium Compounds in Garlic (*Allium sativum*): Recent Findings

Eric Block

Numerous reports have appeared concerning the medical properties of garlic and related *Allium* species. Most of these papers discuss the virtues of consumption of fresh plants or use of commercial products derived from plants (mainly garlic) in the prevention of cancer, as natural antibiotics, and in the treatment of cardiovascular disease and hypoglycemia, among other conditions. Parallel research activity has occurred in the analysis, characterization, and synthesis of the unique compounds present in the fresh plants and in extracts and distillates derived from them. As these various pure chemical components (and sensitive analytical techniques for their detection) have become available, research activity to determine the *in vitro* and *in vivo* biological activity of these products has accelerated. Recent developments and trends in these areas are evaluated in this chapter.

The flavor of freshly cut garlic, generally associated with the compound allicin, *S*-2-propenyl 2-propenethiosulfinate (*3*), results from action of alliinase enzymes on precusor compounds such as alliin, (+)-*S*-2-propenyl *L*-cysteine *S*-oxide (*1*). On heating, or even standing, allicin is converted to a number of other compounds including ajoene, vinyl dithiins, and various di- and poly-sulfides. The compounds formed from crushed garlic are best characterized by mild procedures such as HPLC and LC-MS. Volatile organoselenium compounds from garlic preparations can be identified using the technique of atomic emission detection GC (GC-AED). When fresh garlic is subjected to cooking, or commercial processing by such methods as freeze-drying, maceration in oil, or pickling, among others, the sulfur compounds undergo a variety of changes whose nature must be understood in determining the value, if any, of the resulting products as health supplements. The purported health benefits of garlic are considered both from a historical perspective as well as in terms of the latest findings on antibiotic, cardiovascular, and cancer preventative activity, among other claimed attributes and effects, both desirable and undesirable, of the fresh and processed herb. Because of its reputation as an herb with numerous medicinal properties, garlic is a top selling food supplement, with U.S. sales in excess of $100 million annually and with a variety of different brands of garlic products on the market. Garlic has even been added to well established lines of vitamin supplements marketed by major pharmaceutical houses. Among the myriad garlic products, often with significant price tags, we find pearls, soft gels, gelatin capsules, tablets (with and without enteric coating), and liquids. While "aspirin" is always acetylsalicylic acid, what does "garlic" mean on a label? Does the herb itself and any of the commercial garlic products truly offer any health benefits? If so, how is this documented? To answer these questions, it is necessary to understand what compounds are present both in the intact plant and following processing, to evaluate the appropriateness of the methodology for quantitative analysis of these compounds and determination of their biological activity, and to judge the relevancy and validity of results from *in vitro* and *in vivo* animal and human testing and epidemiological studies.

BACKGROUND

It is well known that the "natural flavor" of garlic (*Allium sativum*) and other *Allium* species, like those from many other common vegetables and fruits, is not present as such in the intact plants but is formed when the plants are crushed or cut. When the cells rupture, rapid chemical reactions occur when the (separated) flavor precursors and enzymes commingle (1-3). Specifically, it is known that in intact garlic cloves (+)-*S*-2-propenyl *L*-cysteine *S*-oxide (*1*) ("alliin") and related *S*-alk(en)yl-*L*-cysteine *S*-oxides (aroma and flavor precursors) are located in the cytoplasm while the C-S lyase enzyme alliinase is located in the bundle sheaths, usually one cell layer thick, close to the phloem (4). Alliinase activity is ten times higher in the bulb of a mature plant than in the leaves and stems (5). Disruption of the cells results in release of alliinase and subsequent, α,β-elimination of the sulfoxides, ultimately affording volatile and odorous low molecular weight organosulfur compounds such as *S*-2-propenyl 2-propenethiosulfinate (*3*) (allicin) via the intermediacy of 2-propenesulfenic acid (*2*) (Scheme 1). Alliinase has been purified to homogeneity and characterized as a dimer of subunits of MW 51.5 kDa each, with a pH optimum of 6.5. Surprisingly, alliinase becomes rapidly inactivated following its interaction with alliin and/or allicin (5).

Allicin, and related symmetrically substituted thiosulfinates, are easily synthesized by peracid oxidation of the corresponding disulfide, e.g. diallyl disulfide (*4*). Garlic also contains two other sulfoxides, *S*-(*E*)-1-propenyl- and *S*-methyl *L*-cysteine *S*-oxides (*5* and *6*, respectively; see Scheme 2). Earlier reports of the presence of *S*-propyl *L*-cysteine *S*-oxide have proven to be incorrect. Also present in garlic and other *Allium* spp. are 24-γ glutamyl peptides of sulfur amino acids. These are considered to

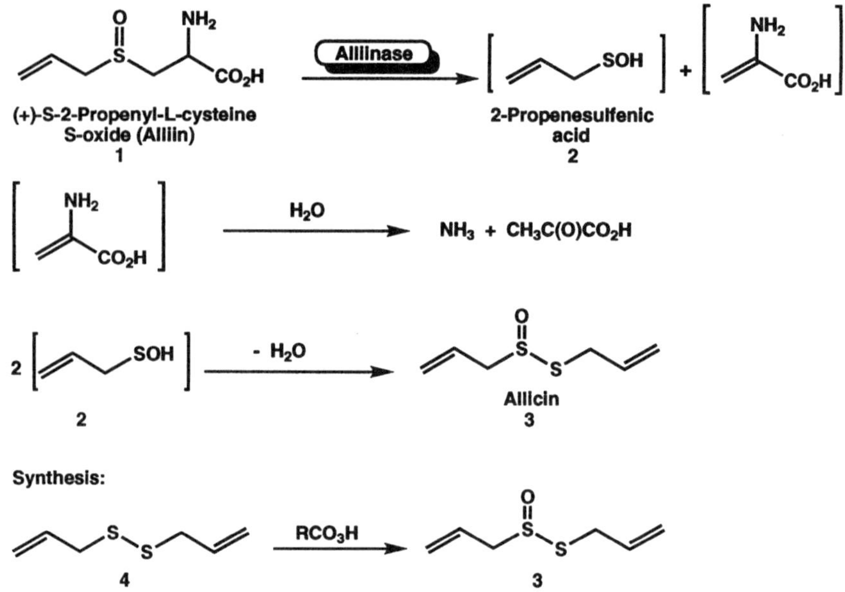

Scheme 1

function as storage compounds of nitrogen and sulfur (precursors to plant chemical defense agents?) and may have a role in transport of amino acids across cell membranes (2). It is uncertain as to whether γ-glutamyl cysteine derivatives in garlic are immediate precursors of alliin or are formed in parallel (6,7). With a total sulfur content of 3.5 mg/g fresh weight (1% of dry weight), garlic has a higher sulfur content than most other common vegetables. The level of selenium in garlic (0.28 g/g fresh weight), although much lower than that of sulfur, is also relatively high compared to other common vegetables (8). The sulfur compounds in garlic are ultimately derived from soil sulfate; similarly the selenium compounds originate from soil selenite (SeO_3^{2-}) or selenate (SeO_4^{2-}). Scheme 2 shows possible biosynthetic pathways for alliin, γ-glutamyl cysteine derivatives, and selenocysteine (a selenium compound in fresh garlic; see below).

During food preparation involving garlic, additional flavors are formed through thermal breakdown of the initial enzymatically-produced flavorants, either in an aqueous or non-aqueous

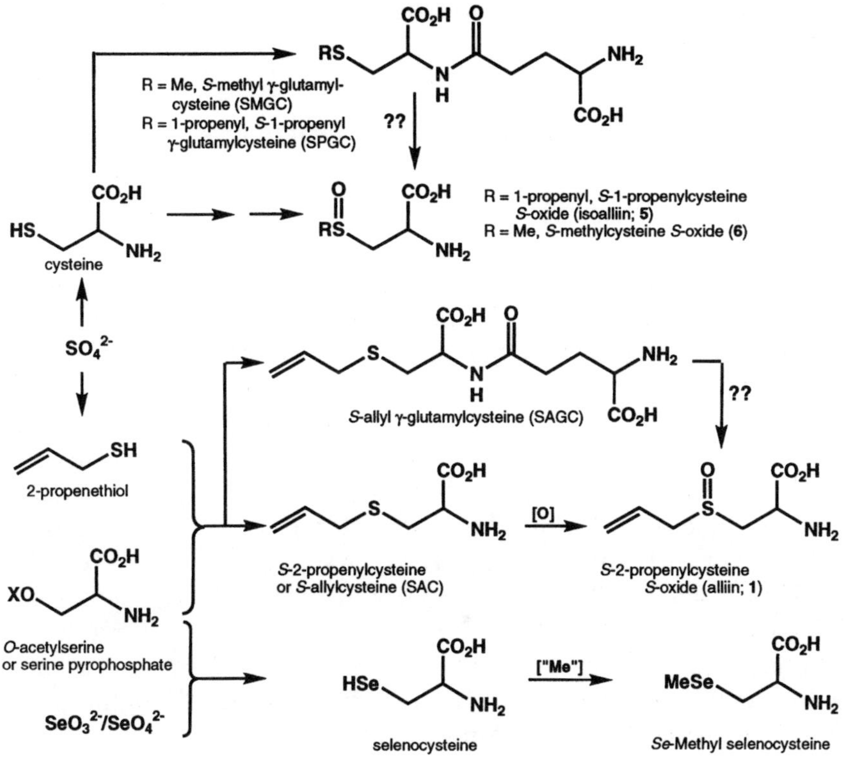

Scheme 2

(e.g. cooking oil) medium. Some of these compounds may be lost though evaporation. Heating in an aqueous medium can lead to products of hydrolysis. If the breakdown products themselves are unstable, further compounds can be formed which may also make important aroma and taste contributions, particularly if these substances have low taste thresholds. Because of the instability and reactivity of many of the *Allium*-derived organosulfur compounds, it can sometimes be difficult to distinguish the genuine flavorants, as defined above, from artifacts formed by the analytical methods and sampling techniques (9, 10). Allicin (*3*), which possesses the characteristic aroma and taste of fresh garlic, is quite reactive and unstable, undergoing hydrolysis on heating in water giving diallyl disulfide (*4*), diallyl trisulfide and the corresponding polysulfides (*3* is moderately stable in water at room temperature due to the protective action of hydrogen bonding).

RECENT WORK ON *ALLIUM* SPP. FLAVORANTS

Particularly efficient isolation of the thiosulfinate flavorants of fresh, crushed garlic is achieved by the technique of supercritical fluid extraction (SFE) using liquefied CO_2 (11). Thus, if 2-3 g fresh, peeled garlic is homogenized with 5 mL water using a commercial tissue homogenizer at room temperature, and the homogenate, after standing for 10 minutes, is extracted at 35 C with 40 mL supercritical CO_2 using a solid-phase trap system with effluent trapping at 0 C and desorbtion using 1.5 mL methylene chloride, normal phase Si HPLC analysis indicates the presence of a total of 2.8 mg/g fresh garlic of the thiosulfinate flavorants AllS(O)SAll (*3*) (72.2%), AllSS(O)Me (16.2%), AllS(O)SMe (6.3%), AllS(O)SCH=CHMe-(*E*,*Z*) (2.5%), AllSS(O)CH=CHMe-(*E*) (1.2%), MeS(O)SMe (1.9%) and trace amounts of MeS(O)SCH=CHMe-(*E*,*Z*). This mild extraction procedure is 25% more efficient than a procedure involving methylene chloride as the extraction solvent. Identity of all compounds was confirmed using authentic synthetic standards and by using various LC-MS techniques under reversed phase C18 conditions (thermospray, atmospheric pressure chemical ionization (APCI)). These data are in good agreement with other published studies (12,13). There is no evidence from the above HPLC studies for the presence in fresh garlic extracts of significant quantities of the polysulfides and thiophenes claimed by prior GC-MS analyses. It is probable that the latter sulfur compounds are artifacts associated with decomposition of thermally unstable thiosulfinates containing the allyl group under the GC-MS conditions. Fresh garlic, when crushed, typically releases 9.4 mg/g fresh weight -glutamyl cysteines (*S*-allyl, SAGC; *S*-1-propenyl, SPGC; *S*-methyl, SMGC), in addition to 3.7 mg/g allicin (*3*), and 1.7 mg/g of other thiosulfinates, with the total weight of all sulfur compounds being 15.9 mg/g (ca. ± 24-30% in each case) (21).

Chromatography of solutions prepared by soaking chopped garlic in methanol afforded allicin (*3*), diallyl di-, tri-, and tetrasulfide, allyl methyl trisulfide, 3-vinyl-4*H*-1,2-dithiin (7), and 2-vinyl-4*H*-1,3-dithiin (*8*), along with two isomeric polar compounds, termed (*E*)- and (*Z*)-ajoene (based on the Spanish word for garlic, ajo, pronounced "aho"), ultimately characterized as (*E*,*Z*)-4,5,9-trithiadodeca-1,6,11-triene 9-oxide (*9*) by spectroscopic and synthetic methods (Scheme 3)(14,15). When synthetic *3* was refluxed with 3:2 acetone:water for 4 h, (*E*,*Z*)-*9* could be isolated in 34% yield. Other products included *7* and *8*, in a 1:4.4 ratio, and diallyl di- and trisulfide. Isolation of *7* and *8* from decomposition of *3* and the identity of the *7*:*8* ratio to that observed from dimerization of thioacrolein (*10*) suggests that the first step in the decomposition of *3* involves intramolecular

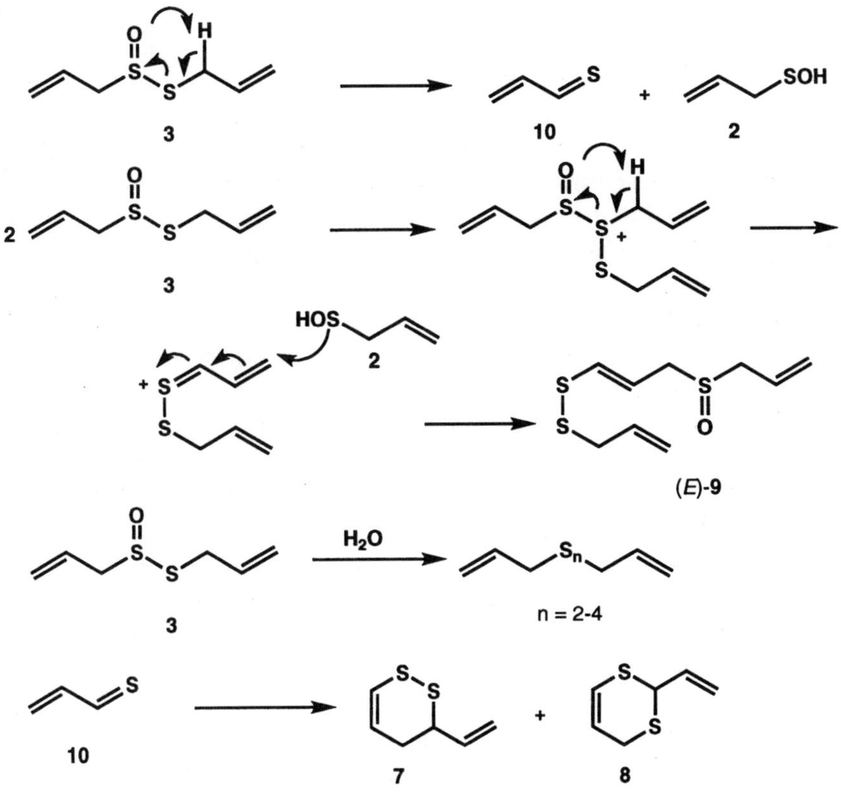

Scheme 3

elimination to 2-propenesulfenic acid (*2*) and *10* (Scheme 3). This postulate finds additional support in the observation of the characteristic sapphire blue color of *10* when *3* is distilled into a liquid nitrogen cooled trap. Since other thiosulfinates of structure $RS(O)SCH_2CH{=}CH_2$, such as $MeS(O)SCH_2CH{=}CH_2$ and $MeCH{=}CHS(O)SCH_2CH{=}CH_2$, are found in garlic extracts, and since these thiosulfinates can also give thioacrolein by the mechanism of Scheme 3, formation of the two dithiins *7* and *8* cannot be used to assay for allicin alone.

Support for the proposed mechanism of thermal decomposition of allicin *3* was obtained by supercritical fluid chromatography-mass spectrometry (SFC-MS) of a fresh garlic extract (*16*). Initial open-tubular SFC data showed two chromatographic peaks. Using an interface to the mass spectrometer equipped with a variable temperature restrictor tip through which the supercritical CO_2 expands into the MS source, it was observed that at 115 C restrictor tip temperature the most abundant ion of the major chromatographic peak was m/z 163, representing the MH^+ for *3*. The minor chromatographic peak was identified by its mass spectrum as a mixture of unresolved isomers of allyl methyl thiosulfinates ($MeS(O)SCH_2CH{=}CH_2$ and $MeSS(O)CH_2CH{=}CH_2$). When the restrictor tip temperature was increased to 165 C, the m/z 163 ion of *3* disappeared and was replaced by the base ion m/z 73 and another major ion at m/z 91, in addition to ions at 145, 129, 115 and 99, indicative of formation of thioacrolein dimers. The m/z 73 and 91 ions correspond to protonated thioacrolein (*10*-H^+) and protonated 2-propenesulfenic acid (*2*-H^+), respectively, both originating from the thermal decomposition of allicin (*3*) shown in Scheme 3. With a different SFC-MS interface, the abundance of the m/z 145 ion relative to the m/z 73 base peak was greatly reduced, suggesting that in this case sufficient energy is provided in the interface to completely decompose *3* under unimolecular conditions before substantial amounts of the thioacrolein dimers *7* and *8* can form.

As indicated above, gas chromatography, as typically performed with elevated injector and column temperatures cannot be used for analysis of thiosulfinate garlic flavorants since they decompose under the analytical conditions. Immediately after the thiosulfinates from crushed garlic are produced, they slowly undergo hydrolysis by the water that is present. The volatile hydrolysis products, along with the more abundant but less volatile thiosulfinates such as allicin, are responsible for the aroma of freshly cut garlic. By sampling the "headspace" above cut plants, headspace gas chromatography (HS/GC) can be used to detect aroma components other than thiosulfinates. Through the use of the extremely sensitive technique of atomic emission detection HS/GC (HS/GC-AED), as well as HS/GC-MS, a variety of organosulfur compounds as well as smaller quantities of organoselenium and mixed organoselenium-sulfur compounds have been found. Sulfur compounds found include: allyl methyl sulfide, allyl methyl disulfide, diallyl sulfide, diallyl disulfide, dimethyl disulfide, diallyl trisulfide, dimethyl trisulfide, and allyl methyl trisulfide. Selenium-containing compounds, present at levels ca. 10^4 less than that for sulfur compounds, include: dimethyl selenide (Me_2Se), allyl methyl selenide (AllSeMe), methanesulfenoselenoic acid methyl ester (MeSeSMe), 2-propenesulfenoselenoic acid methyl ester (MeSeSAll), dimethyl diselenide (MeSeSeMe), bis(methylthio)selenide (MeSSeSMe), and (allylthio)(methylthio)selenide (AllSSeSMe) (17). What is the origin of the headspace organoselenium compounds from garlic? By using the GC-AED technique after derivatizing the amino acids present in whole garlic with $ClCO_2Et$, selenocysteine, $HSeCH_2CH(NH_2)COOH$, was unequivocally identified. Analysis of Se-enriched garlic, prepared by fertilizing growing garlic with selenite or selenate, revealed that *Se*-methyl selenocysteine, $MeSeCH_2CH(NH_2)COOH$, was now the major selenoamino acid, along with small quantities of selenomethionine and selenocysteine (18).

While thiosulfinates are most likely the *primary* flavorants of *Allium* spp., disulfides and other compounds formed by hydrolysis or other reactions of the primary compounds are important as aroma and flavor components of distilled oils of *Allium* spp. and as substances produced when *Allium* spp. are cooked or otherwise processed. Particularly interesting chemistry is associated with the major disulfides from garlic, diallyl disulfide *4*. Upon heating, it undergoes a complex sequence of reactions leading both to diallyl polysulfides as well as to a series of acyclic and heterocyclic compounds resulting from generation and reaction of thioacrolein (*10*) and radical species $CH_2{=}CHCH_2S_n{}^*$ with precursor diallyl polysulfides (Scheme 4; 19). The majority of these compounds have been detected in distilled oil of garlic and may be assumed to arise from thermal breakdown of diallyl disulfide *4*.

COOKED GARLIC

What is the effect of typical cooking procedures on the sulfur compounds in fresh garlic? Frying garlic converts alliin to allyl alcohol and cysteine (20). When chopped garlic is stir fried in hot oil for one minute, 16% of the sulfides but no thiosulfinates remain (21). When garlic is homogenized with a mixture of water and soybean oil and the mixture is steam distilled, con-

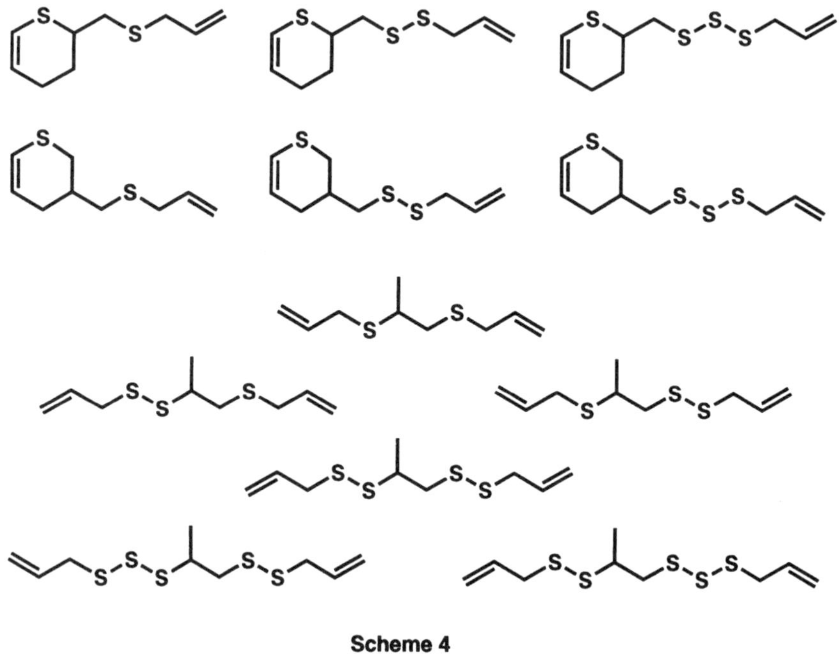

Scheme 4

siderable allicin (*3*) survives. When the soybean oil is omitted, the major sulfur-containing products are diallyl disulfide and trisulfide. It is concluded that allicin is protected by soybean oil during heat processing. This suggests that, when an edible oil is used in cooking garlic, considerable allicin (*3*) may survive *moderate* heating (22). Fried garlic was found to be on a par with raw garlic with regard to its fibrinolytic activity (see below; 23). Heating crushed garlic in boiling water for twenty minutes in a closed container converts allicin (*3*) to diallyl trisulfide; in an open container 97% of the sulfides had evaporated although 7% of thiosulfinates remained (21).

COMMERCIAL AND EXPERIMENTAL GARLIC PRODUCTS

Chopped fresh garlic or fresh garlic juice are unstable to storage. Products of greater stability can be produced from the fresh plant by dehydrating to produce a powdered ("freeze-dried") product, treating with steam to produce a distilled oil, chopping in vegetable oil to afford a "macerate", crushing and shaking with ether to give an ether extract, aging in alcoholic solvents, or pickling in vinegar. Most (Table 16.1) of these garlic products are available commercially, generally in tablet or pill form. A recent report gives representative analyses for several brands of commercial garlic products and shows that there is quite a variation in levels of sulfur compounds from product to product (24). Of the various products analyzed, the aged garlic extract is lowest in content of allicin (on mixing with water), *S*-methyl γ-glutamylcysteine (SMGC), *S*-allyl γ-glutamylcysteine (SAGC), and *S*-*trans*-1-propenyl γ-glutamylcysteine (SPGC) while dehydrated garlic powder, sold for culinary use at substantially lower prices than the health food products, was quite comparable to the other products in the content of the various sulfur compounds.

Powdered Garlic Products

A dry, powdered form of garlic can be prepared by freezing peeled garlic in dry ice or liquid nitrogen, cold pulverizing, and then directly lyophilizing (vacuum drying), or extracting with

TABLE 16.1. SELECTED COMPONENTS (MG/G) OF POWDERED COMMERCIAL GARLIC PRODUCTS[a]

Sample[b]	Allicin	SAGC[c]	SPGC[c]	SMGC[c]	SAC[c]
dg	3.8	20.5	16.7	2.2	0.39
p1	3.3	8.3	5.1	0.82	0.23
p2	5.1	6.4	5.4	0.61	0.17
p3	2.5	7.7	5.5	0.83	0.17
p4	1.1	20.7	17.7	1.2	0.38
p5	0.3	6.8	5.9	1.1	0.12
p6	2.8	15.0	12.5	1.9	0.26
p7	1.1	4.75	4.5	0.69	0.16
p8	3.8	7.4	7.0	1.0	0.21
p9 (aged)	n.d.[d]	0.67	0.64	0.26	0.53

[a]Data provided by the Center for Science in the Public Interest.
[b]dg stands for a name brand dehydrated garlic product used for cooking; p9 (aged) represents an "aged garlic extract" manufactured in Japan; products p1-p8 are manufactured in the U.S. or Germany. The identity of all products may be found in the *Nutrition Action Healthletter*, July/August 1995, volume 22, issue number 6, Center for Science in the Public Interest (Washington, DC).
[c]*S*-Allylcysteine, SAC; *S*-methyl-glutamylcysteine, SMGC; *S*-allyl-glutamylcysteine, SAGC; *S-trans*-1-propenyl-glutamylcysteine, SPGC (see Scheme 2 for structures).
[d]not detected.

acetone. As described by Cavallito, a powder prepared by acetone extraction is odorless until mixed with water, whereupon the typical odor of garlic results (25). Commercial garlic powders and garlic salt for culinary use, prepared in some cases by oven drying chopped garlic, can have a significant garlic odor due to formation of allicin and decomposition products during processing. Powders for incorporation into tablets or gelatin capsules for nutritional and health uses are prepared by drying slices of peeled (rather than chopped) garlic at temperatures up to 60 C. Some thiosulfinates are still formed and lost during the drying process.

A few garlic powder products are prepared by spray drying homogenized garlic cloves, which can result in complete loss of alliin as well as an increase in odor of the powdered product, due to entrapped allicin decomposition products such as diallyl di- and trisulfide. Inert fillers are added to the garlic powder, roughly equivalent to the weight of water originally present in the fresh clove (65%). Thus, garlic powder tablets are said to represent about an equivalent weight of garlic and on dissolving in water release a level of allicin [e.g. possess an "allicin potential"] comparable to that of fresh garlic (21). Garlic powder products retain almost all of their allicin potential for several years as long as the residual moisture in the powder is minimized. Garlic tablets are often enteric coated to prevent inhibition of alliinase, known to immediately occur at the low pH levels found in the stomach. In these cases, since allicin is generated in the small intestines rather than the mouth and esophagus, there would be some differences in absorption and activity, with the absence of any possible antibiotic effect on the stomach microflora. A variety of factors can affect the amount of allicin that is actually released in the body by a particular garlic powder capsule or tablet.

Pearls and Soft Gels: Macerates, Distilled Oil, Solvent Extract

These formulations typically contain oils of processed garlic, which may be steam distilled garlic oil (volatile garlic oil), prepared by steam distilling chopped and crushed garlic, or oil prepared by crushing and macerating garlic in a vegetable oil, or more rarely, the evaporated residue from solvent (e.g. ether) extraction of crushed garlic. These oils would generally be diluted with inert carriers prior to encapsulation.

Steam distillation of garlic was first reported in 1845 (2) although it is probable that this process was carried out much earlier, as with the isolation of essential oils from diverse plants. The major components of steam-distilled oil of garlic are diallyl di-, tri- and tetrasulfides and allyl methyl di-, tri-, and tetrasulfides (All_2S, 2%, All_2S_2, 26%, All_2S_3, 18%, All_2S_4, 8%, All_2S_5, 2%, AllSMe, 1%, $AllS_2Me$, 13%, $AllS_3Me$, 15%, $AllS_4Me$, 6%, $AllS_5Me$, 2%, MeS_2Me, 1%, MeS_3Me, 3%, MeS_4Me, 1%) (26). Since these compounds are formed by hydrolysis and decomposition of allicin and other thiosulfinates, in turn formed when garlic is cut or crushed, it is incorrect to refer to this mixture of compounds as the "essential oil of garlic", since the term essential oil is usually reserved for odoriferous compounds present in the intact plant. The typical content of sulfur compounds in commercial steam-distilled garlic oil for human consumption is 4.4 mg sulfides and polysulfides (composition listed above), diluted to one gram with vegetable oil. The dilution stabilizes the polysulfides and decreases the strong odor of the undiluted oil (21).

Products prepared by chopping or macerating fresh garlic in edible plant or fish oils have been used for culinary purposes for centuries and are commonly available in grocery stores (see cautionary note below concerning the risk of botulism for unacidified garlic in oil products). The encapsulated, clear liquid from oil-maceration of garlic is also available as a health product. The overall yield of sulfur transformation products is optimized if the clove is crushed first, maximizing allicin production, before adding the oil, and then allowing the allicin in oil solution to stand at least 24 hours before use (27). The typical composition of garlic macerates (given as mg sulfur compounds per g of oil-macerated product) is: sulfides and polysulfides, 0.16; vinyl dithiins, 0.60; ajoene, 0.10; total sulfur compounds, 0.86 (21,26). In gelatin capsules, the ajoene content decreased 22% after 18 months at room temperature (63% after 37 months) while the 1,3-vinyldithiin decreased only 3% (8% after 37 months) and the 1,2-vinyldithiin, 1% after 37 months (21). Refrigeration should improve the long term stability of oil-macerated garlic.

As used by Bordia in his animal and clinical studies, crushed garlic was extracted with ether, and the ether was evaporated providing an "ether-extracted oil of garlic". More than 24 hours may be required for conversion of initially formed allicin to the ultimate products, vinyldithiins and ajoene. Analysis of a representative evaporated ether extract showed 5.7 mg/g vinyldithiins, 1.0 mg/g ajoenes, 1.4 mg/g diallyl di- and trisulfides, and total sulfur compounds, 8.1 mg/g (21).

Garlic Aged in Aqueous Alcohol

This type of commercial product, generally imported from Japan, is produced by aging garlic in ca. 1:5 ethanol:water for

20 months, followed by filtration and concentration, and in some cases, evaporation to dryness. The final liquid product contains 12% v/v ethanol, 0.05% total sulfur, and 0.29% total nitrogen, which is considerably less sulfur and nitrogen than found in fresh garlic (0.35% [1% dry weight] and 1.1% [3.1% dry weight], respectively) (21). The typical content of sulfur compounds in alcohol aged garlic, in the form of a liquid or solid commercial product (mg/g product; mean for six lots purchased at local stores): γ-glutamylcysteines (*S*-allyl, *S*-1-propenyl, *S*-methyl), 0.34; *S*-alkyl cysteines, 1.0; alliin, 0.32; cycloalliin, 0.34; *S*-allylmercaptocysteine, 0.14; cystine, 0.01; total sulfur compounds, 2.14 mg/g (21).

Pickled Garlic

Garlic cloves pickled in vinegar have been known for centuries, e.g. in the form of "vinaigre des quatre voleurs" ("Four Thieves' Vinegar") (1), and are still popular in many cultures today. The low pH (ca. 3.5) of the 5% acetic acid solution deactivates the alliinase so that no allicin is formed upon chewing, diminishing the pungency (28), while at the same time preserving the garlic against acid-sensitive bacteria such as that causing botulism (see below). Otherwise, the constituents are similar to those found in fresh garlic, e.g. *S*-allyl cysteine *S*-oxide (alliin), *S*-allyl cysteine, and S-allyl γ-glutamylcysteine as the major products (21).

BIOLOGICAL ACTIVITY OF GARLIC AND ITS DERIVED COMPOUNDS

General Comments

Ideally, all garlic products sold for their health benefit should be validated using randomized, double-blind, placebo-controlled clinical trials with well-defined biological endpoints. Such studies, few of which have been reported in the United States (46), should employ analyzed ingredients together with marker compounds, along with evaluation of product safety. Statistical analysis in these trials should be based on "between group comparisons" and differences should be presented with confidence intervals. Blinding is of course a problem in garlic trials because of its strong odor. Long term studies present the added difficulty of controlling the patients' diets and other habits, with the consequence that the outcome of the studies may reflect differences in various uncontrolled factors (29). Health claims based on *in vitro* data need to be tempered by considering the effects of realistic human doses expected for the consumption of fresh garlic (estimated U.S. per capita consumption of garlic is only 0.5 kg/year! (30)) and various garlic-derived compounds, rather than larger doses given to laboratory animals. Raw garlic, as well as dehydrated garlic products that are reconstituted with water, are best consumed with food to minimize digestive tract upset and "heartburn", although in some cultures sliced raw garlic cloves dipped in sauces are routinely consumed without any apparent ill effects.

Antibiotic Activity

For centuries, garlic preparations have been employed as antibiotics: in India for washing wounds and ulcers, in China for fever and cholera, in Africa (by Albert Schweitzer) for amoebic dysentery, in World Wars I and II as antiseptics in the prevention of gangrene, as well as in epidemics of typhus, diphtheria, and tuberculosis (1,2). Laboratory investigations reveal both antifungal and antibacterial activity. Aqueous and organic solvent garlic extracts as well as allicin show good activity against the fungi *Candida albicans*, *Aspergillus fumigatus*, *Cryptococcus neoformans*, *Histoplasma capsulatum*, among others (31-35). In many of these cases the antimycotic activity of garlic was superior to that of nystatin, griseofulvin and amphotericin B. The growth of both gram-negative and gram-positive bacteria (e.g. *Streptococci*, *Staphylococci*, *Eberthella typhosa*, *B. Dysenteriae*, *B. enteritidis*, and *Vibrio chlorae*), including antibiotic-resistant strains, are inhibited by allicin even at 1:100,000 dilution. Garlic extracts are also reported to inhibit the *Mycobacterium avium* complex from AIDS patients (36). Limited evidence exists for the antiviral activity of garlic. Commercial garlic extracts, including diallyl trisulfide, have been given intravenously with success in the Peoples' Republic of China to treat fungal and viral infections and cryptococcal meningitis (33,37). Ajoene inhibits the growth of pathogenic fungi and bacteria such as *Paracoccidioides brasiliensis* (38), among others (39-41).

Based on the observation that the antimycotic and antibacterial activity of aqueous garlic extracts is reduced upon addition of cysteine, glutathione, or other thiols, it is assumed that the SS(O) group of allicin is essential for antibiotic activity. The thiosulfinate linkage is thought to inhibit sulfhydryl-enzymes by sulfenylating or oxidizing the SH group. No antibiotic activity is shown by *S*-allyl-glutamylcysteine (SAGC). Allicin has antibiotic activity on direct contact with microorganisms (on skin or in the gastrointestinal tract) but it is probable that this activity would be rapidly lost on *in vivo* exposure to cysteine and other thiols found in most cells and body fluids. While allicin itself is unlikely to show systemic antibiotic (or other) activity, metabolites of allicin do appear to be active both intestinally and systemically.

Cardiovascular Activity

Dioscorides, chief physician to the Roman army in the first century A.D., wrote "garlic doth cleaneth the arteries." In 1979, an epidemiological study in India compared three populations consuming different amounts of garlic and onions. The subjects were all vegetarians in the Jain community who ate garlic and onions in liberal amounts (at least 50 g of garlic per week), in smaller amounts (no more than 10 g of garlic per week), or never in their lives. The group of garlic and onion abstainers proved to have the shortest blood-coagulation time and to also show the highest blood-plasma level of the protein fibrinogen (see below). The mean fasting cholesterol values for the three groups were 159, 172 and 208 mg%, respectively, while total triglycerides for the three groups were 52, 75 and 109 mg%, respectively, showing that lipid levels are lowest in the garlic consuming group (42). Other studies have demonstrated an inverse correlation between average garlic consumption and coronary heart disease in different populations and that populations with a high average garlic consumption are protected from coronary heart disease (43).

In studies employing the human liver cell line HepG2, allicin and ajoene, but not alliin, diallyl disulfide or 2-propenethiol (CH_2=$CHCH_2SH$), are found to inhibit cholesterol biosynthesis. The IC_{50} values of 7-9 μM are about one hundredth the level where cytotoxicity begins. Inhibition is exerted at the level of HMG-CoA-reductase (44), presumably by reaction with the mercapto group of the CoA. Serum levels of cholesterol and triacylglycerols in rats and rabbits were decreased on long-term exposure to water-soluble garlic extracts (44). In man, long-term intake of garlic powder tablets led to a reduction in blood cholesterol while in other studies, commercial powdered garlic tablets were found to be as efficient as the hyperlipidemic drug bezafibrate in reducing total cholesterol, LDL cholesterol and increasing HDL cholesterol in patients with primary hyperlipoproteinaemia (45). Human blood serum taken two hours after an oral administration of a 300 mg garlic powder tablet caused substantially less cholesterol accumulation in smooth muscle cells cultured from atherosclerotic plaques of human aorta (46).

In controlled clinical trials involving either fresh garlic or freshly made extracts, it was found that in five out of six trials serum cholesterol was lowered, fibrinolytic activity was increased and platelet aggregation inhibited. High levels of garlic, equivalent to at least 7 cloves per day (e.g. ca. 28 g garlic), were used in a number of studies published prior to 1989 (29). In recent studies, more realistic levels of garlic (3-10 g) were used with significant results (21). In another controlled clinical trial, treatment for 12 weeks with a commercial dried garlic tablet (900 mg/day) was found to produce a significantly greater reduction in serum total cholesterol and low density lipoprotein cholesterol than placebo (47). Meta-analyses indicates that consumption of one-half to one clove of garlic per day reduces cholesterol levels by approximately 9% (48). If commercial products are used to lower blood lipid levels, it is recommended that the allicin potential of these products should be high (the suggested dose of allicin which would be effective for these purposes is 0.07 mg/kg body weight per day (21)).

While an earlier review argued that simply because a substance lowers cholesterol levels, inhibits platelet aggregation and changes fibrinolytic activity, "it does not necessarily follow that it is good for general health" (29), more recent work links elevated levels of serum cholesterol with increased mortality from heart disease (49a). Considerable data is also available from uncontrolled human studies and from animal studies which suggest that the above summarized cardiovascular activity holds also for processed garlic (21,43). An earlier review had also concluded that "conclusive clinical trials [on platelet aggregation inhibitory and antihypertensive actions of garlic] . . . however, are missing" and "although the results of a number of investigations into the actions of garlic indicate a dose-dependent effect, the minimal dose required to obtain such changes is not clear at present and it would seem advisable to use high-dose treatment regimens" (43). A meta-analysis of the effect of a commercial dried garlic powder preparation on blood pressure noted: "The results suggest that this garlic powder preparation may be of some clinical use in subjects with mild hypertension. However there is still insufficient evidence to recommend it as a routine clinical therapy for the treatment of hypertensive subjects. More-rigorously designed and analyzed trials are needed" (49b).

In healthy blood function, blood coagulation is physiologically balanced by fibrinolysis (enzymatic splitting of the fibrous protein fibrin). Impairment of the fibrinolytic activity enhances blood clotting and thrombosis, with the attendant risk of myocardial and cerebral infarction. Platelet aggregation also plays a key role in coagulation and in hemostasis (stoppage of bleeding) (43). Garlic juice or oils have been found to enhance fibrinolysis, based on both clinical and epidemiological studies (43). Garlic inhibits platelet aggregation in animals and in humans (50). A variety of substances from garlic inhibit platelet aggregation including ajoene (14,15,51), dithiins, and diallyl trisulfide and allyl methyl trisulfide (21,52). On the other hand *S*-

allylcysteine has no activity (21). Ajoene inhibits platelet deposition on severely damaged arterial walls in a *in vivo* porcine experimental model (51). Both aqueous and ethanolic extracts of garlic stimulate nitric oxide synthetase, which is associated with hypotensive activity. Since ethanol is known to denature alliinase, preventing allicin formation, it would appear that allicin cannot be responsible for the hypotensive activity of garlic (53a). *S*-Allyl-glutamylcysteine has good *in vitro* activity toward inhibiting the blood pressure-regulating angiotensin converting enzyme (ACE) (53b). In this manner fresh or processed garlic could lower blood pressure.

While there has been considerable interest in the effect of ingestion of garlic on adhesion and aggregation of blood platelets (antithrombotic activity), the studies have mostly been *in vitro*, or *in vivo* in animals, involving extracts and other processed forms of garlic, as well as pure compounds isolated from garlic. More than 50 human clinical studies have been reported. Most of the studies suggest that consumption of moderate amounts of fresh garlic and certain commercial garlic products has a favorable effect on blood lipids (cholesterol, HDL, LDL), blood pressure, fibrinolysis, and blood circulation in animals and humans (21,43,54). In animals fed garlic homogenates or ether extracts, elevated levels of blood lipids are lowered. In humans, some clinical studies have shown that fresh garlic consumption inhibits spontaneous platelet aggregation while also increasing capillary circulation.

According to one review, a lipid-lowering effect of garlic is to be expected at a daily dose of about 900 mg garlic powder containing an allicin equivalent of 5.4 mg (55). The German Federal Bureau of Health indicates a daily dosage of 4 g fresh garlic (about one clove; equivalent to 1.4 g dehydrated garlic) or its processed equivalent (with higher quality tablets, 1 to 2 tablets/day), recommended for prevention of thromboses and arteriosclerosis (55). Consumption of a clove or two of fresh garlic per day, or equivalent amounts of processed forms of garlic, is reported to reduce cholesterol and triglycerides by 10 to 30%. In clinical studies in India, of 432 patients who had experienced prior heart attacks, each given either 0.1 mg/kg/day of an ether extract of fresh garlic (mainly dithiins and ajoene) or a placebo, there was a 35% reduction in new heart attacks and a 45% reduction in total deaths compared to the placebo group along with a considerable reduction in serum lipids (56). Rats fed freeze-dried garlic powder at a level of 2% of their diet showed increased HDL levels, which effect was absent at 0.5 and 1% dietary levels of garlic powder (57).

Cancer Preventative Activity

Allicin and ajoene have been found to be cytotoxic to three different fast-growing cancer cell lines, with EC_{50} values in the micromolar range (58), but less so by two to three orders of magnitude to various liver cells (44). The low cytotoxicity of both compounds in liver cells is said to be in accord with the observation that garlic consumption even in high doses is well tolerated (44). *S*-Methyl cysteine sulfoxide and its metabolite methyl methanethiosulfinate, MeS(O)SMe, at respective levels of 0.5 and 0.05 mmol/kg body weight, inhibited the formation of benzo[a]pyrene-induced micronucleated polychromatic erythrocytes (MPCEs; an indicator for genotoxicity) by 31-33%, compared with control mice. Higher doses of MeS(O)SMe (0.5 and 1.0 mmol/kg body weight) were toxic to the mice. It is suggested that the inhibition of experimental genotoxicity by these two sulfur compounds may, in part, be responsible for the anticarcinogenic effect of vegetables containing these compounds (59).

The oil-soluble allylic sulfur compounds diallyl sulfide, disulfide and trisulfide were found to markedly inhibit the growth of canine mammary tumor cells, with diallyl trisulfide being the only compound that was cytotoxic; in contrast the water soluble compounds *S*-allyl cysteine and related compounds had little effect on these cells (60). These same oil-soluble sulfur compounds have also been shown to inhibit the promotion phase of carcinogenesis in skin tumors induced by DMBA (61,62) and, in the case of diallyl sulfide, carcinogen-induced nuclear damage to colon epithelial cells *in vivo* (63). Depression in the incidence of skin tumors is accompanied by suppression in the activities of epidermal lipoxygenase and ornithine decarboxylase (61). It is reported that "[at 3-12 g/mL] DATS [diallyl trisulfide] can augment the activation of T cells and enhance the anti-tumor function of macrophage, suggesting that DATS may be potentially useful in tumor therapy". Furthermore, 1-100 g/mL diallyl trisulfide was found to inhibit production of NO by macrophages (64).

Oil-soluble *S*-allyl compounds are reported to have greater anticancer activity on the *in vitro* growth of human colon tumor cell line (HCT-15) than water-soluble *S*-allyl cysteine or *S*-propyl or *O*-allyl compounds (65); *Se*-allyl compounds seem to be even more active (Table 16.2) (66,67). In connection with the latter work on cancer preventative properties of selenium compounds, Ip and coworkers found *Se*-enriched garlic to show promising activity (68). The anticancer activity of these compounds may variously be associated with induction of cellular glutathione, a major intracellular antioxidant, stimulation of glutathione-*S*-transferase (69,70), an enzyme which can detoxify and dispose of harmful chemicals, inhibition of ornithine decarboxylase, an enzyme important in DNA synthesis, whose unregulated activity occurs in neoplasms, or by other activity of these compounds as antioxidants or nucleophiles to provide defense against peroxides and alkylating agents. Glutathione peroxidase, a key enzyme involved in destruction of peroxides, contains selenium in the form of selenol (-SeH) at its active site.

Antibacterial properties of garlic may inhibit bacterial conversion of nitrate to nitrite in the stomach, thereby limiting formation of carcinogenic nitrosamines (71). Alternatively, garlic sulfur compounds may inhibit *N*-nitrosation by rapidly forming

TABLE 16.2. COMPARISON OF MAMMARY CANCER CHEMOPREVENTION BY DIALLYL SULFIDE AND DIALLYL SELENIDE (66,67)

Treatment	Dose (mol/kg b.w.)	Tumor incidence	Total tumor yield
Control	none	av. 84%	av. 70
All_2S	0.3×10^{-3}	20/25 (80%)	68
All_2S	0.9×10^{-3}	16/25 (64%)	50
All_2S	1.8×10^{-3}	13/25 (52%)	42
All_2Se	0.6×10^{-5}	10/30 (33%)	16
All_2Se	1.2×10^{-5}	9/30 (30%)	14

S-nitrosothiols or thionitrites and nitric oxide; the *S*-nitroso compounds would then decompose giving disulfides (71). Since high doses of diallyl trisulfide, allyl methyl trisulfide and related sulfur compounds have been found to *promote* diethylnitrosamine-induced neoplasia in rat livers, it is argued that "in evaluating relationships between diet and cancer, it is appropriate to consider not only the possible protective role of garlic and onions but also their enhancing effects" (72). However, one should also consider whether the high doses given the test animals are meaningful in evaluating possible human dosage: the equivalent of 100 mg/kg body weight/day of a trisulfide given to a test animal would be an absurdly high daily human dose of 5.9 L of commercial distilled garlic oil.

A number of studies have documented the anti-oxidant and free radical scavenging properties of fresh garlic extracts and commercially available garlic products (73-77). The apparent radical-scavenging behavior has also been demonstrated in vitro by synthetic samples of *S*-allyl γ-glutamylcysteine, *S*-allylcysteine and *S*-allylmercaptocysteine, although the effects are quite weak (78). A study of the effect of "aged garlic extract" on human metabolism of acetaminophen, which generates a reactive electrophilic metabolite, led to the conclusion that such a garlic extract "has limited potential as a chemopreventative agent (79). Pretreatment of human carcinoma cell lines with *S*-allylcysteine followed by *cis*-platin was found to significantly enhance the cytotoxic effect of *cis*-platin; SAC alone had no effect on cell growth (80).

To date, reports have appeared on the results of nine epidemiological studies relating garlic consumption with diminished risk of gastrointestinal cancer (21). For example, in a study of 564 stomach cancer patients and 1131 controls in Shandong Province in the People's Republic of China, a significant reduction of stomach cancer risk was found to be associated with increasing consumption of allium vegetables including garlic, scallions and Chinese chives (81). In a related study comparing the death rate from stomach cancer in two large groups in Shandong Province of China, it was found that those living in the province's Cangshan County had a lower death rate (3/

100,000) than those living in Qixia County (40/100,000). The residents of the former county eat ca. 20 g raw garlic/day while those in the latter county rarely eat garlic. The most striking finding of an epidemiological study of the incidence of colon cancer among 41,837 Iowa women aged 55 to 69 years over a period of 5 years was the 35% lower risk observed associated with consumption of one or more servings of garlic per week (82). Because of the low levels of garlic consumption in this latter study, questions have been raised that "garlic consumption in this group of middle- and older-aged Midwestern women is simply a surrogate of some other variable, perhaps not even diet related" (83). This criticism could, of course, be raised about any epidemiological study.

Epidemiological studies involving 120,852 men and women aged 55 to 69 years over a period of 3.3 years concluded that garlic supplement use, or consumption of onions or leeks, was not associated with lower risks of lung carcinoma or of female breast carcinoma (84,85). In the absence of specific information on the nature or composition of the garlic supplements used by participants in the study, it is difficult to judge the significance of the conclusions *vis-a-vis* garlic usage.

Enhancement of Thiamine Absorption

The effectiveness of garlic in treatment of beriberi, a vitamin B_1 deficiency disease, was noted by Japanese researchers in the 19th century (21). The basis for action of garlic on vitamin B_1 was elucidated in Japan in the 1950's. It was discovered that thiamine reacts with allicin forming allithiamine which is absorbed in the gastrointestinal tract more easily than thiamine itself. In animals and humans, garlic therefore increases the blood levels of thiamine (86, 87).

Insecticidal and Other Repellent Effects

Garlic oil components/metabolites diallyl disulfide and trisulfide are toxic to mosquito and other insect larvae at levels of 2 ppm (88) and are repellant to *Ixodes ricinus*, the tick which carries the encephalitis virus (89). These observations are consistent with the traditional use of garlic and other *Allium* spp. oils to repell insects, and the claim that those who eat garlic suffer fewer insect bites than those who don't. Legend has it that vampires shun garlic (90). In an effort to provide complete documentation on the diverse physiological effects of garlic, the following abstract from a Norwegian journal is offered *in toto*, without additional comment (91): "Vampires are feared everywhere, but the Balkan region has been especially haunted. Garlic has been regarded as an effective prophylactic against vampires. We wanted to explore this alleged effect experimentally. Owing to the lack of vampires, we used leeches instead. In strictly standardized research surroundings, the leeches were to attach themselves to either a hand smeared with garlic or to a clean hand. The garlic-smeared hand was preferred in two out of three cases (95% confidence interval 50.4% to 80.4%). When they preferred the garlic the leeches used only 14.9 seconds to attach themselves, compared with 44.9 seconds when going to the nongarlic hand ($p < 0.05$). The traditional belief that garlic has prophylactic properties is probably wrong. The reverse may in fact be true. This study indicates that garlic possibly attracts vampires. Therefore to avoid a Balkan-like development in Norway, restrictions on the use of garlic should be considered."

Attractive Effects

The third century Babylonian Talmud (Baba Kama 82a) decrees "that they [the Jews in Judea] should eat garlic on the Sabbath eve because of the time [for performing conjugal cohabitation]." It is further observed that garlic "satiates and warms [the body] and makes the face shine and increases semen . . . and some say it instills love and eliminates jealousy." There does not appear to be any scientific documentation for the activity of garlic as an aphrodisiac.

Metabolism and Effect on Breath and Body Odor

2-Propenethiol is initially detected in garlic breath but disappears after about one hour (17,92). Other sulfur compounds which have been found include allyl methyl sulfide and disulfide, diallyl sulfide and disulfide, dimethyl disulfide, diallyl trisulfide and hydrogen sulfide (17,92). The major organoselenium compound found in garlic breath is dimethyl selenide (Me_2Se), along with lesser amounts of allyl methyl selenide (MeSeAll), methanesulfenoselenoic acid methyl ester (MeSeSMe), and 2-propenesulfenoselenoic acid methyl ester (MeSeSAll) (17). It is likely that 2-propenethiol is a primary metabolite of most garlic-derived compounds. *In vitro* reaction of protein-bound and free cysteine with various sulfur-containing garlic derived compounds such as allicin, diallyl disulfide or trisulfide rapidly gives *S*-allyl mercaptocysteine, AllSSCyst, "SAMC" (13). Such reactions are also likely to occur *in vivo.* Ajoene gives "ajo-cysteine", AllS(O)CH_2CH=CHSSCyst, in addition to SAMC (13). Allicin has never been found in blood after garlic consumption, presumably because of rapid conversion to SAMC. Neither γ-glutamylcysteines nor their metabolites are found in blood after garlic consumption, suggesting that they are hydrolyzed by transpeptidases to *S*-allyl cysteine (SAC), which is converted *in vivo* to *N*-acetyl-*S*-allylcysteine, NASAC, found in human and animal urine after garlic consumption (93). The apparent metabolic transformation from allicin to SAMC to 2-propenethiol (some of which is excreted) may extend to oxidation products of the latter, including 2-propenesulfinic acid, which would readily lose SO_2 forming propene. It remains to be established which of these transformation products shows the greatest physiological activity and which might therefore explain the biological activity of garlic.

About 10% of the sulfur-containing compounds from garlic, and compounds derived therefrom, are excreted through the lungs while smaller amounts are excreted through the skin (55). By analogy to dimethyl sulfoxide, garlic components such as allicin apparently possess the ability to penetrate skin. This would explain the bizarre observation that if you rub garlic on the soles of your feet (or put a garlic clove in your sock!) you will soon develope garlic breath.

Hazards

While a variety of health benefits are associated with garlic, there are a few hazards as well (apart from social problems associated with garlicky odors). Chopped garlic in olive oil without chemical or acid additives, not properly refrigerated, was responsible for three cases of botulism. Researchers found high concentrations of *Clostridium botulinum* in the pH 5.7 garlic product, as often occurs for vegetable tubers or roots which grow in soil where botulinum spores are common. The FDA now requires that microbial inhibitors or acidifying agents be added to garlic in oil products (94). There have been several reports of allergic response following inhalation and ingestion of garlic, particularly in the form of garlic powder and the resulting dust. (95,96). In concentrated form, allicin is strongly irritating to the skin and other membranes (97). For this reason it would be unwise to consume significant portions of raw garlic in the absence of food as a diluent and buffer. When properly diluted, the irritant effects of garlic would be minimized, although some individuals may have lower tolerance levels than others, particularly the elderly. Thus, an 87 year-old man who reportedly consumed four cloves of garlic per day developed spontaneous spinal epidural hematoma with associated platelet dysfunction (98). In animals, high doses of 1- and 2-propenyl disulfides (the human equivalent of 8.6 L or ca. 15,000 capsules per day of distilled garlic oil!) have been found to cause hemolytic anemia, with the α,β-unsaturated 1-propenyl compounds being significantly more toxic than the 2-propenyl isomers (99).

Acknowledgments

I thank my colleagues, whose names are listed in the references, for contributing to the work reported herein, and Clement Ip, Larry Lawson and David Schardt for helpful discussions and use of unpublished material. I gratefully acknowledge support from the National Science Foundation, the NRI Competitive Grants Program/USDA (Award No. 92-37500-8068), and McCormick & Company, Inc.

BIBLIOGRAPHY

1. BLOCK, E. *Sci. Am.* 1985, *252*, 114-119.
2. BLOCK, E. *Angew. Chem., Int. Ed. Engl.* 1992, *31*, 1135-1178.
3. BLOCK, E. In *Food Phytochemicals for Cancer Prevention,* ACS Symposium Series 546, Huang, M.-T.; Osawa, T.; Ho, C.-T.; Rosen, R. T., Ed., American Chemical Society: Washington DC; 1994, pp. 84-96.
4. ELLMORE, G. S.; FELDBERG, R. S. *Am. J. Botany* 1994, *81*, 89-94.
5. RABINKOV, A.; ZHU, X.-Z.; GRAFI, G.; GALILI, G.; MIRELMAN, D. *Appl. Biochem. Biotechnol.* 1994, *48*, 149-171.
6. EDWARDS, S. J.; BRITTON, G.; COLLIN, H. A. *Plant Cell, Tissue and Organ Culture* 1994, *38*, 181-188.
7. OHSUMI, C.; HAYASHI, T.; SANO, K. *Phytochemistry* 1993, *33*, 107-111.
8. CAI, X.-J.; UDEN, P. C.; BLOCK, E.; ZHANG, X.; QUIMBY, B. D.; SULLIVAN, J. J. *J. Agric. Food Chem.* 1994, *42*, 2081-2084.
9. BLOCK, E. *J. Agr. Food Chem.* 1993, *41*, 692.
10. BLOCK, E.; CALVEY, E. M. In *Sulfur Compounds in Food,* ACS Symposium Series 564, Mussinan, C. J.; Keelan, M. E., Ed., American Chemical Society: Washington DC; 1994 pp. 63-79.
11. CALVEY, E. M.; MATUSIK, J. E.; WHITE, K. D.; BETZ, J. M.; BLOCK, E.; LITTLEJOHN, M.; NAGANATHAN, S.; PUTMAN, D., *J. Agric. Food Chem.* 1994, *42*, 1335-1341.
12. BLOCK, E.; NAGANATHAN, S.; PUTMAN, D.; ZHAO, S. H. *J. Agric. Food Chem.* 1992, *40*, 2418-2430.
13. LAWSON, L. D.; WOOD, S. G.; HUGHES, B. G. *Planta Med.* 1991, *57*, 263-270.
14. BLOCK, E.; AHMAD, S.; JAIN, M. K.; CRECELY, R. W.; APITZ-CASTRO, R. *J. Am. Chem. Soc.*, 1984, *106*, 8295-8296.
15. BLOCK, E.; AHMAD, S.; CATALFAMO, J.; JAIN, M. K.; APITZ-CASTRO, R. *J. Am. Chem. Soc.*, 1986, *108*, 7045-7055.
16. CALVEY, E. M.; ROACH, J. A. G.; BLOCK, E. *J. Chromatogr. Sci.*, 1994, 32, 93-96.
17. CAI, X.-J.; BLOCK, E.; UDEN, P. C.; QUIMBY, B. D.; SULLIVAN, J. J. *J. Agric. Food Chem.* 1995, *43*, 1751-1753.
18. CAI, X.-J.; BLOCK, E.; UDEN, P. C.; ZHANG, X.; QUIMBY, B. D.; SULLIVAN, J. J. *J. Agric. Food Chem.* 1995, *43*, 1754-1757.
19. BLOCK, E.; IYER, R.; SAHA, C.; GRISONI, S.; BELMAN, S.; LOSSING, F. *J. Am. Chem. Soc.* 1988, *110*, 7813-7827.
20. YU, T.-H.; LIN, L.-Y.; HO, C.-T. *J. Agric. Food Chem.* 1994, *42*, 1342-1347.
21. a) LAWSON, L. D. In *Garlic: The Science and Therapeutic Applications of Allium sativum L. and Related Species*; Koch, H. P.; Lawson, L. D., Ed.; Williams and Wilkins: Baltimore, MD, 1995.
    b) LAWSON, L. D.; RANSOM, D. K.; HUGHES, B. G. *Thrombosis Res.* 1992, *65*, 141-156.

c) Lawson, L. D. In *Human Medicinal Agents from Plants*; Kinghorn, A. D.; Balandrin, M. F. Ed.; ACS Symposium Series 534; American Chemical Society: Washington, DC, 1993, pp. 306.
22. KIM, S. M.; WU, C. M.; KUBOTA, K.; KOBAYASHI, A. *J. Agric. Food Chem.* 1995, *43*, 449-452.
23. CHUTANI, S. K.; BORDIA, A. *Atherosclerosis* 1981, *38*, 417-421.
24. SCHARDT, D.; SCHMIDT, S. *Nutrition Action Healthletter*, July/August 1995, *22*, (6), Center for Science in the Public Interest (Washington, DC).
25. CAVALLITO, C. J.; BAILEY, J. H.; BUCK, J. S. *J. Am. Chem. Soc.* 1945, *67*, 1032.
26. LAWSON, L. D.; WANG, Z.-Y. J.; HUGHES, B. G. *Planta Med.* 1991, *57*, 363-370.
27. IBERL, B.; WINKLER, G.; KNOBLOCH, K. *Planta Med.* 1990, *56*, 202-211.
28. KIM, M. R.; YUN, J. H.; SOK, D. E. *J. Korean Soc. Food Nutrit.* 1994, *23*, 805-810 (*Chem. Abstr.* 1995, *122*, 131,529).
29. KLEIJNEN, J.; KNIPSCHILD, P.; TER RIET, G. Br. *J. Clin. Pharmac.* 1989, *28*, 535-544.
30. PUTNAM, J. J.; ALLSHOUSE, J. E. *Food Consumption, Prices and Expenditures, 1970-1990.* U.S. Department of Agriculture, Economic Research Service: Washington, D.C.; Statistical Bulletin No. 840, August 1992.
31. APPLETON, J. A.; TANSEY, M. R. *Mycologia* 1975, *67*, 882-885.
32. BARONE, F. E.; TANSEY, M. R. *Mycologia* 1977, *69*, 793-825.
33. DAVIS, L. E.; SHEN, J.; ROYER, R. E. *Planta Med.* 1994, *60*, 546-549.
34. GHANNOUM, M. A. *J. Gen. Microbiol.* 1988, *134*, 2917-2924.
35. PAI, S. T.; PLATT, M. W. *Lett. Appl. Microbiol.* 1995, *20*, 14-18.
36. DESHPANDE, R. G.; KHAN, M. B.; BHAT, D. A.; NAVALKAR, R. G. *J. Antimicrobial Chemotherapy* 1993, *32*, 623-626.
37. DAVIS, L. E.; SHEN, J.-K.; CAI, Y. *Antimicrobial Agents and Chemotherapy* 1990, *34*, 651-653.
38. SAN-BLAS, G.; MARINO, L.; SAN-BLAS, P.; APITZ-CASTRO, R. *J. Med. Vet. Mycol.* 1993, *31*, 133-141.
39. a) HUGHES, B. G.; LAWSON, L. D. *Phytotherapy Res.* 1991, *5*, 154-158.
b) REIMERS, F.; SMOLKA, S. E.; WERRES, S.; PLANK-SCHUMACHER, K.; WAGNER, G. *J. Pl. Di. Protect.* 1993, *100*, 622-633.
40. a) SINGH, U. P.; PANDEY, V. N.; WAGNER, K. G.; SINGH, K. P. *Can. J. Bot.* 1990, *68*, 1354-1356.
b) SINGH, U. P.; PANDEY, V. N.; WAGNER, K. G.; KUMAR, A. *Mycologia* 1992, *84*, 105-108.
41. YOSHIDA, S.; KASUGA, S.; HAYASHI, N.; USHIROGUCHI, H.; MATSUURA, H.; NAKAGAWA, S. *Appl. Environ. Microbiol.* 1987, *53*, 615-617.
42. SAINANI, G. S.; DESAI, D. B.; GORHE, N. H.; NATU, S. M.; PISE, D. V.; SAINANI, P. G. *Indian J. Med. Res.* 1979, *69*, 776-780.

43. ERNST, E. *Pharmatherapeutica* 1987, *5*, 83-89.
44. GEBHARDT, R.; BECK, H.; WAGNER, K. G. *Biochim. Biophys. Acta* 1994, 1213, 57-62.
45. HOLZGARTNER, H.; SCHMIDT, U.; KAHN, U. *Arzniem.-Forsch./Drug Res.* 1992, *42*, 1473-1477.
46. OREKHOV, A. N.; TERTOV, V. V.; SOBENIN, I. A.; PIVOVAROVA, E. M. *Ann. Medicine* 1995, *27*, 63-65.
47. JAIN, A. K.; VARGAS, R.; GOTZKOWSKY, S.; MCMAHON, F. G. *Am. J. Med.* 1993, *94*, 632-635.
48. a) WARSHAFSKY, S.; KAMER, R. S.; SIVAK, S. L. *Ann. Intern. Med.* 1993, *119*, 599-605.
    b) SILAGY, C.; NEIL, A. *J. Royal Coll. Physicians of London* 1994, *28*, 39-45.
49. a) VERSCHUREN, W. M. M.; et al. *J. Am. Med. Assoc.* 1995, *274*, 131-136.
    b) SILAGY, C. A.; NEIL, H. A. W. *J. Hypertension* 1994, *12*, 463-468.
50. BORDIA, A. *Atherosclerosis* 1978, *30*, 355-360.
51. a) APITZ-CASTRO, LEDEZMA, E.; ESCALANTE, J.; JAIN, M. K. *Biochem. Biophys. Res. Commun.* 1986, *141*, 145-150.
    b) APITZ-CASTRO, ESCALANTE, J.; VARGAS, R.; JAIN, M. K. *Thrombosis Res.* 1986, *42*, 303-311.
    c) APITZ-CASTRO, R.; BADIMON, J. J.; BADIMON, L. *Thrombosis Res.* 1994, *75*, 243-249.
52. ARIGA, T.; OSHIBA, S.; TAMADA, T. *Lancet* 1981, 150-151.
53. a) DAS, I.; KHAN, N. S.; SOORANNA, S. R. *Curr. Med. Res. Opinion* 1995, *13*, 257.
    b) SENDL, A.; ELBL, G.; STEINKE, B.; REDL, K.; BREU, W.; WAGNER, H. *Planta Med.* 1992, *58*, 1-7.
54. KIESEWETTER, H.; JUNG, F.; JUNG, E. M.; BLUME, J.; MROWIETZ, C.; BIRK, A.; KOSCIELNY, J.; WENZEL, E. *Clin. Investig.* 1993, *71*, 383-386.
55. REUTER, H. D.; SENDL, A. In *Economic and Medicinal Plant Research.* Wagner, H.; Farnsworth, N. R., Ed. Academic Press: New York, 1994, pp. 56-113.
56. BORDIA, A. *Dtsch. Apoth. Ztg.* 1989, *129*, (Suppl. 15), 16-17.
57. KAMANNA, V. S.; CHANDRASEKARA, N. *Lipids* 1982, *17*, 483-488.
58. SCHARFENBERG, K.; WAGNER, R.; WAGNER, K. G. *Cancer Lett.*, 1990, *53*, 103-8.
59. MARKS, H. S.; ANDERSON, J. A.; STOEWSAND, G. S. *Food Chem. Toxicol.* 1993, *31*, 491-5.
60. SUNDARAM, S. G.; MILNER, J. A. *Cancer Lett.* 1993, *74*, 85-90.
61. BELMAN, S.; SOLOMON, J.; SEGAL, A.; BLOCK, E.; BARANY, G. *J. Biochem. Toxicol.* 1989, *4*, 151-160.
62. DWIVEDI, C.; ROHLFS, S.; D. JARVIS, D.; ENGINEER, F. N. *Pharm. Res.* 1992, *9*, 1668-1670.
63. WARGOVICH, M. J.; GOLDBERG, M. T. *Mutation Res.* 1985, *143*, 127-129.

64. FENG, Z. H.; ZHANG, G. M.; HAO, T. L.; ZHOU, B.; ZHANG, H.; JIANG, Z. Y. *J. Tongji Med. Univ.* 1994, *14*, 142-147.
65. SUNDARAM, S. G.; MILNER, J. A. *FASEB J* 1995, *9*, A869; 1994, *8*, A426.
66. IP, C. 1995, personal communication.
67. EL BAYOUMY, K.; IP, C.; CHAE, Y. H.; UPADHYAYA, P.; LISK, D.; PROKOPCZYK, B. *Proc. Ann. Meet. Am. Assoc. Cancer Res.* 1993, *34*, A3322.
68. a) IP, C.; LISK, D. J.; STOEWSAND, G. S. *Nutr. Cancer* 1992, *17*, 279-286.
    b) IP, C.; LISK, D. *J. Nutr. Cancer* 1993, *20*, 129-137.
    c) IP, C.; LISK, D. *Carcinogenesis* 1994, *15*, 1881-1885.
69. SPARNINS, V. L.; MOTT, A. W.; WATTENBERG, L. W. *Nutr. Cancer* 1986, *8*, 211-215.
70. SPARNINS, V. L.; BARANY, G.; WATTENBERG, L. W. *Carcinogenesis* 1988, *9*, 131-4.
71. a) MEI, X.; WANG, M. C.; XU, H. X.; PAN, X. P.; GAO, C. Y.; HAN, N.; FU, M. Y. *Acta. Nutr. Sinica* 1982, *4*, 53-58.
    b) SHENOY, N. R.; CHOUGHULEY, A. S. U. *Cancer Lett.* 1992, *65*, 227-232.
72. NOBUYASU, T.; MATSUDA, T.; OTOSHI, T.; YANO, Y.; OTANI, S.; HASEGAWA, T.; NAKAE, D.; KONISHI, Y.; FUKUSHIMA, S. *Cancer Res.* 1994, *54*, 2895-2899.
73. YANG, G. C.; YASAEI, P. M.; PAGE, S. W. *J. Food Drug. Anal.* 1993, *1*, 357-364.
74. LEWIN, G.; POPOV, I. *Arzneimittel-Forschung* 1994, *44*, 604-607.
75. POPOV, I.; BLUMSTEIN, A.; LEWIN, G. *Arzneimittel-Forschung* 1994, *44*, 602-604.
76. REKKA, E. A.; KOUROUNAKIS, P. N. *Pharmazie* 1994, 49, 539-540.
77. TOEROEK, B.; BELAGYI, J.; RIETZ, B.; JACOB, R. *Arzneimittel-Forschung* 1994, *44*, 608-611.
78. IMAI, J.; IDE, N.; NAGAE, S.; MORIGUCHI, T.; MATSUURA, H.; ITAKURA, Y. *Planta Med.* 1994, *60*, 417-420.
79. GWILT, P. R.; LEAR, C. L.; TEMPERO, M. A.; BIRT, D. D.; GRANDJEAN, A. C.; RUDDON, R. W.; NAGEL, D. L. *Cancer Epidemiol., Biomark. Prev.* 1994, *3*, 155-160.
80. YELLIN, S. A.; DAVIDSON, B. J.; PINTO, J. T.; SACKS, P. G.; QIAO, C.; SCHANTZ, S. P. *Cancer Lett.* 1994, *85*, 223-232.
81. YOU, W. C., BLOT, W. J., CHANG, Y. S., ERSHOW, A., YANG, Z. T., AN, Q., HENDERSON, B. E., FRAUMENI JR., J. F., AND WANG, T. G. *J. Natl. Cancer Inst.* 1989, *81*, 162-164.
82. STEINMETZ, K. A., KUSHI, L. H., BOSTICK, R. M., FOLSOM, A. R., AND POTTER, J. D. *Am. J. Epidemiol.* 1994, *139*, 1-15.
83. BALLARD-BARBASH, R.; KREBS-SMITH, S.; SUBAR, A.F. *Am. J. Epidemiol.* 1995, *141*, 84-85.
84. a) DORANT, E.; VAN DEN BRANDT, P. A.; GOLDBOHM, R. A. *Cancer Res.* 1994, 54, 6148-6153.

b) DORANT, E.; VAN DEN BRANDT, P. A.; GOLDBOHM, R. A. *Breast Cancer Res. Treat.* 1995, 33, 163-170.
85. DORANT, E.; VAN DEN BRANDT, P. A.; GOLDBOHM, R. A.; HERMUS, R. J. J.; STURMANS, F. *British J. Cancer* 1993, *67*, 424-429.
86. FUJIWARA, M.; NATATA, T. *J. Biochem.* 1954, *41*, 29-39.
87. YOSHIMURA, M. *Bitamin* [Kyoto] 1958, *14*, 640-646.
88. AMONKAR, S. V.; BANERJI, A. *Science* 1971, *174*, 1343-1344.
89. CATAR, G. *Bratisl. Lek. Listy* 1954, *34*, 1004-1010; *Chem. Abstr.* 1955, *49*, 2002.
90. STOKER, B. *Dracula*, 1897.
91. SANDVIK, H.; BAERHEIM, A. *Tidsskr Nor Laegeforen* 1994, *114*, 3583-3586.
92. RUIZ, R.; HARTMAN, T. G.; KARMAS, K.; LECH, J.; ROSEN, R. T. In *Food Phytochemicals for Cancer Prevention*, ACS Symposium Series 546, Huang, M.-T.;Osawa, T.; Ho, C.-T.; Rosen, R. T., Ed., American Chemical Society: Washington DC; 1994, pp. 102-119.
93. NAGAE, S.; USHIJIMA, M.; HATONO, S.; IMAI, J.; KASUGA, S.; MATSUURA, H.; ITAKURA, Y.; HIGAS, Y. *Planta Med.* 1994, *60*, 214-217.
94. MORSE, D. L.; PICKARD, L. K.; GUZEWICH, J. J.; DEVINE, B. D.; SHAYEGANI, M. *Am. J. Public Health* 1990, *80*, 1372-1373.
95. LYBARGER, J. A.; GALLAGHER, J. S.; PULVER, D. W.; LITWIN, A.; BROOKS, S.; BERNSTEIN, I. L. *J. Allergy Clin. Immunol.* 1982, *69*, 448-454.
96. FALLERONI, A. E.; ZEISS, C. R.; LEVITZ, D. *J. Allergy Clin. Immunol.* 1981, *68*, 156-160.
97. KAPLAN, B.; SCHEWACH-MILLET, M.; YORAV, S. *Int. J. Dermatol.* 1990, *29*, 75-76.
98. ROSE, K. D.; CROISSANT, P. D.; PARLIAMENT, C. F.; LEVIN, M. B. *Neurosurgery*, 1990, *26*, 880-882.
99. MUNDAY, R.; MANNS, E. *J. Agric. Food Chem.* 1994, *42*, 959-962.

Index